FemTech

Lindsay Balfour
Editor

FemTech

Intersectional Interventions in Women's Digital Health

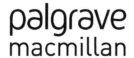

Editor
Lindsay Balfour 🆔
Centre for Postdigital Cultures
Coventry University
Coventry, UK

ISBN 978-981-99-5604-3   ISBN 978-981-99-5605-0   (eBook)
https://doi.org/10.1007/978-981-99-5605-0

This Palgrave Macmillan imprint is published by the registered company Springer Nature Singapore Pte Ltd.

The registered company address is: 152 Beach Road, #21-01/04 Gateway East, Singapore 189721, Singapore

Paper in this product is recyclable.

Acknowledgement

This book would not have been possible without the support of the Centre for Postdigital Cultures at Coventry University and the Postdigital Intimacies research cluster. Moreover, the team at Palgrave, including Marion Duval and Karthika Devi, have provided much appreciated guidance, administrative support and patience as this volume came together. To all of the authors who have contributed chapters here—thank you for your tireless work researching and revising, and for your commitment to safe and inclusive access to healthcare worldwide.

To my family and colleagues—past and present—as well as those in the FemTech industry whose insights and expertise continue to guide my thinking and writing, thank you. Scott, Aidan and Cordelia—thank you for sacrificing your own time with me for another book project; you are my first loves and with you I have it all.

This volume is dedicated to the millions around the world suffering under gendered injustice and healthcare systems that have failed to provide. I hope that this collection sparks a conversation, and then a change, in the way that we develop digital health tools for those who need them most.

Contents

Notes on Contributors

Sara Al Derham is an award-winning documentary filmmaker and a post-graduate researcher at Newcastle University in Media, Culture, and Heritage. She is currently researching Instagram usage and wellbeing among young women in Qatar. Her research interests primarily focus on media, culture, and women in the Middle East and the Arab Gulf in particular. Alderham is also a lecturer at Qatar University, and was the developer and previous manager of *Alkass Digital*, a digital media platform, based within Alkass Sports Channels in Qatar covering sporting news across the MENA region.

Farah Azhar is an assistant professor in the Department of Mass Communication at Minnesota State University. Dr. Azhar graduated with a PhD in Media and Communication Studies from the University of Oregon's School of Journalism and Communication. She holds a Master's in Economics from Lahore University of Management Sciences, Pakistan, and a Master's in Social Policy from the University of Pennsylvania. Her research is at the intersection of health communication, technology, gender, and development. She has over five years of international experience working with the central bank and nonprofit organizations.

Lindsay Balfour is Assistant Professor of Digital Media in the Centre for Postdigital Cultures at Coventry University. She is an experienced researcher, public speaker, and author with international experience in the nonprofit sector and formal academia. She has held grants from the Social Sciences and Humanities Research Council of Canada and the Andrew W. Mellon Foundation. She holds a PhD from the University of British Columbia. Her research draws on Feminist Science and Technology Studies to examine the relationship between Feminine Technologies ("FemTech") and the forms of knowledge and experience produced by and about women's bodies. She is PI on a project in development that researches access and inclusion in FemTech, and the efficacy of digital interventions for gender-based violence and Co-I on several projects related to FemTech and online safety regulation. Her work offers wider benefits concerning the global health of women, such as those outlined in the UN Sustainable Development Goals regarding Women and Girls, and in particular targets focusing on sexual and reproductive health.

Stefano Canali is a researcher in philosophy of science, with particular interests in the philosophy of data, medicine, and technology. Currently, he is a postdoc at the Department of Electronics, Information and Bioengineering (DEIB) and META—Social Sciences and Humanities for Science and Technology at the Politecnico di Milano, with a project on the epistemology and ethics of wearable technology for health. Stefano received a PhD in Philosophy at Leibniz University Hannover, an MSc from the Science and Technology Studies Department of University College London, and a BA from the Department of Philosophy of the University of Milan.

Marisa Cohn is an associate professor and codirector of ETHOS Lab, a feminist methods lab in the Business IT Department at the IT University of Copenhagen. She conducts ethnographic research into feminized forms of engineering labor and temporalities of technological change.

Ally Day is Associate Professor of Disability Studies at the University of Toledo. Her book, *The Political Economy of Stigma: HIV, Memoir and Crip Positionalities* (2021), addresses the complicated interactions between those living with HIV and AIDS Service providers. She is currently working on her second book project, *Gestational Ableism: Disability, Pregnancy and Radical Crip Futures*.

Chris Hesselbein is an ethnographer of science and technology who focuses on how the production and consumption of technoscience—both digital and more mundane—inform, and often naturalize/normalize, our understandings of embodiment, materiality, and esthetics. He is currently a postdoc in the Department of Management Engineering and at META – Social Sciences and Humanities for Science and Technology at the Politecnico di Milano where he studies alternative funding schemes for scientific research, such as crowdfunding and entrepreneurial philanthropy. Chris received his PhD in Science and Technology Studies at Cornell University, an MSc in Cultures of Arts, Science, and Technology (CAST) from the University of Maastricht, and an MA in History of Modern Politics and Culture from the University of Utrecht.

Niktalia Jules is a third-year master's student at the University of Wisconsin, Milwaukee. She uses they/she pronouns and identifies as a non-binary femme. A coordinated degree seeker at UWM, they are a pupil of both the women and gender studies and library information science departments. She currently holds a Bachelor of Science in sociology from Stephen F. Austin State University. Their research interests expand across topics of race, gender, sexuality, spirituality, anti-capitalism, archives/libraries, and information studies. Overall, her academic scholarship focuses largely on the nexus of Black queer studies, Black femmes, and archival representation.

Ravinder Kaur is Professor of Sociology at the Department of Humanities and Social Sciences, Indian Institute of Technology, Delhi. She has been engaged in the study of gender-biased sex selection (GBSS) for over two decades, examining the causes and consequences of GBSS in India with a comparative focus on China. She has been part of projects funded by ActionAid and the SIDA (Swedish International Development Cooperation Agency), on the same topic. Her research examines the intersections between reproduction (including fertility and infertility), family, education, work, state policies on family planning and population control as well as new technologies shaping the management of reproductive processes such as menstruation, pregnancy, and birth.

Khawar Latif Khan is a PhD student in the Communication, Rhetoric, and Digital Media program at North Carolina State University. Khawar completed his MS in Technical Communication in the year 2019 under the Fulbright Scholarship. His research interests include UI/UX design, digital humanities, and online information design.

Paro Mishra is Assistant Professor of Social Anthropology at the Department of Social Sciences and Humanities, Indraprastha Institute of Information Technology, Delhi (IIITD). Her core research interests lie at the intersection of Gender and Technology—New Reproductive Technologies and Information/Digital Technologies. Paro has received several fellowships and grants from the Netherlands Institute for Advanced Studies, University Grants Commission, Indian Institute of Technology, Delhi, and the Indian Council of Social Science Research. Her select publications include special issue coeditorship for *Asian Bioethics Review* (2021; 13(1)) and in Journals like *Asian Journal of Women's Studies* (2022), *Anthropology and Aging* (2021), *The Sociological Review* (2020), *Society and Culture in South Asia* (2015), and *Economic & Political Weekly* (2013).

Rebecca Monteleone is Assistant Professor of Disability Studies at the University of Toledo. She is coeditor of *Disability and Social Justice in Kenya: Scholars, Policymakers and Activists in Conversation* (2022) and is currently working on a book project, *Cure and Control: Disability, Authority and Medical Technology in the Twenty-First Century*. She has obtained recognition as a Fulbright Scholar, a Mirzayan Science and Technology Policy Fellow at the National Academy of Sciences, Engineering and Medicine, and an IGERT Fellow with the National Science Foundation.

Lara Reime is a PhD Fellow in the Technologies in Practice research group at the IT University of Copenhagen. Her interdisciplinary research project combines design and ethnographic methods to explore sociotechnical entanglements of infertile bodies, with focus on bodily and embodied practices of fertility tracking. Building on feminist theories of bodies and embodiment, her research explores critical, material, and speculative approaches to self-tracking and reproduction. Her work puts forward an understanding of reproductive bodies that goes beyond the female body and encompasses interpersonal and more-than-human relations as well as experiences of male, nonbinary, trans*, and infertile bodies.

Rachel D. Roberson has a PhD in Education Policy & Organizations at the University of California, Berkeley, with a specialization in Higher Education Administration. Rachel's scholarship compliments a decade-long career working with education-related nonprofits, schools, and colleges in various spaces and places from California to Texas, Colorado, and Minnesota. As a scholar/educator, Rachel leverages Black feminist praxis and community-based methods to build toward collective liberation, uniquely positions her to fill an urgent need within higher education scholarship. Their expertise and conceptual mastery of the intersections of race, gender, and sexuality, surveillance studies, and political economy of the body enables them to evaluate a wide range of complex social phenomena, including but not limited to institutions of higher education, sport in society, and ethics of biometrics. While Rachel's work maintains an ardent commitment to interdisciplinarity, they center three primary questions: (1) how Black bodies are regulated and controlled, (2) why these regulatory tools are enforced, and (3) how an awareness of structural relations to power enables institutional disruption and moves toward liberation?

Georgia M. Roberts teaches in the Interdisciplinary Arts and Sciences at University of Washington, Bothell. Roberts' current project explores the intersection between cultural representations of humanoid AI as feminine hairlessness and the emergent grammar of "smoothing" in data science/predictive analytics.

Sarah Seddig works at the intersection of women's sexual and reproductive health, technological innovation, and social entrepreneurship in emerging markets. Interested in the distribution of power, she researches modes of control and empowerment by following digital infrastructures, innovative technologies, and their data. Specifically, her PhD project "Bodies of Data. The Power of Female Technology in Sexual and Reproductive Health in Kenya's 'Silicon Savannah'" traces how commodification practices targeting healthcare disparities and socio-economic inequalities resurface in a new data-driven and gender-specific context. "Bodies of Data" is independently funded by the Independent Research Fund Denmark (2020–2023), hosted by the Danish Institute of International Studies (DIIS), and affiliated to the Department of Anthropology at the University of Copenhagen. Sarah is part of the DIIS' research unit Peace and Violence and "DIIS Tech," a research initiative on Technology and Power.

Rik Smit is an assistant professor and program coordinator at the Center for Media and Journalism Studies at the University of Groningen. His research focuses on the intersections of memory studies, software studies, and critical data studies and appeared in journals such as *New Media & Society, Convergence,* and *The Journal of Media History.* He is part of the international editorial team for the journal *Memory, Mind and Media.* Currently, he is working on a project on algorithmically generated memories.

Lisa Stuifzand is a graduate student at the Center for Media and Journalism Studies at the University of Groningen, holding a BA in Media Studies and an MA in Datafication & Digital Literacy. Currently, she is part of the policy research staff at the Parliament fraction of pan-European political party Volt. Her previous research focused on algorithmic discrimination, digital literacy, and political advertising in relation to Irish pro-choice and pro-life movements.

Vasiliki Tsaknaki is an assistant professor at the IT University of Copenhagen, in the Digital Design department. Her research combines material experiences, computational crafts, and somatic design methods. Through practice-based studies, she investigates intersections of these areas with a feminist theoretical commitment, aiming to trouble and dissolve binaries between body/mind, body/material, and human/ nonhuman.

Shambhawi Vikram is a PhD candidate at the Jawaharlal Nehru University (JNU), Delhi. She also has an MPhil in Women's studies from

JNU. Her research explores on contemporary debates around menstruation in urban spaces, where she used historical feminist perspectives to examine the deployment of discourses of health and hygiene in the context of menstruation by Activists, the State, and the Development Industry. She has also been a coresearcher in a project relating to Discrimination Relating to Non-Normative Genders and Sexualities at the Tata Institute of Social Studies, where she carried out research on the evocation of discourse and imaginaries of Sexual Violence in Student Politics.

Hannah L. Westwood is a PhD researcher in the Centre for Postdigital Cultures at Coventry University, on a fully funded trailblazers studentship. She is investigating the FemTech industry, and how it can become more equitable, accessible and inclusive, with a particular focus on digital fertility trackers and digital contraception such as Natural Cycles. Hannah graduated with an MA in Women's Studies from the University of York in 2022.

List of Figures

1

Introduction: Who Is FemTech For?

Lindsay Balfour

In 2016, Ida Tin, the founder of Clue, a digital Danish menstruation application coined the term "FemTech," a portmanteau of "feminine" and "technologies" that refers to the wide range of products designed with women's digital health in mind. Prior to this, investments in feminine technologies totalled a mere 100 million (USD) worldwide (FemTech Analytics). In 2019, however, just three years after the phrase entered our vocabulary, FemTech was valued at 18.75B. FemTech now includes both hardware, such as wearable, ingestible, and embeddable devices, along with software; for example, digital applications and web-based platforms. These products are designed to reach a range of women's health needs, including menstruation and ovulation tracking, diet and fitness, sexual health, pleasure, and wellness, contraception and maternal health, and, less frequently, tools for conditions such as endometriosis, polycystic ovary syndrome (PCOS), menopause, and mental health. The industry is predicted to be worth 60 billion dollars (USD) by 2027

L. Balfour (✉)
Centre for Postdigital Cultures, Coventry University, Coventry, UK
e-mail: ad5341@coventry.ac.uk

© The Author(s), under exclusive license to Springer Nature Singapore Pte Ltd. 2023
L. Balfour (ed.), *FemTech*, https://doi.org/10.1007/978-981-99-5605-0_1

(Emergen, 2020). Yet while FemTech is a rapidly evolving and expanding global market, there remains very little research into the relationship between FemTech and health inequalities that arise as a result of social factors such as race, class, sexuality and ability, not to mention the vast geographical differences between dominant and emerging markets. In the academic literature, for example, little critique is given to how these forms of marginalization intersect but are overlooked in products that largely assume a white, heterosexual, affluent, childbearing, and able-bodied user.

This is, perhaps, understandable, given that women's health in general has been often been overlooked. In Spring 2021, for instance, the UK government launched a Call for Evidence for a new digital strategy for women's health, arguing: "For generations, women have lived with a health and care system that is mostly designed by men, for men. This has meant that not enough is known about conditions that only affect women, or about how conditions that affect both men and women impact women in different ways" (Thomas, 2021). In the United States, women of child-bearing age were effectively "banned" from participating in clinical trials—an omission that was only remedied in 2010 (FemTech Analytics, 2021). Less than three years later, the first smartphone apps for tracking menstruation became available (FemTechAnalytics, 2021), reflecting the myriad ways in which technology has often outpaced responsible research. Indeed, in a 2014 piece written for MIT's *Technology Review*, Vivek Wadhwa questions the "codes we lie by, laws we follow, and computers that move too fast to care,"[1] suggesting that innovation often codes not occur without ethical consequences. The implications of this for gendered forms of inequality are exacerbated and expose what is often referred to as the "gender data gap" (Criado Perez, 2019). Despite women being roughly 50% of the global population, there has yet to be significant acknowledgement of the ways in which the "male by default" systems of healthcare have led to misdiagnosis, minimal acknowledgement of women's pain and symptoms, delays in treatment, and a lack of diversity in clinical trials (Thomas, 2021). Moreover, women are

---

[1] https://www.technologyreview.com/2014/04/15/172377/laws-and-ethics-cant-keep-pace-with-technology/

routinely living longer than men (UK Census, 2021), requiring comprehensive, high-quality, and targeted later-in-life care. More than ever, and in an era where regular access to doctors and pharmacies has been limited (i.e. during the COVID-19 pandemic), women are more often turning to technology for their health needs.

Landscapes of Investment and Surveillance

It would be tempting to assume that the growth of the FemTech industry over the last decade might ameliorate some of the challenges in women's health and health innovation to date. Digital health is a significant investment opportunity and has been since the advent of wearable fitness trackers such as FitBit and the AppleWatch. Yet the investment landscape remains skewed away from products designed by and for women. A cumulative 2 billion dollars was invested in women's digital health worldwide between 2013 and 2020, yet that represents less than 3% of total digital health investments (Das & Das, 2021), despite the fact that women make up 80% of the healthcare workforce, are responsible for 80% of healthcare decisions in their household, and spend 29% per capita more than men on general health (Shah & Epker, 2021). Moreover, while FemTech is a global market, most of the investment and research focus remains on the United States, with some attention being turned now to the UK and European markets, and very little towards either the Australia-Pacific (APAC) region or Middle East and North Africa (MENA). Regardless of geographic orientation, the industry remains skewed towards white and affluent users in the Global North, and women in general are rarely involved at higher levels of design, investment, or consultation when it comes to the digital products paradoxically designed for them. The challenges of this one-size-fits-all investment model are clear—women's health is not yet seen as a viable economic venture under the normative wealth accumulation strategies of patriarchal capitalism, leaving digital tools for marginalized women critically under-funded, under-regulated, and under-governed.

Beyond the gaps in investment, women's health technologies and the data produced by them are under-scrutinized, not rigorously tested, often not medically accurate, and do not capture the diversity of women's experience. In fact, CEO of the Organisation for the Review of Care and Health Applications (ORCHA), Liz Ashall-Payne, recently announced that only 15% of FemTech apps currently meet quality thresholds (Thomas, 2021). Moreover, FemTech products often fail to offer an accessible data management strategy or commitment to protect women's data from being sold to consumer-driven marketing schemes. In December 2018, for instance, London-based charity Privacy International reported that many well-known menstruation apps were regularly sharing user data with social media channels. Of the 36 applications they tested, more than 61% immediately transferred data to Facebook when a user opened the app. This is not just a challenge for FemTech startups. Indeed, in 2021, the ovulation app Flo reached a settlement with the Federal Trade Commission after allowing the data accumulated by its almost 100 million users to be shared with third party companies, including advertisers (Singer, 2021). More recently, with the overturn of Roe v. Wade in the United States, digital reproductive applications have come under fire for not protecting their users' data in the face of increased scrutiny over women's reproductive and sexual health practices. Where then, is the balance? We know that during the pandemic, women turned more than ever to technology for their health needs and now, with the fears around accessing reproductive services in traditional settings, FemTech still has a critical role to play in bringing digital tools to the women who need them most. This volume tackles the above challenges and more to offer a critical lens on the current women's digital health landscape, while questioning the extent to which such tools are truly innovative or not.

Intersectionality and Access

While the growth of women's health technologies is accelerating at a rapid pace, it is often approached without much critical attention to issues such as equitable access, data privacy, and quality thresholds. And while the most utilized and profitable FemTech products include ovulation and fitness trackers and reproductive technologies, this only represents a small fraction of intimate health concerns affecting women.

Although the availability of FemTech has been increasing over the last decade, the COVID-19 pandemic has accelerated the need for discreet, portable, and accessible digital tools that can be used in a self-monitoring capacity as a response to an absence of access to regular healthcare. Yet while COVID-19 has facilitated the growth of FemTech, it has also exacerbated and exposed significant gaps in the industry that include: a) inconsistent policies and regulatory frameworks, particularly around quality control and data privacy, b) a void of STS and social science research and theorization of emerging markets, and c) social barriers to access based on race, class, sexuality, ability, and other protected characteristics. As such, FemTech leaves out a significant portion of the global female population, despite its potential to positively affect the health and well-being of women around the world. These inequalities are further exacerbated in the emerging markets of the Global South, where women's sexual and reproductive health is not only often controlled and stigmatized, but where FemTech investments across the entire region that includes South Asia, Africa, and South America account for only 11% of the global market (FemTech Analytics, 2021). While a recent report released by Australia's FemTech Collective (2021) acknowledges that "women are much more than their reproductive capabilities, and women's health goes beyond the needs of fertility and reproduction," more needs to be done to limit the barriers many women face in accessing these products due to a diversity of marginalizations based on race, socioeconomic status, non-conforming gender and sexuality, (dis)ability and neurodiversity, and so on.

These gaps, of course, have disproportionate effects for marginalized and underserved women, who already suffer within an inequitable healthcare system that does not meet their diverse needs. Ultimately then, this volume asks: What are the gaps in research in the FemTech industry, with regards to race, socioeconomic status, sexuality, ability and neurodiversity, and other marginalizations? In other words, who is FemTech for? This project, then, brings Feminist Science and Technology Studies (FSTS) and the sociology of health and gender into conversation with digital culture and intelligent healthcare to respond to the gaps in women's access to self-monitored technologies of well-being, and in consideration of intersectional marginalizations within both the health and technology sectors where racialized and low-income women suffer disproportionately. By addressing the gaps in FemTech research and sociocultural barriers to access, this volume will critique the forms of knowledge and experience produced through medical and cultural discourses regarding women's bodies to both highlight the inequalities in women's digital health and imagine alternative models which optimize technology for women in a way that is safe, accessible, and inclusive.

FemTech and Science and Technology Studies

This volume progresses through several layers of the FemTech eco-system, each section, and chapter, building off the one before. At its core, it is informed by the concepts and values of FSTS. Whether a lack of critical literacy around digital health, design and aesthetic impediments, the reality that women's symptoms and pain are not taken seriously, or the fact that most FemTech products still presume a white, middle class, heterosexual, reproductive, and able-bodied user, it is problematic that women (particularly those in underserved or emerging markets) still have unequal access to basic reproductive healthcare and women's health technologies (Wiese, 2021). Moreover, the FemTech industry as a whole exposes a more widespread and systemic series of gaps within STEM (Science, Technology, Engineering, and Mathematics). This volume aims to explore FemTech within the context of FTST, whereby the entanglements of race, class, gender, ability, sexuality, and other social and cultural identities are brought to the fore. If STS is inherently the consideration of the creation, development, and consequences of science and technology in their historical, cultural, and social contexts, then this collection asks, to borrow in part from Sara Díaz, "what role can technoscience play in the movements to achieve gender justice?" and how are the operations of power and privileged exacerbated and challenged within the women's digital health milieu? (2020).

Feminist theory has long critiqued traditional intersections of gender and science, drawing attention to the social contexts in which scientific studies take place, the absence of women researchers, assumptions about "woman" and "femininity" as "natural," and displacing truth and objectivity as privileged forms of knowledge. The contributions of STS have been an instrumental force in recognizing not only interdisciplinarity but the historical, social, and cultural consequences of science and technology. The addition of feminist theory to this field of study has been to emphasize the construction of gender, technology, and science and further what Donna Haraway has called a "successor science project that offers a more adequate, richer, better account of a world, in order to live in it well and in critical, reflexive relation to our own as well as others' practices of domination and the unequal parts of privilege and oppression that make up all positions" (Haraway, 2013). We need Feminist Science and Technology Studies particularly in healthcare, and now digital health, as a way of critiquing and responding to the one-size-fits-all model of healthcare that has seen women's health needs go under-governed, under-researched, and under-funded for centuries. As Jutta Weber (2013) describes:

> Feminist science studies scholars now want to challenge boundaries and to refigure concepts and frames of thought by inventing powerful stories and different socio-material practices. To strive for more liveable worlds beyond the hegemonic tales of progress, of technoscience as biological, and technological determination means also to reinterpret what counts as nature, as sex, or as gender. The central premises of recent feminist science and technology studies are that science and culture are deeply interwoven, that facts are theory laden, and that theories are not neutral but can better be seen as stories.

True to the founding principles of FSTS and feminist technoscience then, this volume considers the social constructivist and situation creation of knowledge (see Wajcman; Haraway; Harding), and through its varying analyses of the FemTech ecosystem, argues that the social and material intersect in the relationship between humans and technology.

Moreover, this collection adds to the field of FSTS by considering its evolution not only in a new era of digital health intervention but also in its attention to intersectional marginalizations, surveillance studies and data security, and emerging markets of technoscience innovation. In other words, this volume neither celebrates FemTech unequivocally nor does it take lightly the concerns of its critics. As a body of work poised on the edge of an industry and set of innovations primed for explosion, the collection here unfolds as a survey of the current industry landscape, but also as a cautionary tale and a call for FemTech for develop in a way that holds true to feminist principles of inclusion, access, and accountability. The book is organized, thus, into three sections. The first offers critical commentary and contextualization of feminine technologies, exploring current debates and theories in the study and development of women's digital health. The second section turns to the "margins" in order to examine specific points of intervention where FemTech is being deployed, particularly in emerging markets and in the forgotten corners of women's health. The final section then takes up the question: what now? What are the lingering and future challenges for FemTech?

Part I Theories and Contexts: "Constructing a Critical FemTech Discourse"

Embodied technologies operate on a threshold between the familiar and foreign, where the body itself becomes a platform for knowledge (see Pedersen & Illiadis, 2020). As products that simultaneously require intimate access and produce intimate results, wearable, implantable, and ingestible technologies are both desired and feared. The knowledge produced by these devices allows us to experience technology at the level of the body in a way that seems safe, intimate, and helpful. Digital or not, the process still connects deeply to biology and users can often feel it working. Embodied technologies allow users to feel at ease in a sea of devices that manage schedules, music, spending practices, data storage, and surveillance. In comparison to this ubiquity—what we might now call our "postdigital"[2] times—FemTech products seem discreet, small, and convenient. They produce a knowledge of what we refer to as the

---

[2] "Postdigital" in this sense is an understanding that the digital is no longer a separate domain of culture but in every sphere of social, cultural, and political life. It delineates a context where the digital is invisible and naturalized in how we think, act, know, and feel.

Quantified Self[3] (Lupton, 2017; Esmonde, 2020) that is equal parts reassuring and alarming, using the familiarity and comfort of the body itself to assuage fears about both the digital and the medical unknown.

FemTech functions, thus, as a form of "excarnation" (Kearney, 2014), whereby the body no longer registers, through its own interpretation, how it "feels" but how the machine feels it. This excarnation takes on more resonance when viewed through the lens of gender and the forms of embodied biotracking that manage, "improve," and surveil women's intimate processes (Lupton, 2017). In this case, such technologies mimic culture and prove not so new after all—women have always been taught to feel estranged from their own bodies. They have, of course, also been taught to aspire to particular standards of beauty and perfection. There is no doubt that FemTech products often risk subscribing to biometric tracking in ways that enforce a standard of "perfection" that, particularly for women and people of colour, is a constantly moving target. In her article, "Notes on the Perfect: Competitive Femininity in Neoliberal Times," Angela McRobbie warns against the dangers of a feminism subsumed by neoliberalism vis a via women's self-regulation of their own bodies. She writes of the technologies that have long brought "the perfect into life, or [have] vitalise[d] it as an everyday form of self-measurement. How well did I do today? Did I manage to eat fewer calories? Did I eat more healthily? Did I get to the gym? Did I achieve what I aimed to achieve at work?" (2015). As new trackers and technologies hit the market daily, they are bolstered by the same questions women have had for generations—about their performance in the home, the workplace, and within their own bodies and, as such, must be newly situated within the framework of what McRobbie terms "competitive feminism" as it has re-emerged through a discourse of the quantified self (QS).

As an industry, FemTech has sought to close the gaps in women's health by offering digital solutions that target a host of issues, with ovulation, fertility, and contraception tools accounting for almost 75% of

---

[3] Quantified self refers both to the cultural phenomenon of self-tracking with technology and to a community of users and makers of self-tracking tools who share an interest in self-knowledge through numbers. Quantified Self practices overlap with other trends that incorporate technology and data into daily life, often with the goal of improving physical, mental, and/or even social performance.

products currently on the market (Fermata, 2020). Somewhat related, menopause apps are beginning to gain traction in the digital health market—at roughly 7.5%—while mental health finds its way into less than 1% of FemTech's realm of products (Fermata, 2020). The women's digital health industry is growing, to be sure, yet remains stymied by a series of gaps that range from investment, to quality control, to access and equality. Part I of this collection considers this existing landscape, and its gaps, and offers a series of critical theories and contexts for thinking about how FemTech operates, its relationship to power relations of gender and the extent to which it actively excludes, particularly through its reliance on somewhat fixed notions of sexual and gender difference and its tacit assumption about what a "woman" is and means—in this case, cis-heterosexual and reproductive-capable. As Bethany Corbin points out, "through the use of personas, forms, default settings, and design assumptions, FemTech developers have created products that categorize women and limit their data input to a range of normal values, even if the woman's unique, personal biology falls outside the artificial normal range" (Corbin, 2020). It is this kind of normative focus that prompts the chapters in this section to explore contemporary FemTech in consideration of a larger and historicized health milieu that ascribes to conventional narratives of gender, beauty, and femininity. Niktalia Jules, for instance, explores discourses of hysteria in the self-monitoring and control mechanisms in period-tracking apps. In "Hysteria Under Watch: Biological Essentialism and Surveillance in Menstrual Tracking Applications," Jules positions FemTech within the larger cultural history of attempts to "control" menstruation through the use of biometric technologies. Hannah Westwood's "Reinventing the Beauty Myth? FemTech's Cost to the Consumer" further develops and explores how technologically-enabled social emancipation dovetails with problematic beauty expectations in the commercialization of FemTech. Westwood extends Naomi Wolf's theory of the "beauty myth" and mass media consumerism into the realm of FemTech, offering an astute observation on the challenges of FemTech within regimes of commodification and menstrual surveillance capitalism. In the final chapter of Part I, Lara Reime, Marisa Cohn, and Vasiliki Tsaknaki examine how bodies are shaped through technologies in "Fertile Becoming: Reproductive Temporalities with/in Tracking Technologies."

Through the lens of posthumanism and feminist new materialism, they question the social-technological imaginary of the fertile body as bound by time, by developing a queer understanding of human–non human bodily entanglements.

Overall, this section aims to initiate a series of debates critical for thinking through the question at the heart of this collection: Who is FemTech for? The FemTech industry theoretically offers almost unprecedented access to intimate health tools for anyone with a smartphone and a Wi-Fi signal. But the majority of women do not find themselves represented with the narrow category that the majority of such tools seeks to regulate and/or improve (i.e. able bodies, reproducing, cis-female, heterosexual, white, and middle class). In her important book, Whipping Girl, Julia Serano (2007) describes the nuanced forms of exclusion even within a health industry marketed to women. As she points out, trans women have often had to act more "feminine" to access care within traditional health settings. More broadly speaking, the term "Fem" Tech suggests products only for those for those who identify as "femme" or feminine, as though femininity is synonymous with having a uterus and ovaries. Such naming tends to reinforce rather than disrupt assumption about sex and gender, assumptions that are not helped by the often colour-coded marketing of "FemTech" products, represented in ads through swatches of pink, red, and purple. Thus, the critical theorization and historicization of gender and health offered in these first three chapters is a crucial baseline from which to interrogate the more precise forms of exclusion experienced by those in the Global South and in other invisible or underserved corners of social and cultural life, as it relates to women's healthcare.

Part II Materialities and Case studies: "FemTech at the Margins"

Following the above discussion of the FemTech ecosystem and in a series of provocative and nuanced chapters, this second section gives specific insight into a range of niche challenges facing the FemTech industry. It provides depth and close analysis of specific contexts in which FemTech is emerging amongst marginalized or underserved populations. This section disrupts the dominant modes of FemTech and calls for a more expansive understanding of digital health that addresses both the gender data gap as well as the lack of investment and challenges faced by potential users in the Global South. In this way, the section follows through on Haraway's challenge to think about multiple nodes and intersections of bodies, technologies, positionings simultaneously. Thinking about the specific contexts and challenges of FemTech within this section helps to expand an understanding of equity and inclusion in the sector overall. In Haraway's words, "Feminist embodiment, then, is not about fixed location in a reified body, female or otherwise, but about nodes in fields, inflections in orientations, and responsibility for difference in material-semiotic fields of meaning" (2013). The material-semiotic, here, is of course the acknowledgement that the social is not separate from the material, within an understanding that epistemological (ways of knowing), ontological (ways of being), ethical (ways of seeing) and politics (ways of acting) are interrelated planes. Each chapter here, thus, operates from the starting point that experiences with FemTech are neither "good" nor "bad" but are contingent, whether in rural Pakistan or in an American collegiate gymnasium. As a cohesive section, these contributions offer an analysis of FemTech that focuses on intersectional marginalization. Geographically, however, these case studies span the globe, from Kenya to South Asia, to Europe and America, all giving specific attention to the operations of race, class, and sexuality. Together, they address challenges such as menstrual taboo, sports performance tracking, chronic illness, and sexual and reproductive health and rights.

FemTech is represented across all continents, but with disproportionate impact and, in the Global South, FemTech remains an emerging market. While 51.9% of FemTech companies operate within North America, this number falls to 23.5% across Europe, 13.9% in Asia, approximately 4.5% in both Australia and South America, and just 1.6% in Africa (FemTech Analytics, 2021). FemTech Investment from these regions yields similar figures, with investments from Africa, Australia, and Latin America combined representing less than 3% of total global investments (FemTech Analytics, 2021). The point here, is not to analyse the quantitative metrics of the FemTech industry, but rather to point out the reality that both investment and availability of women's digital health is skewed towards the wealthy and industrialized regions of the Global North. Looking at the distribution of funds and resources, it is hard not to ask again, as the title of this volume suggests, "who does FemTech truly serve?"

While often analysed in terms of a lack of investment opportunity, the emerging markets of the Global South also need to be understood in terms of a complex intersection of cultural knowledge and power relations. The use of sexual and reproductive healthcare products, such as contraception, for example, carry different consequences in many parts of African, South Asia, and the Middle East. This is not to suggest, of course, that women's healthcare is not also under threat in heavily industrialized and capitalist countries such as the United States and Great Britain. Chikako Takeshita (2013) outlines the importance of remembering that, in many cultures, menstruation prevents women from undertaking normal household work, including cooking, or visiting temples, making the need for period-tracking intensely important, but also private. Such technologies also offer critical potential interventions to ameliorate maternal morbidity and gender-based violence. In 2021, the UN Population Fund's (UNFPA) estimated, another six months of disruptions in health services due to the COVID-19 pandemic could lead to a worldwide increase in unintended pregnancies by 7 million and at least 31 million cases of gender-based violence—disruptions that could be remedied, in part, by increased digital access. The need is clearly present; the FemTech industry has the potential to revolutionize healthcare access for those who need it most, especially in emerging markets. The chapters that follow explore these possibilities in detail.

This section, then, responds to this challenge in both innovative and precise ways. To begin, Paro Mishra, Ravinder Kaur, Shambhawi Vikram's contribution, "One Size (doesn't) Fit All: A Closer Look at FemTech Apps and Datafied Reproductive Body Projects in India" explores how "datafied body projects" develop users' sense of selfhood. They critique the W.E.I.R.D. demographics in traditional FemTech design (Western, Educated, Industrializes, Rich, and Democratic) and argue instead for a greater understanding of intersectionality, including gender identity, class, caste, ethnicity and region, in apps produced for the South Asian demographic. Georgia Roberts then turns a lens on chronic illness and immunodeficiency, in her chapter "Artificial Intelligence and Reproducing Female Hairlessness as Social Stigma." Here, Roberts advocates for the use of AI and data tracking as a way to close the gender data gap in autoimmune disorder research and suggests that FemTech has a pivotal role to play in developing technologies for chronic illness. Next, Rachel D. Roberson surveys the role of fitness and sleep tracking in the athletic experience of black women. "Hoop Dreams or Hoop Nightmares: Athletics, Fitness Tracking, and the Surveillance of the Black Body" draws on histories of the surveillance of black bodies to question the often-overlooked connection between FemTech, race, and biometric tracking in professional athletics. In Khawar Latif Khan and Farah Azhar's chapter "FemTech and taboo topics: Raaji as a tool for educating women in Pakistan," we return to South Asia, with an exploration of menstrual taboo in Pakistan. This chapter looks specifically to "Raaji," a FemTech-inspired chat bot, designed to provide education and empowerment amongst women in Pakistan, in order to assess the extent to which digital tools "on the margins" can provide a space for women in the Global South outside the powers of capitalism and neoliberalism. Finally, Sarah Seddig turns our attention to sub-Saharan Africa and the role of the digital in sexual and reproductive rights. Seddig's emphasis on health inequalities in Kenya (including 'unwanted' pregnancies, sexual and gender-based violence, and maternal and infant mortality) acts as a springboard from which to unpack the balance between the need for data in these matters, and the subsuming of such data into surveillance regimes, an interface that is of critical importance in the development of emergent FemTech markets, including what Seddig terms "the Silicon Savannah".

If Feminist Science and Technology Studies asks "how and for whom knowledge, technologies, agents, and hybrids have been employed so far and continue to be employed" (Weber, 2013), then FemTech, as an industry and movement, needs to follow suit. These chapters diligently address this challenge—neither to admonish nor exonerate the FemTech industry but, rather, to address the ways in which equitable and inclusive

FemTech must take into consideration the entanglements of materiality, innovation, place positionality, and identity formation that render such technologies alternately effective, or moot.

Part III Challenges Still to (Over)come: "Technoselves and Data Sovereignty"

Part III casts a look both backwards and forwards, to consider how the FemTech landscape has evolved, and to turn ahead to some of the debates and concerns that will continue to challenge FemTech as the industry grows. At the same time, as feminine technologies are products of the social and cultural relations in which they are produced, so too do they give us opportunity to pause and reflect on how FemTech products and discourses can become agents of change themselves. As Weber (2013) recognizes, "On the one hand, relations of domination are becoming more complex and opaque. On the other hand, the reshaping of central categories through technoscientific practices opens up new options for refiguring gender, nature, and sociotechnical systems." FemTech may do just that—and the chapters that form this third section ask those hard questions about how the ecosystem can adapt as it confronts the challenges to come. These questions are the ones that often get missed in the rush to innovate and expand the reach of digital health tools. Questions such as: what we do with data? How are identities produced through the archiving of such date? And how can research adopt different methods to offer new insights into women's digital health? As products that simultaneously require intimate access and produce intimate results, wearable, implantable, and ingestible technologies should be desired, but with caution. The knowledge produced by these devices allows users to experience technology at the level of the body in a way that seems safe, intimate, and helpful but the biometric practices of such devices risk subscribing to gendered and patriarchal norms of knowledge and surveillance capitalism. Indeed, the histories of Science and Technology Studies, and Feminist STS in particular, tell us that women—and especially women of color—have often been excluded from the medical discourses paradoxically conceived around them. As Jourdan Webb (2020) stresses, "In considering the role of women in the QS movement, and the impact of self-tracking technologies on female health, selfhood and embodiment, it is necessary to understand wearables' role as a mechanism for both neoliberal and post-feminist patriarchal surveillance".

The first contribution to this section, then, picks up on the state of FemTech in our current political, cultural, and social paradigm—at the end of a global pandemic. In "Wearing Danger: Surveillance, Control and Quantified Healthism in American Medicine," Rebecca Monteleone and Ally Day explore how consumption and surveillance dovetail in the discourses of "healthism" perpetuated by fitness tracking and particularly through Electronic Medical Records. Such forms of FemTech, they argue, must avoid participating in a medical industrial complex that creates inequitable "sociotechnical" identities of gender and ableism. Following this, Lisa Stuifzand and Rik Smit examine the relations of power within the "normative design" framework of menstrual tracking in "Between Liberation and Control: Mixing Methods to Investigate How Users Experience Menstrual Cycle Tracking Applications." They argue for a mixed methods approach to unpack the complex web of user engagement with FemTech products and the dual forces of liberation and control experienced by women who use tracking technologies. Finally, Stefano Canali and Chris Hesselbein's chapter "Using and Interpreting FemTech data: (Self-)knowledge, empowerment, and sovereignty" argues for new methods of analysis that resists privileged access to data. As they suggest, the emancipatory and feminist potentials of wearable FemTech are limited by the failure to recognize users as capable of interpreting or acting upon their own data. Together, these three chapters offer both critique and caution, in consideration of the development of a women's digital health ecosystem that might operate outside the normative regimes of medical and biological science and technology.

Throughout this volume, the terms woman, women, womxn,[4] menstruators, and more will be used. While it is the collective feeling among

---

[4] "Womxn" is used often in intersectional feminism as an alternative spelling to woman. It is done so in objection of assumed sexism and/or gender hierarchies that can be reproduces vis a vis the sequencing of m-a-n and m-e-n. It is also used to be more inclusive of trans and nonbinary women.

authors here that the experience of intimate health, particularly that taken up in an intersectional context, is not confined to any particular gender, we recognize that both "women" and "fem" are the dominant language of the FemTech and women's digital health industries. Thus, while other terms are used, we often refer to "women" to designate the target user of this ecosystem, but we do not do so unproblematically. If anything, the volume critiques the narrow focus of the industry which must be made inclusive for all genders, along with other marginalized characteristics such as race, class, and ability.

Indeed, through its unique focus on the FemTech ecosystem, and the relations of power there within, this volume asks a question that has been lost in the rush to innovate and advance medical research: Who is FemTech for? The chapters here also remind us of the dangers of techno-liberalism in a society that proposes digital life as an antidote to inequality. In their book, *Surrogate Humanity* (2019), Neda Atanasoski and Kalindi Vora define technoliberalism as "the ideology that technology advances human freedom and postracial futurity by asserting a postlabour world in which racial difference, along with all other human social difference, is transcended." As an ideology, in other words, technoliberalism advances beyond our reality—as a society we are neither post-racial, post-gender, nor post-labour, and the surrogate effect of FemTech is often a reproduction of longstanding, inequitable power relations between humans. The phenomenon of tracking and biometrics and the forms of embodied computing—wearables, ingestibles, and implantables—that are marketed to "help" women regulate intimate bodily processes are certainly nothing new.

Yet under neoliberalism, "health" has become not only tracked, but individualized where self-reliance and control are emphasized. And we know that this neoliberal regime disproportionately disadvantages women and people of colour, not to mention other "non normative" bodies and lifestyles (i.e. neurodiverse, queer, alternately abled). As Dolezal and Oikkonen (2021) argue, "self-tracking practices feed into the production of highly normative bodies, extending the neoliberal and patriarchal regulatory mechanisms of the wellness, health, beauty, and fashion industries into increasingly self-managed, self-regulated, and intimate domains." The intersectional and genealogical analyses of FemTech in this volume offer a critical intervention into how race, class, and region (along with other marginalized oppressions) interact in the representation, design and manufacturing of FemTech products. At the same time, they are instructional in terms of how we might move forwards in utilizing the potential of feminine technologies for equitable health and well-being.

References

Atanasoski, N., & Vora, K. (2019). *Surrogate humanity: Race, robots, and the politics of technological futures.* Duke.

Census. (2021). National life tables – life expectancy in the UK: 2018 to 2020. *Office for National Statistics.* https://www.ons.gov.uk/peoplepopulationand-community/birthsdeathsandmarriages/lifeexpectancies/bulletins/nationallife tablesunitedkingdom/2018to2020

Corbin, B. (2020). Digital micro-aggressions and discrimination: FemTech and the 'Othering' of women. *Nova Law Review, 44.* https://ssrn.com/abstract=3630435

Criado Perez, C. (2019). *Invisible women: Exposing data bias in a world designed for men.* Harry N. Abrams.

Das, R., & S. Das. (2021). FemTech Collective Market Report. 29–38.

Díaz, S. (2020). In N. Naples (Ed.), *Science, technology and gender. Companion to women's and gender studies.* Wiley Blakwell.

Dolezal, L., & V. Oikkonen. (2021). Introduction: Self-tracking, embodied differences, and intersectionality. *Catalyst: Feminism, theory, technoscience.*

Esmonde, K. (2020). 'There's only so much data you can handle in your life': Accomodating and resisting self-surveillance in women's running and fitness practices. *Qualitative Research in Sport, Exercise and Health, 12*(1), 76–90. https://www.tandfonline.com/doi/abs/10.1080/2159676X.2019.1617188

FemTech Analytics. (2021). FemTech Industry Landscape Overview. https://www.femtech.health/femtech-overview-q4-2021

FemTech Collective Market Report. (2021). www.femtechcollective.com

Femtech Global Market Map. (2020). Fermata Inc. https://sg.hellofermata.com/blogs/blog/femtech-global-market-map-released-by-fermata-inc-nov-2020

Haraway, D. (2013). Situated knowledges: The science question in feminism and the privilege of partial perspective 1. In M. Wyer et al. (Eds.), *Women, science, and technology: A reader in feminist science studies* (3rd ed., pp. 456–472). Routledge.

Kearney, R. (2014, August 30). Losing our touch. *New York Times*. https://opinionator.blogs.nytimes.com/2014/08/30/losing-our-touch/

Lupton, D. (2017). The diverse domains of quantified selves: Self-tracking modes and dataveillance. *Economy and Science, 45*(1), 101–122. https://www.dhi.ac.uk/san/waysofbeing/data/data-crone-lupton-2016e.pdf

McRobbie, A. (2015). Notes on the perfect competitive femininity in neoliberal times. *Australian Feminist Studies, 30*(83), 3–20.

Pedersen, I., & Illiadis, A. (2020). *Embodied computing: Wearables, Implantables, Embeddables, Ingestibles*. MIT Press.

Serrano, J. (2007). *Whipping girl: A Transsexual Woman on Sexism and the Scapegoating of Femininity*. Seal Press.

Shah, K., & Epker, E. (2021). Investment and fundraising in the Femtech industry. *FemTech Collective Market Report*, 56–67.

Singer, N. (2021, January 13). Flo settles F.T.C. charges of misleading users on privacy. *New York Times*. https://www.nytimes.com/2021/01/13/business/flo-privacy.html

Takeshita, C. (2013). 'Keep life simple': Body/technology relationships in racialized global contexts. In M. Wyer et al. (Eds.), *Women, science, and technology: A reader in feminist science studies* (3rd ed., pp. 242–261). Routledge.

Thomas, J. (2021). *FemTech has a key part to play in women's health strategy*. Digital Health London. https://www.digitalhealth.net/2021/06/femtech-has-a-key-part-to-play-in-womens-health-strategy/

Webb, J. (2020). The quantified (female) self examining the conceptualisation of female health, selfhood and embodiment in Fitbit strategic communication campaigns. In B. Cammaerts, N. Anstead, & R. Stupart (Eds.), *Media@LSE working paper series* (pp. 1–53). LSE.

Weber, J. (2013). From science and technology to Feminist Technoscience. In M. Wyer et al. (Eds.), *Women, science, and technology: A reader in feminist science studies* (3rd ed., pp. 543–556). Routledge.

Wiese, J. (2021). Femtech in emerging markets. In *FemTech Collective Market Report*, pp. 39–54.

Part I

Constructing a Critical FemTech Discourse

2

Hysteria Under Watch: Biological Essentialism and Surveillance in Menstrual Tracking Applications

Nik'Talia Jules

Reproductive justice struggles against the state have historically shown the varied ways body surveillance interacts with intersections of race, class, ability, and sexuality. Reoccurring struggles for bodily autonomy have shown the limits blasé responses to medical and political reproductive interventions. For instance, the U.S. Supreme Court's overturn of Roe V. Wade effectively renounced abortion access as a constitutional right. Its dissolution during the summer of 2022 reintroduced how far the state will seek to intervene in the lives of women and birthers. In fact, this decision essentially took place in spite of months of protests, walks, and gatherings carried out by a wide range of reproductive justice communities due to its premature leakage. Additionally, Roe's actual repeal fittingly incited a flurry of concerns about reproductive justice, bodily autonomy, and fundamental rights. Similarly, popular pundits and scholars alike have weighed in on the dystopian-like effects of dismantling abortion rights, especially with regard to the use of digital menstrual

N. Jules (✉)
University of Wisconsin-Milwaukee, Milwaukee, WI, USA
e-mail: njules@uwm.edu

trackers. Various internet blogs and new journals reports on data selling lawsuits taken against menstrual tracking apps such as Flow hark to a new age criminalization of birthing bodies via their menstrual data. Digital menstrual trackers then were immediately met with suspicion as reproductive rights advocates urged menstruators to delete these apps to avoid future incrimination.

While this public outcry came from various parties, some cis women who took to social media in protest of the United States Supreme Court's anti-abortion decision also complained about trans inclusive reproductive labels for other genders affect by Roe's overturning. Phrases such as birthing people, menstruators, and people with vaginas were seen equally worthy of condemnation as federal dismantling of Roe V. Wade. This reductive framing of abortions and reproduction as solely a woman's issue undergirds those logics behind U.S. Supreme Court as Roe's undoing— as well as most menstrual tracking apps. Then it should be apparent by now that this turn in legislation will have varying negative effects on all marginalized identities. Yet, intersectional feminism once again must meet these simplistic "sisterhood of womanhood" and woman empowerment motifs with critiques of biological essentialism. Therefore, it is worth reiterating Bobel's (2010) argument that "not all women menstruate [and] not just women menstruate" to refuse patriarchal oppression which relies on the reification of biological essentialism by cis women (p. 158). Bobel's caution is also an important reminder that the exclusionary and normative discourse within menstrual tracking apps are not menstrual tracking apps are not just a by-product of Roe V. Wade overturn; instead, biological essentialism is written into the foundation of western medicine and its inherent menstrual stigmatization. What follows is a discussion that explores an intersectional critique of menstrual tracking apps as tools of the white phallocentric medical system and analyzes the *Stardust Period Tracker* app to do so.

Surveillance, Intersectionality, and Hysteria

Western health science discourse has roots that undergird the American government's entrenchment upon reproductive rights of birthing bodies and people of color. Such discourse manifests as untrue and outdated beliefs about sex, gender, race, and other identities that have and still continue to frame modern medicine. It is not surprising then that sexism and racism appear in spite of the seemingly neutral façade that health science purports. The perceived objectivity of medicine persists in the face of well-documented examples that expose health science ability to reifying systemic oppressions. Kelly Hoffman and others (2016) for instance expose misconceptions of higher pain tolerance amount African Americans as a form of medical racism (p. 4296). Another example involves medical sexism wherein women overall are likely to receive diagnoses and prescriptions relating to psychological issues for physical illnesses invoking notions of instability and hysteria that this chapter will unpack in what follows (Bueter, p. 5).

In our hyper-technological age, reproductive surveillance through menstrual tracking data might represent a new mechanism of control but criminalization and surveillance of menstruating bodies are as old as the institution of slavery (or perhaps older). Misconceptions about menstruation and reproductive routinely engendered a form of white paternalism that necessitates state interventions on menstruators' bodily autonomy. Histories of reproductive injustice experienced by women and people of color speak to the ways in which birthing abilities become targeted by the state in violent and strategic ways. Applying intersectionality as an analytical tool, in this respect, proves useful to dissect the experiential differences felt by menstruating and birthing bodies under the power of state and western medical science, as a critical Black Feminist framework with a lineage dating to early Black American abolitionist thought (Cooper, p. 6). Such an intersectional lens here aims to lay bare the varying means by which medicine and the state collude to constrict reproductivity among white and Black menstruating bodies. This is evident in the vast amounts of documentation on bodily experimentation and reproductive surveillance imposed upon varying races, genders, and other identities.

Taking this into account, I argue that the American government and medical authorities' surveillance of menstruating bodies centers on discourses of sex-selective hysteria positioning the menstruating people as in of constant supervision. And as a consequence, Femtech technologies, specifically menstrual tracking apps, later emerge to reify a necessity of surveillance and supervision.

The intersections of racism and sexism in medicine, in both historical and contemporary American culture, enable the stigmatization of menstruation and subsequently menstruating bodies. As part of the burgeoning industry known as "FemTech" or feminine technologies, menstrual tracking apps operate as modern-day tools of reproductive and gender surveillance which maintain menstruation as a pathologized biopsychological process. These digital menstrual trackers use "women-centered" themes and empowerment narratives to position themselves as progressive feminist business endeavors. The overall premise of emphasizing women's health is central to menstrual tracking technologies marketing as uplifting if not necessary for a woman wellness. Therefore, in this following section, I aim to unravel this misconception and argue, instead, that mainstream Femtech health tools are the benefactors of unreckoned histories of reproductive surveillance. I begin by tracing discourses of premenstrual syndrome in the nineteenth and twentieth centuries and highlight the ways in which these histories dovetail with American female reproductive injustices. Moreover, I later argue that hysteria emerges as means of population management in differing ways by drawing on Foucault's notions of biopower, biopolitics, and panoptical gaze as tools that reinforce the hysterization of menstruating bodies. Ultimately, I suggest that hysteria still persists as a present-day tool and organizing principle within tracking applications through which menstruators individually and collectively are subjected to imaginative and normative conceptions of health and gender performance. All in the aim to reconceive simplistic notions of women empowerment and digital health tools as neoliberal mechanism that retool older interventions upon bodily autonomy.

Hystories of PMS

Origins of menstrual medicalization can be found in early western thought. These philosophies built the foundations of modern medicine while reifying subjugation of various populations. Reviewing ancient beliefs surrounding hysteria, we can observe their progression well into America's nineteenth and twentieth-century medical knowledge. One of the first recognizable references to hysteria dates to ancient Egyptian times (Tasca et al., p. 110). Yet it is oft-cited ancient Greek figures such as Aristotle and Hippocrates' hypotheses on uteri, menstruation, and hysterical behaviors that undergird phallic superiority appearance in modern-day western medicine (Delaney et al., p. 45). Treatment for such reproductive pathology back then would entail yielding directly to men. As time progressed, such phallocentric interventions still continued their advancement into the nineteenth century just by more dispersed and subtler means. Laura Briggs, for example, explains that nineteenth-century physicians believed that hysteria, as a disease of "overcivilization," could not afflict other races but rather maintain the biological prestige of wealthy white women (p. 246). Yet, further on she reveals that medical discourse on hysteria circumscribed not only bodies of middle and upper-class white women but the "uncivilized" populations within Eurocentric cultures (p. 247). Discursive usages of hysteria in the west were then meant to maintain race, class, gender, and sexual hierarchies among an increasingly diverse population. As a running theme to date, sexist usage of medicalization that appears to surveil one population also seeks to discipline other identities. In this sense, hysteria specifically functioned to impose differing modes of subjugation for menstruators depending on their identities.

Histories of hysteria suggests its prescriptive purpose upon menstruation and their menstruating bodies visible in past and present applications of women's health discourse. An insidious paradox, women's health derives from a set of ideologies which tends to justify subjugation for irrational menstruating bodies while constructing said volatility as its inherent norm. Hysterical narratives thus came to mirror other discourses that presented non-normative behavior as mental illness. This specifically meant that white women became pathologized for their minds in addition to their reproductive system especially if the subversion of gender norms characterized the irrational behavior (Foucault, p. 103). It is no surprise, then, that women more often than men were diagnosed with hysteria. Likewise, these gendered forms of hysterical representation often combined with class division introduced differing terminology depending on societal status. Neurasthenia, for instance, was deployed as a more respectable term for the same condition rather than the designation "hysteria" that was more likely to be applied to lower class status (Henning, p. 22). The emergence of hysteria in these stratified ways highlights not only its gendered but deeply classed and racialized capabilities. Re-thinking nineteenth-century hysteria through the lens of intersectionality suggests that the forms of oppression that operate in modern-day digital health technologies continue to draw on multiple interlocking oppressions that target certain bodies for control and regulation. Indeed, what emerges from histories of hysterical medicalization are the varying forms of reproductive surveillance exercised via narratives of pathology that seek to control not only white women, but other marginalized populations as well. In other words, contemporary tracking practices wrought through digital technology remain tethered to latent discourses of slavery, colonialism, and white supremacy under which low-income women of color have always been disproportionately scrutinized.

Gender and reproductive surveillance has long since been a distinct response to all birthing bodies seeking their own reproductive autonomy. Janet Farrell Brodie (2001) explains that the United States in the nineteenth century saw a significant decline of "children born to native-born, married white couples… between 1800 and 1900" due to white women's variegated menstrual interventions such as period tracking and ingesting herbal mixtures (p. 40). However, at the same time that women were empowered to take ownership over their reproductive health, physicians of the latter 1800s admonished against female patients seeking out emmenagogic herbal prescriptions for abortive purposes rather than to merely induce menstruation (Brodie, p. 48). Women's health here present the interests of regular menstruation as health while denying menstruators the reproductive health rights to abortions. Just as menstruators nowadays seek Femtech apps to control their reproductivity, mid-nineteenth-century bourgeoise white women too were seeking to prolong and/or resist their "biological duties" of birthing and mothering as well as undermining societal condemnation of abortions at the time. Likewise, heighten public emphasis on the bioscientific model during the nineteenth century unfortunately only saw a repackaging of those "discarded" circular moralizing logics about women, menstruation, and birthing from prior to the Enlightenment era (Briggs, p. 261). Arguably, medical discourse on hysteria then emerges to quell women's resistance to motherhood under a growing trend of medicalization. This process of rendering women as medically pathological paired well with rationales for reproductive surveillance and state interventions. These narratives perpetuated biological essentialist ideologies of an innate inferiority among any person who was not white and male. Indeed, the foundations of western medicine that emerged from these revamped Eurocentric heteronormative phallocentric beliefs laid the groundwork for binaries of normative and pathological bodies that continues to persist in the twenty-first century.

In terms of racialization of medicine, Deirdre Cooper Owens and Sharla M. Fett (2019) suggest that white nineteenth-century physicians were intent on "medicalizing Blackness," Black bodies became inherently pathological and thus subject to the mercies of physicians seeking to extract medical knowledge (p. 1342). Enslaved Black women, too, of the mid-1800s felt the effects of contemporary gender and reproductive surveillance especially as related to capitalism. Yet, gender surveillance of enslaved Black women did not entail maintenance of normative feminine values rather the purpose of this racialized reproductive control served to perpetuate wealth for wealthy white slaveholders. Black birthing and childrearing consequently underwent continuous aims to align with the economic interest of slaveholder. Consequently, as Marie Jenkins Schwartz (2009) describes, antebellum era physicians were sought out to extract as much capital from Black women's fertility as possible. She writes further: "Medical intervention began with puberty and followed women throughout their reproductive years. Slaveholders and doctors alike considered the slaveholder's willingness to provide this medical care as evidence of a benevolent concern for a slave women's well-being" (1). Such a system is reminiscent of contemporary reproductive technologies that explicitly market themselves to young women and menstruators to capitalize on their internalization of menstrual stigma such as premenstrual syndrome. In a similar form of benevolence, Femtech apps freely provide users knowledge about their bodies and minds through daily logging of biometric data only to sell it covertly and profit from companies using said data to stigmatize menstruating bodies. All in all, reproductive surveillance evidenced the nexus of menstruating people during the mid-nineteenth century. Here, we specifically observe how white wealthy Victorian women saw oppressive medicalization vis a vis burgeoning hysterical perception of their psychosomatic disobedience (Owens & Fett, p. 1343) while enslaved Black birthing bodies—too impure to be socially reformed—were subjected to consistent medical intervention and surveillance (Washington, p. 54). These medical histories continued to feed into our current understanding of women's health discourse.

Moreover, during the early twentieth century, racial and gender tensions framed biomedical thought in ways that still shape Femtech's reductive emphasis on women's health. This medical discourse oftentimes implies that menstruators only face sexist oppression. However, Dorothy E. Roberts' in *Killing the Black Body* (1999) discusses white American fears of "race suicide," or what could be considered as racial hysteria, during the early 1900s and its connection to Margaret Sanger and her initial "feminist" birth control initiative (p. 72). Roberts writes how this once progressive endeavor for "expand[ing] women's reproductive options was marked by racism from its very inception" with "the spread of contraceptives to American women hing[ing] partly on its appeal to eugenicists curtailing the birthrates of the 'unfit' including Negroes" (Roberts, p. 67). Similarly, Femtech apps operate on logics of progressive "feminist" ideals that actual only seek to support a certain identity type (read: cis women, feminine, and heterosexual) regardless of violence it might perpetuate towards other genders and races. Likewise, Harriet Washington (2007) also attests to the use of eugenics to "scientifically validate" Black births as innately producing unfit offspring and thus in need of reproductive surveillance ranging "from involuntary sterilization to Norplant to 'the shot'" (p. 146). As a result of eugenics, both menstruating people and people of color felt a growth of surveillance around their sexual reproductivity. Eugenics policies were enacted on state levels then to monitor and control increases in population between white Americans and other races. Such legislation included negative eugenics, or the "efforts to prevent the propagation by less desirable groups," for example as well as positive eugenics which both had filtered into state policy (Hill-Collins, p. 76). Fears about Black menstruators and their offspring became a growing hysterical issue in need of medical and governmental intervention as white female hysteria began fading into other empirical supported clinical disorders.

Indeed, the continuation of reproductive surveillance into the latter half of twentieth century for American menstruators meant condemnation of their bodies and minds. A growing fissure between psychological and neurological research advancements fragmented hysteria into several specific clinical disorders such as depression and anxiety (Winstead, p. 73). Though, not too long after hysteria's dispersion, premenstrual tension (PMT) emerges in 1931 followed by premenstrual syndrome (PMS) a few years later (Stein & Kim, p. 63). These conditions both represent a means of scientifically documenting the inferiority of menstruating bodies. Ovaries and hormones become linked to the mental processes of menstruators making them certifiably unreliable and hysterical. Premenstrual syndrome, since its inception, continues to reinscribe limits onto femininity and women due to anecdotal menstrual stigma that western medicine validates. Likewise, physician Katharina Dalton's coining of PMS also foreshadows profiting of menstrual stigma that echo contemporary Femtech applications. In the 1980s, for example, premenstrual syndrome gained more recognition due to the sensationalizing of three court cases regarding assault charges presenting Dalton's diagnosis as their defense argument. In fact, two of the three cases were acquitted based on this rationale with testimonies from Dr. Katharina validating this menstrual discourse of psychopathology among menstruators and women (Chrisler et al., p. 239). All the while, an era of neoliberal feminism too growing alongside burgeoning post-feminist ideologies of the nineties. The convergence of these events produced a plethora of self-help/advice, dieting, and menstrual cycle literature inundating bookstores for women's constant self-improvement (Stein & Kim, p. 69). These nascent markets of women's health are traceable to the privatization of healthcare and the warping of gender equality rhetoric as calls for personal responsibility under neoliberal regimes. So, it is unsurprising to note that another psychiatric disorder similar to its other hysteria-like predecessors, premenstrual dysphoric disorder (PMDD), appeared in the 2013 DSM-V to continue the legacy of medicalized biological essentialism (American Psychiatric Association, 2013). And now neoliberalism along with a technologically advanced surveillance state converges to readdress the hysterical woman along with menstruators of all genders.

Foucault and Menstrual Stigma in "Stardust Period Tracker"

History has shown hysteria exists in multiple manifestations. Its persistence lies within a lineage visible largely through the inherent pathologizing of menstruating bodies. The very root of menstrual stigma surges from the same ancient (and misogynist) scientific narratives of previous decades.

Yet such discourse is not limited to the past and continues to manifest in state surveillance and disciplining of menstruators and reproduction vis a vis new forms of technology. Subsequently, this means that modern menstruators are likely to still suffer the effects of hysteria. Indeed, menstruating people continue to encounter hysterical attempts to supervise their bodies by what Michel Foucault calls the process of "hysterization" (p. 103). In his well-known text, *History of Sexuality* (1978), "hysterization" is specified as a function which the act of medical science concurrently genders and pathologizes the female sexed body during nineteenth century (Foucault, p. 103). Such a process meant that women were subjected to varying forms of state institutionalization and social discipline. Today, most menstruators face less overt interventions by the state and social networks to conform their bodies and minds into appropriate gender conventions. Still, the effects of hysterization on menstruating bodies are very much present in another permutation—one that fits in the palm of your hand. Now in mobile form, stigma about menstruation and menstruators follows the same processes of imposing pathology upon certain biological organs and processes. In what follows, I will explore the phenomenon of menstrual trackers, using the example of Stardust—a cycle tracker based on lunar-menstrual synchronicity—and through the lens of biopower and panopticism as initiated by the work of Michel Foucault.

Hysterization, as Foucault writes, began as a process that realigns the "feminine body" for its proper function in society, the family, and repro-duction (p. 104). It is closely associated with menstrual stigma and together operate as technologies of power that seek to make all menstrua-tors conform to modern-day values of neoliberal capitalism and hetero-normative gender roles. More than ever, these processes intend to utilize digital means that render the histories of reproductive surveillance and control as disconnected from contemporary tracking practices that claim to be post-race and even post-gender but actively—in a Foucauldian sense—leverage the self and the body in the service of the surveillance apparatus. In a paradoxical fashion, advancements in reproductive tech-nology then have positioned (self) surveillance as ahistorical (or rather ahysterical) and as something one now does for their own benefit regard-less of race, gender, or sexuality. Indeed, the same mechanism undergird-ing the hysterization of women during the nineteenth such as an emphasis on confession, surveillance, and charges of pathology inform contempo-rary menstrual tracking apps. Deborah Lupton (2014), for example, dis-cusses how digital self-tracking technologies offer their users qualifiable means of knowing the self and body. Specifically, Lupton writes that reproductive and sex tracking apps relate to women (and I might add menstruators) by "further medicalis[ation] via the practices of intensive documentation and self-management" (p. 10). Digital menstrual track-ers, however, only permit knowledge about oneself and body insofar as users first perceive their bodies as foreign, irrational objects that only through surveilling and confessing its inferiority on menstrual tracking apps might one acquire greater autonomy. Digital menstrual trackers then trivialize the histories of hysteria and reproductive surveillance in their technologies. This subdues public awareness of previous encroach-ments of state interventions upon menstruating bodies.

Thinking about the *Stardust* through the lens of intersectional surveil-lance then offers a deeper understanding of the menstrual tracking apps and reflects more general calls for an intersectional investigation of

Femtech industry. For example, Caroline A. Figueroa and others (2021) found an array of shortcomings in digital health apps such as "biases in app designs and algorithms" and "increased security risks," which were located using an intersectional lens. Released in 2018, *Stardust* like most digital health apps falls under the "health and fitness" category seeking to digitalize individual responsibility for wellness. Yet, an intersectional lens here might insert that not all identities can claim individual responsibility for their own wellness because various systems of oppression make their survival inherently dependent upon state welfare and community members. By emphasizing personal responsibility, *Stardust* and other digital menstrual trackers seem to frame their apps to be not only devoid of contemporary and historical vestiges of systemic prejudices but specifically advocating against feminist tenets citing empty woman empowerment arguments. This is to say, Femtech apps such as *Stardust* deploy woman-centered narratives that denounces a mythical homogenous patriarchal oppression that does not attest to the ways in which sexism has been historically stratified across various marginalized identities in the states and around the world. However, such findings are not unsurprising since data science nor western medicine—as two knowledge systems interconnected in the creation of menstrual tracking application—have done very little to resolve the many systemic biases embedded into their logics. Nonetheless, it is necessary then to consider intersectionality as pertinent to assessing Foucault's hysterization process of menstruators as a varied experience.

Namely, *Stardust* claims that it "integrates science, astronomy, and artificial intelligence to predict your menstrual lunar synchronicity" presents a nuanced version of hysterization (*Stardust Period Tracker*), one that, intentionally or unintentionally, reaffirms the lunacy of menstruating bodies. The app glorifies what other menstrual tracking apps attempt to covertly exploit: the historical (and hysterical) medical discourse about menstruating bodies. For example, research done by another digital menstrual tracker, the Clue app, and a team of data scientists declares that "the menstrual cycle **does not sync** with the lunar cycle" [their emphasis] (*Clue app*). *Clue* proclaims that it routinely receives requests from users to include lunar cycles to the app which prompted this research (*Clue app*). And while this digital menstrual tracker's usage of science here is meant to elucidate on the irregularity of menstruation as a proverbial monkey wrench in other studies and anecdotes about moon and menstrual cycle symbiosis, Clue also capitalizes on the notion of the menstrual cycle as lunacy. For instance, one testimony from a user on the main page of Clue's website graciously thanks the app as it "helped [them] to see patterns in [their] cycle" of their irregularity (*Clue app*). Just the same, other studies conducted on mental health and moon cycles mostly found no correlation between the two variables. Therefore, why exactly were there several studies preceding Clue's hellbent on linking menstruation to moon cycles? Returning to the Briggs' piece from earlier, we may find that the answer lie within the dichotomous medical discourse of savagery versus civilization in nineteenth-century America. This savage/civilized binary emerges to subjugate women, menstruators, working class people, and people of color based upon conjectures of an innate connection to primitive and animalistic essences (Briggs, p. 249). Such discourse has been repetitively deployed in attempts to impose white male paternalistic interventions as well as systemic violence through histories of racial and female hysteria. In effect, white male supremacy uses narratives of certain populations incapacity to properly care for themselves as means to evoke hysterization. Digital menstrual trackers like *Stardust* continue to deploy the hysterization process and its reproductive surveillance now under the guise of fun features and empowerment.

Moreover, *Stardust's* usage of witchcraft and spirituality as an empowerment motif under the guise of capitalist configurations that renders menstruators docile and self-surveilling. The app offers users the ability to "sync your cycle to the moon and stars" and an interpretation of menstruation through a sort of "witchy" spiritualism that makes participation seem harmless yet empowering (*Stardust Period Tracker*). Its emphasis on an innate relationship between menstruation and moon cycles seeks to incite users' daily surveillance. Just as other most menstrual tracking apps, *Stardust* aims to foster an incessant need in users' constant self-surveillance and self-reporting as a result of daily logging of PMS and personal symptoms. We can also argue that these key features represent those mechanisms of hysterization—confession, surveillance, and internalization of one's perceived biological inferiority. For Stardust users, this is accomplished through specific app features such as "specialized daily insights[s]" about one's menstrual cycle via notifications, the ability to log PMS and other menstrual related symptoms every day for "personal predictions," and the capacity for "sharing and syncing [of] periods with friends" that collectively invoke constant surveillance of the self as well as other menstruators (*Stardust Period Tracker*). The subversive histories of witchcraft and spirituality then become retooled to make menstruators aware of their pathology and docile to hysterization. One key problematic component of this app (and others) is its neoliberal feminist marketing strategy. Spirituality and witchcraft are repackaged as simply another selling point to menstruating people. In the case of Stardust, a glossy narrative of witchcraft elides histories of surveillance, institutionalization, and harm done to women and menstruators classified as witches and/or hysterical. America's colonial era specifically showcases how both white and Black women spiritualists/naturalists were met with oppressive forms of surveillance and subjugation (Kocić, p. 2). Such a historical reclamation of spiritual "rebellion" only emptily empowers while largely operating under the same medieval premise of surveilling menstruating bodies. Hysterization continues thus by presenting itself as a fashionable app by which menstruators perform their own oppression without a discernible figure/force.

Biopower, Biopolitics, and Panoptical Figures

Sandra Lee Bartky (1990) uses Foucault's metaphor of the "Panopticon" to argue that women's (self) surveillance stems from the patriarchy. This panoptic figure is always present in the women's actions and represents a "disciplinary power that inscribes femininity in the female body [which] is everywhere and ... nowhere ... everyone and yet no one in particular" (p. 142). This figure too shapes menstruating bodies through pathologizing menstruation thus restricting the behaviors of menstruators. Indeed, menstrual stigma fuels the self-discipling and self-surveilling of menstruators. A parallel can be drawn from Foucault's description of hysterization as "ordering [the female body] wholly in terms of the functions of reproduction and keeping it in constant agitation through the effects for that very function" (p. 153). The phallocentric male panoptic figure requires the constant agitation of menstruators to continue governing over those who menstruate and their reproductivity. Indeed, as Foucault writes in *Discipline and Punish* (1975), the effect of surveillance should have "the inmate ... caught up in a power situation of which they are themselves the bearers" (p. 201). Menstrual stigma functions as this constant agitation that renders menstruator consumed with surveilling their bodies. This stigma represent no singular discernible force but the reappears in the many social arenas subtly with the phallocentric male's historical loathing of menstruation. Yet, if most menstruators recognized menstrual stigma as merely phallicism within western medicine would heighten attention to self-surveillance continue? What makes self-surveillance and self-disciplining so preferable? Femtech apps like *Stardust*, for example, offers neoliberal feminist narratives of self-improvement and female empowerment to those who make up its over 1 million app downloads (Stardust Period Tracker). In this instance, choice functions as an illusory device that suspense menstruators hesitation against reproductive surveillance under the guise of a "feminist" agency. It is likely that the phallocentric male panoptic figure lurks within this reductive pro-woman rhetoric as well.

Subsequently, we can recognize some menstruators' desires for women's health tools as emerging against menstrual stigma and observe that menstrual stigma too creates this reductive emphasis on women's empowerment. Oftentimes, this is paradox is seen in mainstream menstrual products being sold under the rhetoric of female empowerment, agency, and "freedom" despite underlying menstrual stigma (Wood, p. 329). Femtech apps, too, position themselves as offering menstruators (mainly women) freedom from and control over the unpredictability of their periods in addition to making strides towards advancing female health initiatives. Users of the Stardust app specifically meant to gain heighten menstrual health and empowerment through moon-based spiritualism themes. All of these efforts are an attempt at again exulting a simplistic sisterhood narrative opposed to sexist oppression using female empowerment as a rhetorical bandage. However, the overuse of female empowerment to combat sexist oppression in health suggest that the panoptic figure is not merely male but white too. The panoptic represents normative perceptions of women's health which emphasizes a distinct kind of white womanhood. Likewise, hysterization has historically been aimed towards reconditioning rebellious white women for their roles as mothers and wives. As we have seen, hysteria—in its transition into premenstrual tension, premenstrual syndrome, and finally premenstrual dysphoric disorder—has a pathologizing lineage which corresponds with white male supremacy. This is evident in the singular pathologizing nature of premenstrual symptoms in western cultures. Menstruators in non-western countries have been reported sharing similar premenstrual symptoms such as breast swelling, fatigue, and irritability yet the nature pathologization of these symptoms as a disease collectively is not so apparent in these other cultures (Walker, p. 16; Johnson, p. 347; Rodin, p. 55). The white male panoptical figure governs over menstruators by insulating their perceptions of menstruation through feedback loops between western scientific discourse and western mainstream outlets (Usser & Perz, p. 216). Still, menstrual stigma, similar to female hysteria, functions as a totalizing mechanism meaning to regulate all menstruating bodies on a collective scale.

And this is where we might recognize Foucault's notion of biopolitics and biopower. Menstrual stigma leads menstruators of all identities to believe that concealment and surveillance are the only way to engage with one's menstrual cycle. The white male panoptical figure thus organizes this menstrual stigma in a way that effuses throughout western society in an individualized manner. It governs over menstruators by circumscribing their perceptions of menstruation through western media and scientific discourse. Menstrual stigma then becomes internalized and ultimately enacted upon by menstruators themselves. These responses to stigma emerge as consumerist expressions which seek self-help books, therapy, make-up, and menstrual tracking apps to assist menstruators in their ""imperative toward self-examination, self-optimization, and personal responsibility" under surveillance capitalism (Ford et al., p. 49). Menstruators individual and collective internalization of menstrual stigma function as the way that the white male panoptical figure organizes menstruating bodies' biopower and as biopolitical force. These products also act as forms of gender surveillance to ensure that menstruators relate to their bodies as feminine women only. *Stardust* too asks menstruators to surveil their reproduction in a gendered way with witchy spiritualist motifs and overall feminine graphics. In this way, biological essentialism presents itself within Stardust specifically but in most digital menstrual tracker generally. The process starts with the cooptation of reclaimed feminist narratives by Femtech that funnels into their various technologies like menstrual tracking apps. *Stardust* specifically uses spiritual empowerment marketed largely towards women-identified populations with a "women-owned" self-certification (Stardust Period Tracker). By doing so, the app distinctly highlights an ahistorical, post-racial, and neoliberal rendering of feminist narratives to maintain its capitalistic motives. Menstruators then are rendered docile to the influences of capitalism, the patriarchy, and white supremacy through "glamorized norms rather than through gender-based prohibitions" of digital menstrual tracking apps like *Stardust* (Sanders, p. 41). As a result, this gender surveillance ensures heteronormative feedback with most menstrual tracking apps. This again is the hysterization process by which the *Stardust Period Tracker* distinctly employs. It positions menstruation as simultaneously an esoteric experience and a scientifically confirmed result of feminine biology. The essence of menstruating bodies is thus touted as solely feminine and empirically abstruse. Stardust and other digital menstrual trackers become another expression of the white male panoptic figure.

Conclusion: Menstrual-Tracking Apps and Biological Essentialism

A major selling point of menstrual tracking apps is their ability to algorithmically predict menstruation, ovulation, and other components of reproduction seemingly "freeing" users from mental calculation of previous generations, while providing the benefit of knowledge about and over one's body. Over 200 million regular users (and counting) employ digital menstrual trackers to document, manage, and observe their menstrual cycle (Worsfold et al., p. 1). The vast number of users showcases the esteemed view these menstrual tracking apps hold for a plethora of menstruators. It can be deduced that many menstruators then seek to have some authority over their menstrual cycle. Yet are these apps truly the feminist health interventions they purport to be? And if not, what purpose do they serve to menstruators other than surveillance and menstrual stigma? Various researchers have broached digital menstrual trackers as a topic with normative prescriptions of menstruation and menstruators. For example, Adrienne Pichon and others (2021) identify three main gaps of these digital tool in their scholarly examination of menstrual tracking apps: (1) imposition of regular menstrual cycles despite "irregular" periods being a recognized norm; (2) menstruation and menstruators are largely reduced to concealment practices; and (3) the varied users of menstrual tracking apps "are represented as flat with monolithic experiences" (p. 388). Gaps such as these speak to the nature of biological essentialism within these digital tools. Menstrual tracking apps operate on dualistic narratives empowerment and menstrual stigma that worsen the experience for menstruators that do not identify as women nor resonate with mainstream forms of femininity. What follows is the appearance of two main issues concerning menstrual tracking apps—regular/irregular menstruation binary and the gendering of menstruation.

The presence of menstrual stigma within menstrual tracking apps works to reify both notions of a regular/irregular menstrual cycle and menstruation as a gendered biological process. Many of these tools "fluctuate between attempting to empower women by use of self-analysis and strengthening the perception that menstrual cycles represent an unmanageable contemptible process that needs to be handled and suppressed" (Morrison, p. 146). Indeed, ancient narratives of menstruation as messy and hysterical, as we have seen, are at the foundation of menstrual tracking apps. People who menstruate become those hysterical and messy associations of menstruation regardless of a regularly surveilled cycle. For example, many (if not all) menstrual tracking apps presuppose what a normal menstrual cycle represent: 28 days with ovulation by the 14 day and lasts between 2 and 7 days (Worsfold et al., p. 1). This medicalized notion of a regular period cycle shapes the way menstruators and non-menstruators consider the menstruating body. Menstruation then is perceived as an ongoing daily process that always influences the behaviors and emotions of menstruating people irrespective of one time of the month. Thus, menstrual tracking apps serve as health interventions to combat the unrelenting hormonal bombardment menstruating people face—bleeding, ovulating, premenstrual, or otherwise. "Irregular" menstruators also must navigate knowledge about their menstruation solely through rendering their menstrual cycles into regularity/healthiness. For most menstrual tracking apps, this "regular" 28-day cycle is the usual default unless in the beginning users input their own cycle information or the app adjusts after logging one's period a few months in a row. Menstruators perpetually seek to align themselves with a regular cycle that premises menstruation as a process that continuously manipulates menstruators' behaviors and emotions rather than infrequently or irregular one. Menstrual stigma about the mercurial nature of menstruation (and naturally those who menstruate) reify regular/irregular binaries that permit digital menstrual trackers to predict and plan around regular periods while taming irregular cycles to become predictably temperamental. Either way, biological essentialism within regular/irregular menstrual discourse equates irrationality with menstruation itself and especially those that menstruate.

Ultimately, dominant menstrual stigma finds more than one way to incite normative ideals about menstruation, gender, and sexuality. This additional facet of biological essentialism within menstrual tracking apps implies that menstruation relates inherently to mainstream notions of feminine women. Gilman (2021) affirms that most digital menstrual trackers rely on gender stereotypes and biological essentialism, and these apps act "as a gendered surveillance tool… many apps use pink color schemes and graphics, such as flowers and hearts, that reinforce feminine notions of gender performativity… these apps also make stereotypical, gendered assumptions about users and their goals [for using menstrual tracking apps]" (p. 107). Stardust is no exception, either, with an interface that uses pink and purple hues, set off against its "night sky" backdrop. Such imposition of feminine themes, color schemes, and graphics tend to foreclose on the notion that other genders might use digital menstrual trackers. In this sense, most of these digital apps like Stardust also intrinsically relate femininity to a regular/health menstrual cycle by investing in feminine imagery and marketing. What emerges is a fallacious association between menstrual health and femininity which means to surveil and pathologize both. Likewise, feminine women (and arguably feminine people generally) become seen as hysterical due to this mode of biological essentialism. These reified gender constructions within menstrual tracking apps operate at the expense of trans and gender variant folks who witness over and over again the simplification of "menstruation as a phenomenon exclusive to (and universal to) women—ditto the presence of a vagina" with regard to digital menstrual trackers (Spiel et al., p. 6). Menstrual tracking apps then clandestinely reinforce a reductive depiction of menstruation and gender on two fronts.

In sum, both the gender-normative design aesthetics and feminist discourses of empowerment act as a deceptive sleight of hand whereby the more disciplinary operations of gender, race, and surveillance can continue unchecked. The lineage of hysteria and clinical inventions of premenstrual illnesses within western biopsychology discourse are evidence of the pathologized history of menstruating bodies. This oppressive regime continues via the long-standing belief that menstruation—like women and people of color—requires constant supervision. However, menstruating individuals are now tasked with surveilling and silencing any indication of their period/period symptoms, while regimes of biopower, biopolitics, and discipling patriarchal deployment of panopticon refashion nineteenth-century hysterization into modern-day menstrual tracking technologies. What has also emerged in the context of these reproductive digital tracking apps, and the Femtech more generally, is a thin veneer of female empowerment masking decades of menstrual stigma. Menstruators enveloped in this pro-woman technologized hysterization process take on the role of the white male panoptic figure as their own menstrual disciplinarian. Furthermore, those menstruating people that specifically use the *Stardust Period Tracker*, due to its thematic allure of spirituality and astrology, fall prey to perpetuations of sexist (and albeit surreptitiously racist) ideologies of menstruating bodies that hinge on biological essentialism. An intersectional lens offers illumination on the histories of reproductive surveillance tactics still invoked within menstrual tracking apps largely marketed to women. And it is through the recognition of these culminating regimes that menstruators might seek real autonomy over their bodies in the twenty-first century.

References

American Psychiatric Association. (2013). *Diagnostic and statistical manual of mental disorders* (5th ed.). American Psychiatric Publishing.

Bartky, S. L. (1990). Foucault, femininity, and the modernization of patriarchal power. In *Femininity and domination,* by S. L. Bartky, Routledge, pp. 25–45.

Bobel, C. (2010). When 'Women' becomes 'Menstruators'. In *New blood third-wave feminism and the politics of menstruation*, by C. Bobel, Rutgers University Press.

Briggs, L. (2000, June). The race of hysteria: 'Overcivilization' and the 'Savage' in late nineteenth-century obstetrics and gynecology. *American Quarterly, 52*(2), 246–273.

Brodie, J. F. (2001). Menstrual interventions in the nineteenth-century United States. In *Regulating menstruation: Beliefs, practices, interpretations*, by Van de Walle Etienne and E. P. Renne, University of Chicago Press, pp. 39–63.

Bueter, A. (2015). Androcentrism, feminism, and pluralism in medicine. *Topoi, 36*(3), 521–530. https://doi.org/10.1007/s11245-015-9339-y

Chrisler, J. C., & Caplan, P. (2002). The strange case of Dr. Jekyll and Ms. Hyde: How PMS became a cultural phenomenon and a psychiatric disorder. *Annual Review of Sex Research, 13*, 274–306.

Clue Period & Ovulation Tracker with Ovulation Calendar for IOS, Android, and Watchos. (n.d.). *Clue Period & Ovulation Tracker with Ovulation Calendar for IOS, Android, and WatchOS*, Clue, helloclue.com/.

Collins, P. H. (1998). It's all in the family: Intersections of gender, race, and nation. *Hypatia, 13*(3), 62–82.

Cooper, B. (2015). Intersectionality. In L. Disch & M. Hawkesworth (Eds.), *The Oxford handbook of feminist theory* (pp. 385–406). Oxford Academic.

Delaney, J., et al. (1988). *The curse: A cultural history of menstruation.* University of Illinois Press.

Do Periods Really Sync with the Moon? (2021, July 29). *Clue period & Ovulation tracker with ovulation calendar for IOS, Android, and WatchOS.* www.hello-clue.com/articles/cycle-a-z/myth-moon-phases-menstruation

Figueroa, C. A., et al. (2021). The need for feminist intersectionality in digital health. *The Lancet Digital Health, 3*(8), e526–e533.

Ford, A., et al. (2021). Hormonal health: Period tracking apps, wellness, and self-management in the era of surveillance capitalism. *Engaging Science, Technology, and Society, 7*(1), 48–66. https://doi.org/10.17351/ests2021.655

Foucault, M. (1975). Panopticism. In M. Foucault (Ed.), and A. Sheridan (Trans.), *Discipline and punish* (pp. 195–228). Penguin Books.

Foucault, M. (1978). *The history of sexuality* (R. Hurley, Trans.). Pantheon Books.

Gilman, M. E. (2021). Periods for profit and the rise of menstrual surveillance. *Columbia Journal of Gender and Law, 41*(1), 100–113.

Henning, M. (1999). Don't touch me (I'm electric): On gender and sensation in modernity. In J. Arthurs & J. Grimshaw (Eds.), *Women's bodies: Discipline and transgression* (pp. 17–47). Cassell.

Hoffman, K. M., et al. (2016). Racial bias in pain assessment and treatment recommendations, and false beliefs about biological differences between blacks and whites. *Proceedings of the National Academy of Sciences, 113*(16), 4296–4301.

Johnson, T. M. (1987). Premenstrual syndrome as a western culture-specific disorder. *Culture, Medicine and Psychiatry, 11*(3), 337–356.

Kocic, A. (2010). Salem witchcraft trials: The perception of women in history, literature and culture. *FACTA universitatis-linguistics and literature, 8*(1), 1–7.

Lupton, D. (2014, June 11). Quantified sex: A critical analysis of sexual and reproductive self-tracking using apps. *Culture, Health & Sexuality, 17*(4), 440–453.

Morrison, M. (2021). The datafication of fertility and reproductive health: Menstrual cycle tracking apps and ovulation detection algorithms. *Journal of Research in Gender Studies, 11*(2), 139–151.

Owens, D. C., & Fett, S. M. (2019, October). Black maternal and infant health: Historical legacies of slavery. *American Journal of Public Health, 109*(10), 1342–1345. https://doi.org/10.2105/ajph.2019.305243

Pichon, A., et al. (2021). The messiness of the menstruator: Assessing personas and functionalities of menstrual tracking apps. *Journal of the American Medical Informatics Association, 29*(2), 385–399.

Richardson, J. T. E. (1995). The premenstrual syndrome: A brief history. *Social Science & Medicine, 41*(6), 761–767. https://doi.org/10.1016/0277-9536(95)00042-6

Roberts, D. E. (1999). *Killing the black body: Race, reproduction, and the meaning of liberty*. Vintage.

Rodin, M. (1992). The social construction of premenstrual syndrome. *Social Science & Medicine, 35*(1), 49–56.

Sanders, R. (2016). Self-tracking in the digital era. *Body & Society, 23*(1), 36–63.

Schwartz, M. J. (2009). *Birthing a slave: Motherhood and medicine in the Antebellum South*. Harvard University Press.

Spiel, K., et al. (2019). Patching gender. In *Extended abstracts of the 2019 CHI conference on Human Factors in Computing Systems*, pp. 1–11.

Stardust Period Tracker. (2022). Stardust App Inc., Vers. 2.2.3. *Apple App Store*. https://apps.apple.com/us/app/stardust-period-tracker/id1495829322

Stein, E., & Kim, S. (2009). *Flow: The cultural story of menstruation*. St. Martin's Griffin.

Tasca, C., et al. (2012). Women and hysteria in the history of mental health. *Clinical Practice and Epidemiology in Mental Health: CP & EMH, 8*, 110–119.

Ussher, J. M., & Perz, J. (2020). Resisting the mantle of the monstrous feminine: Women's construction and experience of premenstrual embodiment. In C. Bobel et al. (Eds.), *The Palgrave handbook of critical menstruation studies* (pp. 215–231). Palgrave Macmillan.

Walker, A. E. (1997). *The menstrual cycle*. Routledge.

Washington, H. A. (2007). *Medical apartheid the dark history of medical experimentation on black Americans from colonial times to the present*. Paw Prints.

Winstead, B. A. (1984). Hysteria. In C. S. Widom (Ed.), *Sex roles and psychopathology* (pp. 73–96). Plenum Press.

Wood, J., et al. (2020). (In)Visible bleeding: The menstrual concealment imperative. In C. Bobel et al. (Eds.), *The Palgrave handbook of critical menstruation studies* (Vol. 2020, pp. 319–332). Palgrave Macmillan.

Worsfold, L., et al. (2021). Period tracker applications: What menstrual cycle information are they giving women? *Women's Health, 17*, 1–8.

3

Reinventing the Beauty Myth? FemTech's Cost to the Consumer

Hannah L. Westwood

Introduction

More critical engagement is needed with FemTech, as a rapidly expanding industry that is beginning to disrupt the digital health space. In particular, it is necessary to consider issues of access and affordability for the consumer in an industry that is predicted to be worth $60 billion by 2027 (Emergen Research, 2020). While there is no doubt that FemTech is poised to improve the health of women, transgender, and non-binary people, a crucial question remains: what is the true cost of FemTech, and who is it really for? In particular, it is important to consider what cost the consumer assumes in accessing FemTech products and services, and how this cost contributes to the value of the industry. Indeed, the purchasing power of women has a long history of exploitation. From home appliances in the 1950s to beauty products and services in the 1990s and beyond, industries focused on advertising and selling products to women have a complicated history that is inextricably linked to capitalism,

H. L. Westwood (✉)
Coventry University, Coventry, UK
e-mail: westwoodh@uni.coventry.ac.uk

© The Author(s), under exclusive license to Springer Nature Singapore Pte Ltd. 2023
L. Balfour (ed.), *FemTech*, https://doi.org/10.1007/978-981-99-5605-0_3

patriarchy, and oppression (Wolf, 1990/1991). Similarly, the ease with which the benefits of digital health are elided by capitalism is something that must be explored in relation to the FemTech industry, especially when questions of (in)accessibility are linked to forms of economic marginalisation.

This chapter elaborates on the link between (in)accessibility and economics, using Naomi Wolf's theory of the beauty myth as a framework for analysing FemTech. In *The Beauty Myth*, Wolf (1990/1991) theorises that as women have gained social and political emancipation, the beauty and diet industries have grown as a way to keep them covertly, but fundamentally oppressed. This chapter will first unpack Wolf's theory and show that although it has been argued that the beauty myth is less relevant today due to recent body positivity movements, its application to FemTech proves that the myth has reinvented itself within the general health and wellness ecosystem in which FemTech sits (Damelin, 2019; Abraham, 2019; Wolf, 2011). To illustrate how the beauty myth is reiterated within the FemTech industry, I identify three of Wolf's central concerns; advertising, economic marginalisation, and self-surveillance. Each of these concerns is paired with a relevant case study of a FemTech product or company. To begin, I examine the link between advertising and the digital fertility tracker Natural Cycles, analysing the use of influencer marketing to convince new users to purchase a subscription. Next, I offer a reading of reusable menstrual underwear brands Thinx, Modibodi, and WUKA to consider how the economic marginalisation of women is reinforced by companies that make, market, and sell products made primarily for menstruators, a phenomenon often referred to as "menstrual capitalism" (Røstvik, 2022). Finally, I unpack the practice of self-surveillance encouraged by workplace health insurance programs, with a particular focus on those that provide in vitro fertilisation to consider how such practices are common within FemTech, and to show that sharing of self-surveillance data is often the price users must pay to access otherwise unreachable technologies. This unique application of the beauty myth reveals unsafe and inequitable practices within FemTech and can be used to analyse the current landscape of the industry. Thus, this chapter provides a critical theoretical springboard for the case studies examined in Part II of this volume. Additionally, this chapter highlights central concerns with the industry to begin to provide a framework for making FemTech more accessible, equitable, and safe.

The Beauty Myth

Writing a decade after what she sees as the end of second-wave feminism, when women gained access to the workplace and education and improved rights over their bodies and lives, Naomi Wolf (1990/1991, p. 9) asks "a generation on, do women feel free?". The answer, as it transpires, is no. As western women gained rights across many aspects of life, a new oppressor emerged: the beauty myth. Infiltrating all aspects of life, the concept of the beauty myth is leveraged by Wolf to explicate the backlash against the improved rights and freedoms that women in the West gained during the 1970s and 1980s, including improved reproductive rights and equality in education settings and the workplace. Taking this history into account, the beauty myth theorises that as women gained social emancipation, they have, in fact, become increasingly oppressed by stringent beauty standards that dictate how a liberated, responsible, and successful woman should look. This has undermined women's equal participation in their newly gained freedoms in education and the workplace and keeps them covertly oppressed. This oppression involves both strict rules for how to look and dress, and the often hidden cost associated with this, which has been further explored as "aesthetic labour" and "personal care capitalism" (Elias et al., 2017; Røstvik, 2022, p. 6).

Building on the work of other feminist writers including Kim Chernin (1981, 1985) and Sandra Lee Bartky (1988/1997), *The Beauty Myth* provides its readers with a detailed breakdown of exactly how the beauty, diet, and cosmetic surgery industries keep women oppressed.[1] From how

[1] Wolf does not problematise the term woman and *The Beauty Myth* makes no reference to the experiences of trans and non-binary people and how they may be uniquely affected by the beauty myth (for example, rigid gender stereotypes increasing experiences of gender dysphoria). Other issues with the text, including, but not limited to: the lack of attention to how gender intersects with race, class, and sexuality; the Judeo-Christian and western-centric focus of analysis and the use of widely debunked statistics on anorexia (see Schoemaker, 2004) cannot be ignored. *The Beauty Myth* provides an interesting and useful framework to analyse the FemTech industry, but it must be acknowledged that it is not without its problems.

women must look if they want to participate in the workplace, to the positioning of beauty as religion in a secularising society, Wolf provides readers with the critical tools with which to uncover the true motivation of the beauty industry—to keep women oppressed. Most interesting to this analysis are Wolf's first two chapters, "Work" and "Culture". "Work" explicitly relates the beauty myth to the economy by showing that as women's participation in paid labour increased, the beauty myth surfaced in order to keep women financially oppressed by mandating participation in paid beauty work. Wolf (p. 20) shows the permanence of this by linking it to historical conceptions of beauty as currency ("she looks like a million dollars"). This has evolved into valuing women as individual capitalist subjects whose simultaneous participation in and oppression by paid labour and the market is required by neoliberal conceptualisations of feminism (Rottenberg, 2018; Banet-Weiser, 2018). As part of this, women are expected to have a successful career alongside being a mother and presiding over the home. Indeed, in addition to the economic marginalisation of the beauty myth, Wolf's chapter touches on the unpaid domestic work that is disproportionately carried out by women that keeps them time poor, a subject that has been explored in significantly more detail outside of *The Beauty Myth* (Hochschild & Machung, 1989; Budlender, 2004; Breen & Prince Cooke, 2005). These factors compound, Wolf shows, to keep women economically and temporally marginalised, as well as exhausted, in order to ensure they do not challenge the structures that oppress them (p. 53). In the second chapter—"Culture"—Wolf explores the ubiquity of beauty advertising in magazines that contributes to upholding the myth. This chapter reveals how beauty and diet culture advertising revenue is necessary for the survival of women's magazines, which otherwise produce "serious, prowoman content" and spread feminist ideas to the general reader (p. 71). The result of such advertising is that the beauty myth spreads quickly, and readers are influenced into participating in expensive beauty work, which is positioned as necessary by the advertising in women's magazines. This co-opts the feminist content in women's magazines into a form of feminist politics that is profitable to advertisers, in a way "that seems to explicitly recognize that inequality exists while stopping short of recognizing, naming, or disputing the political economic conditions that allow that inequality to be profitable"—in other words, a traffic in feminism (Banet-Weiser & Portwood-Stacer, 2017, p. 886; Banet-Weiser, 2018). These particular sections of *The Beauty Myth* provide much of the framework through which it is possible to analyse the FemTech industry to evaluate its reliance on the messages promoted by the economic marginalisation and advertising present in beauty myth culture.

There is some debate as to whether the beauty myth, as Wolf conceptualised it in her 1990 text, is still relevant today, due to an increase in body positivity movements (Damelin, 2019; Abraham, 2019; Wolf, 2011).[2] Social media, in particular, has been credited with breaking down beauty standards, increasing diversity, and promoting body positivity (Abraham, 2019). Body positivity movements on social media encourage users to reject harmful beauty standards, engage in appreciation of one's own body and share images of "real" bodies, including a diversity in shapes and sizes, and those depicting features including cellulite and stretch marks (Cohen et al., 2021; Rodgers et al., 2022). These movements encourage the dismantling of the strict beauty standards that Wolf details in *The Beauty Myth*, and such practices have even trickled into advertising. For example, Dove's "real beauty" advertising campaign featured a diverse array of women and consulted feminist writer Dr Susie Orbach (2005) in their vision to create a responsible campaign. This has been followed by campaigns that pledge not to retouch models with photoshop and include wider ranges of body diversity in their advertising, such as American Eagle's #AerieREAL. In addition to body positivity movements, the relevance of the beauty myth today has been eroded by the breaking down of the strict gender binaries that Wolf refers to. For example, referring to how women attempted to change the "gray, sexless, and witless" working environments that they began to inhabit, Wolf (p. 45) writes that "men failed to respond with whimsy, costume, or color of their own". However, since *The Beauty Myth's* publication, it has become more accepted for people of all gender expressions to explore dress and makeup if they so wish. Strict gender norms have been replaced

---

[2] While social commentary articles have dismissed the relevance of the beauty myth due to the rise of body positivity, much of the literature recognises the promotion of self-care work as necessary in tandem with loving one's body as simply a new standard in which personal care capitalism can continue to develop. See Riley et al. (2022) and Orgad and Gill (2022).

by growing acceptance of people inhabiting all parts of the spectrum of gender and sexuality and a rejection of traditional gender stereotypes that men and women must follow. In sum, there is a clear argument to suggest that the beauty myth, as Wolf conceptualised it, is simply less relevant today.

However, I aim to show how the concepts of health and wellness have replaced the "beauty" in the beauty myth to the extent that they similarly encourage women's participation in their own oppression vis à vis newly articulated modes of self-management and capitalism. As Wolf (2011) argued in an article evaluating *The Beauty Myth* twenty years after its initial publication, the rhetoric of the beauty myth lives on in discourses of health and wellness; indeed, as the beauty myth has become increasingly less relevant, it has had to reinvent itself. Much as Wolf argued that the beauty myth replaced the oppression of staying in the home that women liberated themselves from in the 1970s, I show that health and wellness has replaced beauty and diet culture in the myth as a way to continue to oppress those who have liberated themselves from traditional gender and appearance norms. This is also conceptualised by neoliberal feminism, under which a woman's role must include the care of their own health and well-being (and often that of their family), typically at a financial cost to them, again requiring capitalist participation (Banet-Weiser et al., 2019, p. 7; Rottenberg, 2018). As an industry that focuses on the health and wellness of women and marginalised genders, FemTech is poised to reject this new iteration of the beauty myth by promoting inclusion and access, and reversing the harmful practices used by the beauty, diet and cosmetic surgery industries that are detailed throughout *The Beauty Myth*. However, such practices can be hard to identify and lurk within the progress that Wolf (pp. 33–34) identifies as social rights achieved by second-wave feminism. Similarly, the FemTech industry represents progress for addressing health concerns unique to women, but this progress can mask the inequitable and inaccessible nature of the industry for many. Therefore, this chapter offers a close reading of several FemTech products and brands, to unpack the ways in which the beauty myth is reproduced in the current landscape of the FemTech industry. In particular, I focus on advertising, economic marginalisation, and self-surveillance as examples of what may be holding FemTech back from its full equitable potential. Ultimately, an awareness of how these challenges have grown out of the beauty myth will allow the industry and its stakeholders to ensure that its products and practices are in line with aims to ensure inclusion and access.

Influencer Advertising and Natural Cycles

FemTech's advertising practices have developed from misleading beauty myth advertising in women's magazines to new forms such as influencer advertising, which is explored in relation to Natural Cycles in this section. Wolf (p. 71) argues that the nature of beauty myth advertising does not allow consumers to make free and informed choices about the purchase of products, and one of her central concerns is the disguising of advertisements as editorial copy. Such advertisements intentionally mislead readers, who can find it difficult to discern what is genuine content and what is beauty myth content published to appease advertisers (p. 74). While print magazines are in decline and are increasingly being replaced by their digital counterparts, Wolf's concerns persist in FemTech advertising. In particular, social media influencer advertising replicates the same issue in which it is difficult for readers to discern whether messages about a product are genuine. Influencer advertising involves partnering with a social media user, typically with a large following, to advertise a product or service in return for monetary compensation (Stubb et al., 2019, p. 110). Influencer marketing is highly effective, with consumers—especially younger consumers—more likely to trust influencer recommendations than brand produced and therefore buy products promoted by influencers (Iskiev, 2022). Social media sites typically employ strict rules about ensuring any sponsorship for a post is disclosed, usually by stating that it is a paid partnership, and by using the hashtag #ad (Stubb et al., 2019). Nonetheless, it can be difficult for consumers to discern whether a social media influencer's comments about a product they are sponsored by are genuine or not, which can be just as misleading to the consumer as its beauty myth predecessor in print magazines. Natural Cycles—a digital fertility tracker primarily marketed as a form of contraception—is a FemTech company that uses influencer marketing across social media sites including YouTube and Instagram. Using influencer marketing lends a legitimacy to Natural Cycles that is hard to achieve through other forms of advertising, but is potentially troubling due to the serious consequences if it fails when used as a contraceptive.

Montana Brown, former Love Island UK contestant with 1.2 million Instagram followers, is partnered with Natural Cycles, advertising its yearly subscription to her followers and offering a discount code. Analysing two of Brown's sponsored Instagram posts reveals Natural Cycles' key messages: the superiority of non-hormonal contraception, the promotion of knowing one's body better through using the app, and simplicity of use. The superiority of non-hormonal contraception is a key marketing message used by Natural Cycles and is evident in Brown's posts. In one post, Brown (2021a; Fig. 3.1) is pictured outside in an underwear set, holding a Natural Cycles-branded thermometer, with a big smile on her face. The accompanying caption reads "my mood when I can use natural cycles instead of putting hormones in my body [partying face emoji]" (Brown, 2021a). In another post, Brown (2022) proclaims "still loving my hormone-free journey". In both images, Brown (2021a, Fig. 3.1; 2022, Fig. 3.2) appears to be wearing little to no makeup, is smiling and is pictured in a natural setting—in one image she is outside with a blue sky in the background, and in another she is posing in front of a plant. This imagery is used to underline the joy of using non-hormonal, "natural" contraception that can be achieved with the purchase of a Natural Cycles subscription. Ironically, the only non-natural imagery in each promotional photograph is the pink Natural Cycles-branded thermometer. This is indicative of the lack of self-awareness that Natural Cycles displays when stressing that their non-hormonal, "natural" methods are better, without acknowledging that it requires the acquisition and use of an expensive technology (Della Bianca, 2021, p. 7). The superiority of non-hormonal contraception is a message that is reinforced across the Natural Cycles website, of which their campaign #hormonefreein2023 is a part (Natural Cycles, 2023a). The hashtag #hormonefreein2023 employs the rhetoric of a new year's resolution, implying that changing to use a non-hormonal contraceptive method with no side effects is aspirational, but possible by purchasing a Natural Cycles subscription.

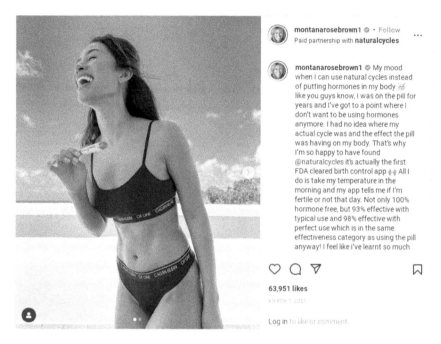

Fig. 3.1 Instagram post from account @montanarosebrown1 advertising Natural Cycles, 7 March 2021. (Brown, M. R. [@montanarosebrown1] (2021a, March 7). *My mood when I can use natural cycles instead of putting hormones in my body* [Image]. Instagram. https://www.instagram.com/p/CMHy038AtZt/)

The second key message that is portrayed through Natural Cycles' influencer campaign partnership with Brown is the assertion that the product can provide users with embodied knowledge about their menstrual cycles and fertility. This is emphasised through the captions on both of Brown's posts analysed here. Brown (2021a) asserts that having used Natural Cycles, "I feel like I've learnt so much about my body and my cycle". In a post ten months later, Brown (2022) elaborates further, stating that "every day it's [Natural Cycles] teaching me new things", and this embodied knowledge has allowed Brown to "reconnect" with her body. Brown's assertions here yet again echo discourse from Natural Cycles' (2023a) website that promises users will "learn the unique pattern of your cycle with tailored updates and insights". However, in neither post does Brown elaborate on what embodied knowledge she has gained

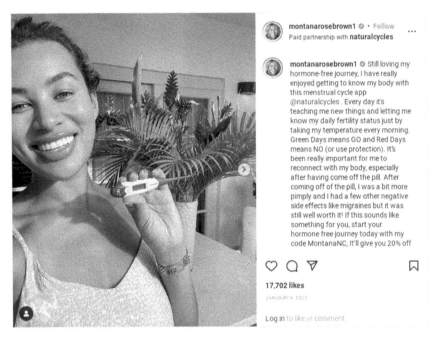

Fig. 3.2 Instagram post from account @montanarosebrown1 advertising Natural Cycles, 9 January 2022. (Brown, M. R. [@montanarosebrown1] (2022, January 9). *Still loving my hormone-free journey, I have really enjoyed getting to know my body with this menstrual cycle app @naturalcycles* [Image]. Instagram. https://www.instagram.com/p/CYgnc3YgPlr/)

through using Natural Cycles, and it remains unclear exactly *how* a user can gain a better understanding of their cycle. Natural Cycles is effectively a digitisation of the fertility awareness method (FAM), a non-hormonal way of tracking fertility by using bodily cues such as basal body temperature (BBT) and cervical mucus (Della Bianca, 2021; Bell et al., 1980). The FAM grew in popularity in the 1970s and groups teaching this method allow menstruators to learn about their bodies and menstrual cycles and determine their fertility status on any given day, to prevent or achieve conception (Bell et al., 1980). Natural Cycles, which simply asks users to input their temperature on a daily basis, streamlines this method by calculating fertility status using its FDA-approved algorithm which tells a user whether they are fertile (red) or not fertile (green) on any given day (Natural Cycles, 2023b). By keeping its algorithm that calculates fertility status proprietary, users are kept in the dark about how their fertility status is calculated and do not understand what temperature changes indicate fertility status. Therefore, it is difficult to see how Natural Cycles empowers users to learn more about their bodies and menstrual cycles.

Finally, Brown's posts promote the ease of use of Natural Cycles. In both posts, Brown (2021a, 2022) highlights that the only thing Natural Cycles needs to determine fertility status is temperature. In one post, Brown (2021a) writes "all I do is take my temperature in the morning and my app tells me if I'm fertile or not that day". The use of the word "all" in particular emphasises the ease of use and the low time commitment involved in using the app. The simplicity of using Natural Cycles is encapsulated by the phrase "Green Days means GO and Red Days means NO", referring to the colour-coded fertility indicators that the app produces to inform users about whether they can have unprotected sex on each given day (Brown, 2022). This messaging disregards the complexity of using basal body temperature (BBT) data to predict fertility status and does not acknowledge the many factors that can influence BBT, including the time the temperature is taken, illness and alcohol consumption. This over-simplification is dangerous, therefore, as it intentionally misleads users into believing that BBT is a perfect indicator of fertility status, which it is not. As shown, the three key messages portrayed in Brown's advertisements; the superiority of non-hormonal contraception, improved embodied knowledge and ease of use reflect Natural Cycles' messaging on their website and in other marketing materials. However, analysing each of the key messages reveals that they do not necessarily reflect the full truth of user experience. This is akin to the beauty myth advertising in magazines critiqued by Wolf in which products such as skin cream exaggerate their anti-ageing results. Furthermore, the advertising constructs a sense of empowerment that is achieved through taking personal responsibility for changing to "natural" contraception. This draws on the neoliberal feminism inherent in beauty myth advertising that implies that the purchase of certain products can lead women to have a successful lifestyle. The misleading advertising intentionally obscures factors that may make Natural Cycles unsuitable for some users, and the use of influencer marketing encourages users to purchase the product without conducting further research or having a full understanding of the risks involved. This is particularly troubling given that if the Natural Cycles app fails, users may experience an unplanned pregnancy, which is undoubtedly emotionally and financially distressing.

Economic Marginalisation and Menstrual Capitalism

In addition to relying on misleading advertising, FemTech also draws from the beauty myth to keep women financially oppressed through the cost of its products, and reusable menstrual underwear provides an interesting case study with which to analyse this. Highlighting how the beauty myth is fundamentally entangled with the economy, Wolf suggests that selling beauty and diet products to women is ultimately about keeping them financially oppressed (p. 20). Specifically, by setting out ever-changing goals for women's appearance, the beauty myth requires the acquisition of expensive beauty products such as moisturisers and cosmetics (p. 29). According to Wolf (p. 113), the timing of the rise of beauty products was no accident: as White middle-class women began to enter the workforce, and for the first time earn a wage, beauty myth advertising convinced them to waste this money on cosmetics, diet books and surgery. In turn, a financial incentive for the purchase and use of such products is created, as women are rewarded (for example through promotions at work) for buying into advertisers' conceptualisations of beauty, thus reinforcing the legitimacy and necessity of the myth (pp. 28–29). Women are typically poorer than men, due to prejudiced hiring and promotions that favour men over women and the gender pay gap, and when what little disposable income they have is spent on beauty products, they become economically marginalised (Wolf, p. 113; Bertrand & Hallock, 2001; Abendroth et al., 2017; Criado-Perez, 2020). In a utopian world in which the beauty myth has been dismantled, Wolf argues that women's money, no longer wasted on beauty products, could be used in any number of positive ways, from funding women's education to safe transport to world travel (p. 113). Indeed, at the crux of the beauty myth is this: if women are kept poorer, exhausted and overwhelmed by the beauty myth, then they simply will not have the power to fight against systems of oppression. The application of economic marginalisation to FemTech is clear. From sexual wellness apps to fitness trackers to menstrual underwear, the overwhelming majority of FemTech products require the purchase of a product and/or subscription. While, unlike the beauty industry, many FemTech solutions address real health issues that many women face, the issue of inaccessibility due to cost is one that undoubtedly must be addressed if the industry is to reject a new iteration of the beauty myth that incorporates health and well-being into its problematic rhetoric. Using reusable menstrual underwear as a case study, in what follows, I interrogate the economic marginalisation inherent within the FemTech industry.

Reusable menstrual underwear utilises new technology that allows thin fabric to absorb menstrual blood and incontinence. The gusset of menstrual underwear consists of many layers of thin, but highly absorbent fabric that means it will not leak. The underwear can be reused once washed, and therefore is attractive to customers trying to reduce their environmental impact. However, for many, menstrual underwear represents a significant investment. Taking Thinx (2023a), Modibodi (2023) and WUKA (2023a) as representative examples, one pair of moderate to heavy flow underwear costs between approximately £12 and £30 for UK shoppers. There are several online tools that calculate the average cost of disposable period products, which can be used to compare the cost with menstrual underwear.[3] Mooncup (2023)—a reusable menstrual cup company—has a savings calculator estimates that disposable period products costs £42.90 per year, while another hosted on the Omni Calculator website and created by two researchers states that the cost is £49.11 for

---

[3]To evaluate the relative cost of period underwear and disposable sanitary products, assumptions were made based on an 'average' menstrual cycle. This is a 28-day cycle (resulting in 13 periods per year), a moderate flow lasting 5 days, using an average of 22 disposable sanitary products per cycle, which costs an average of £45 per year. The figure used for one pair of moderate flow period underwear was £22.50, and it was estimated that a user would need 5 pairs of underwear per cycle. The same assumptions about menstrual cycle length were made when calculating both the cost of the disposable products and menstrual underwear. Clearly, menstrual cycles vary widely and therefore the cost will also vary.

tampons users, and £40.84 for sanitary pads users (Smialek & Zulawinska, 2023). Using the range given above, five pairs of menstrual underwear cost approximately £112.50. Estimations on how long a pair of menstrual underwear lasts vary, but most have a guide of around two years, with the suggestion that this lifespan can be increased by ensuring users care for their underwear properly (Thinx, 2023b; WUKA, 2023b). Thinx (2023b) suggests that their menstrual underwear can withstand 40 washes, which, if washed once per period, means they can last up to three years, while Modibodi (2022) claims their underwear can last 100 washes, providing over seven years of use. Using the lower estimate of a two-year lifespan, the cost of disposable sanitary products is marginally—about £22.50—cheaper than menstrual underwear per year. Underwear with a longer lifespan can therefore be more cost-effective in the long term for people who menstruate than using disposable products. It is also important to note that in the UK, while tax has been removed from disposable sanitary products, menstrual underwear is still subject to value-added tax (VAT), meaning that its cost is higher, although there is currently a campaign to end menstrual underwear tax (Periodpants.Org, 2023). Based on the above calculations, menstrual underwear is an innovative solution for consumers that helps them to make an environmentally conscious choice and have a more comfortable period at a cost that is not significantly above that of alternative sanitary products.

Nonetheless, there are still access barriers that potential users face, including the high upfront cost of obtaining the underwear and regular access to washing facilities. Such access barriers are obscured by the way menstrual underwear products are promoted. Companies such as Modibodi, Thinx and WUKA participate in a kind of greenwashing whereby the environmental benefits of the product are highlighted in a way that obscures access barriers. Additionally, such advertising forefronts feminist portrayals of menstruation that are appropriated to sell products. This continues the tradition of menstrual capitalism that Camilla Mørk Røstvik (2022, p. 17) describes as "the exploitation of menstruators by corporations, advertisers and other for-profit entities". Modibodi's (2020) "The New Way to Period" advertisement is indicative of how menstrual underwear promotion obscures access barriers. The minute-long video features five menstruators of various races, body shapes and gender expressions taking part in mundane activities including eating, showering and doing laundry. The advertisement depicts a bin overflowing with tampons and pads—menstrual products of the past—subtly highlighting the environmental superiority of Modibodi menstrual underwear. The video also depicts pain and menstrual blood, attempting to normalise the actual experience of menstruation, in stark contrast to the advertising of pads and tampons that has historically centred white women and girls smiling, featured outdoor and sporting activities and used blue liquid to symbolise menstrual blood (Røstvik, 2022, p. 168). By all accounts, Modibodi's "The New Way to Period" advertisement depicts an environmentally friendly and feminist period that intentionally distances itself from menstrual advertising of the past. However, despite providing "a new way to period", menstrual underwear nonetheless provides a way to manage menstrual blood in an invisible (and thus societally acceptable) way at a cost to the consumer. Additionally, a salient feature of menstrual capitalism is the use of profits to fund advertising rather than product development that directly benefits the consumer (Røstvik, 2022, pp. 19–20). Therefore, analysed in the context of menstrual management and capitalism, it is clear to see that menstrual underwear advertising deploys feminist and environmentally conscious messaging in order to obscure the access barriers to using the product.

Ultimately, menstrual underwear companies such as Modibodi, Thinx and WUKA continue in the harmful tradition of menstrual capitalism and perpetuate the culture of menstrual management. Thinx, which employs similar marketing strategies to Modibodi, was exposed as having a harmful corporate culture in which bullying, fat shaming and sexual harassment were prevalent, and ultimately resulted in then-CEO and co-founder Miki Agrawal stepping down (Røstvik, 2022, p. 159; Malone, 2017). Despite marketing themselves as a feminist and inclusive brand, Thinx's corporate culture reveals that menstrual companies are just that: companies. Regardless of brand activism and taboo-breaking advertising, reusable menstrual underwear companies are fundamentally following in the footsteps of their predecessors in the single-use menstrual product industry, in which gendered hierarchies, the undervaluing of women workers, and harmful corporate practices were the norm (Røstvik, 2022, p. 123). The use of inclusive and positive advertising of menstrual underwear also tends to obscure the accessibility barriers explored above. While charity campaigns, such as WUKA's (2023c) partnership with refugee charity Choose Love, are beginning to address these barriers, it is clear that more must be done. Such campaigns make use of their typically affluent customer base in order to fund the delivery of their products to people who face access barriers, acknowledging the inequality in the FemTech industry. However, this is just the beginning for dismantling menstrual capitalism and ensuring that menstruators have access to the menstrual products that they need. Therefore, although the cost of menstrual underwear is roughly equal to that of single-use menstrual products, there are undoubtedly still elements of the beauty myth, especially in relation to economic marginalisation of menstruators that reinvented in the reusable menstrual underwear space. This analysis of the economic marginalisation of women through FemTech, and specifically menstrual capitalism begs the question at the heart of this collection: who is FemTech for?

Self-surveillance, Data Privacy, and Workplace Health Insurance

Practices of self-surveillance, which stem from the beauty myth and are now becoming increasingly compulsory, also question who FemTech is for through the inclusion of such practices in workplace health and wellness initiatives. The beauty myth has rendered the intense self-surveillance of bodies normal, paving the way for the digitisation of such practices in FemTech. Indeed, as Wolf (p. 100) shows, beauty myth ideology encourages women to scrutinise their bodies in the mirror to identify flaws including wobbly, dimpled flesh, thick thighs, and a rounded stomach. This self-surveillance operates as an oppressive marketing tactic by which to sell products, from anti-ageing creams to diet books, in order to "fix" the flaws identified. While rituals of self-surveillance have arguably only intensified, the tools have been updated. Indeed, in the final chapter of *The Beauty Myth*, Wolf predicts that "we will be subservient to ever more refined technology for self-surveillance", citing devices such as Holtain's

Body Composition Analyzer, a portable body fat analysis tool (p. 267). This prediction certainly rings true in consideration of contemporary FemTech, as self-surveillance practices rendered normal by women's magazines in the 1990s have paved the way for the digital health industry, allowing users access to more timely and accurate data than ever before. FemTech, as part of the digital health ecosystem, has thus evolved the beauty myth to encourage self-surveillance across health and wellness, positioning it as a way to learn more about one's body in order to continue to sell its products. Fitness trackers, for instance, provide an abundance of data on daily steps, exercise, and sleep; ovulation trackers allow users to record mood, sexual activity, and temperature on any given day; and nutrition trackers ask users to record food intake, calories, and physical activity. It is quite possible to self-surveil almost all aspects of one's life and aggregate the data into what is known as the "quantified self" (Lupton, 2016, p. 102). While many people who take part in the quantified self-movement do so by choice, it is becoming increasingly compulsory across multiple social domains including the workplace, education, and insurance (p. 103).[4] For example, UK-based health, life, and car insurance company Vitality Health (2023) offers rewards and discounts to members that stay active, by using data generated by fitness trackers such as an Apple Watch. The data is used by Vitality to monitor if their customers are leading an active lifestyle in order to reduce (or increase) premiums. This is indicative of the pervasiveness of self-tracking: where it was once confined to the home with the use of the mirror and scales, it is now ever-present through smartphones and activity trackers, and there is increasing pressure to share self-surveillance data to access products and services.

The sharing of self-surveillance data, including that produced by FemTech products, with workplaces is becoming increasingly common due to the rise of workplace health insurance and wellness initiatives (Brown, 2021b). The impetus behind such programs is that if a workplace can help their employees manage their health, then productivity

---

[4] This feeds into discourses of healthism that have expanded the concept health across multiple social domains and iterate health as an individual's responsibility (see Crawford, 1980). A full analysis of how healthism operates within FemTech is beyond the scope of this chapter.

will increase, and the workplace will be more attractive to potential employees. The adoption of FemTech into such workplace initiatives is alarming, as it purports to "solve" the accessibility challenge identified in the above section: the high cost of feminine technologies. It is undeniable that these programs help employees access FemTech products and solutions that may have previously been unreachable, particularly for technologies that are cost prohibitive. However, what appears as altruism on behalf of employers raises a new set of questions for the uptake of FemTech within corporate scenarios, not least of which are concerns that such programs share employee self-surveillance data with their companies, which could lead to discrimination, among other consequences (Brown, 2021b). For example, employers may have access to data that reveals which of their employees are menstruating, trying to conceive, pregnant or experiencing menopause, which could be used to justify business decisions such as eligibility for promotions or pay raises. Still, the ostensible promises of self-tracking through workplace-initiated programs remains attractive. The FemTech industry typically aims to provide health solutions to users for so-called "women's issues" that are not addressed by traditional medical systems, such as management solutions for chronic conditions such as endometriosis. Therefore, there are often few or no alternatives to many of the FemTech solutions that users engage with, leading to a strong incentive to participate in self-surveillance, despite any data privacy concerns such as the sharing of information with workplaces. Therefore, the sharing of self-surveillance data with external bodies, such as an employer, is the price that users must pay in order to access necessary health solutions. Thus, the "cost" of accessing FemTech goes far beyond the literal economic cost, as explored in the previous case study relating to menstrual underwear.

The prominence of workplace health and wellness initiatives is shown through the existence of companies that capitalise on this very niche. One such company is Progyny, a fertility benefits network that enables employers to provide in vitro fertilisation (IVF) to its employees. Progyny's (2023a) website promotes its corporate identity using a smart blue and white colour scheme, and featuring photos of smiling couples, parents with children and photos of ultrasounds. The messaging on the website is strongly aligned with its corporate clients, highlighting that providing

IVF solutions through Progyny can increase employee wellbeing, reduce claims for employers and increase productivity compared to seeking IVF using traditional medical coverage, or out of pocket (Progyny, 2023b). Additionally, there is a strong emphasis on keeping costs for employers low while providing superior care for employees. One of Progyny's (2023a) main messages is that "everyone should be able to pursue their dream of having a family". By providing IVF through Progyny (2023b), employers are given "the ability to tangibly reinforce [their] company's values". In an interview with CNBC, Progyny CEO David Schlanger further reinforces this message, by suggesting that providing Progyny allows employers to "attract and retain top employees" and demonstrate that "you stand for diversity in the workforce, you stand for family-building values" (Zhao, 2018). Furthermore, in true neoliberal feminist fashion, the CEO advocates that providing IVF through Progyny allows employers "to give a message to your female employees that they can both have a very successful career and *actually* not sacrifice on having a family" (Zhao, 2018, emphasis added). The fact that Schlanger mentions a career before a family, and the use of "actually" implies that employers need not be worried that the IVF process will compromise on workforce productivity. Ultimately, Progyny is promoting that benefits and company culture are more important to both current and prospective employees than ever before, and by adding IVF services from Progyny to a company's benefits portfolio will help to attract and retain the best talent (Zhao, 2018). Boasting clients including Facebook and Microsoft, Progyny suggests that use of its services can allow companies to grow and be successful.

This messaging, coupled with the corporate feel of the website, strongly implies that Progyny is on the side of employers and is concerned with providing a cost-effective service for companies, by ensuring the IVF and pregnancy experience for the workforce will not compromise on productivity and the ability to carry out their work efficiently and effectively. By using Progyny to achieve pregnancy, employees are thus expected to continue work as normal throughout their IVF and pregnancy, and, given Progyny's promises to their corporate clients, there is little tolerance for those that are not able to continue work as normal while also undergoing fertility treatment. The benefit can also mean users are unable to leave employment because they are reliant on the fertility services, especially if they are undergoing treatment. In addition to this, it is important to consider concerns surrounding data privacy for employees using Progyny's services (Brown, 2021b). If an employer has access to a list of which of their employees are undertaking IVF, this information may be used to make business decisions based on factors such as the stress and risk associated with undertaking IVF and the possibility of pregnancy. Additionally, it is likely that it will only be the childbearing partner that will be penalised by such decisions, which may lead to gender discrimination. The corporate culture that Progyny promotes is one of family values in which it is expected employees will want to pursue pregnancy, and this may lead to discrimination against employees that choose to be child-free, as they are not considered to align with the company's values. However, despite the potential risks of accessing IVF through an employer by using Progyny, those that want to pursue fertility treatment may have little choice. As Progyny's (2023b) website shows, IVF is expensive and difficult to access, and so if a company provides it to employees, it is often the only financially viable way of accessing it, and the potential risks may be a small price to pay for individuals facing infertility. Therefore, as the collection of self-surveillance data becomes ever more compulsory from insurance to the workplace, so does its sharing, which can lead to discrimination that goes far beyond Wolf's concerns in *The Beauty Myth*. Progyny's marketing strategy and tuned-in corporate messaging suggest that FemTech is ultimately not only for those who can pay for it, but for those willing to consent (even tacitly) to the structures of surveillance leveraged by both employer and FemTech provider.

Conclusion

Using the beauty myth as a critical lens through which to analyse the FemTech industry reveals the ways in which FemTech can be inequitable and harmful. Taking Wolf's conceptualisations of advertising, economic marginalisation, and self-surveillance into account, this chapter highlights harmful traditions out of which the health and wellness industry has grown. Indeed, the beauty myth has grown out of latent discourses of neoliberal feminism and norms of self-improvement that have long been used to sell beauty products and now plague the health and wellness space. Therefore, while the FemTech industry does have the capacity to innovate by widening access and inclusion, as this analysis has shown, it proves not so innovative after all as it continues to keep women beholden to advertising and self-surveillance while simultaneously economically oppressed. Using Natural Cycles, menstrual underwear brands Thinx, Modibodi, and WUKA, and workplace health and wellness benefits such as those offered by Progyny as examples reveal the reinvention of the beauty myth in FemTech. In other words, discourses of consumerism and advertising, economic marginalisation, and self-surveillance do not suddenly appear in the advent of FemTech. Rather, they call on latent narratives that can be traced back to the emergence of the beauty myth following second-wave feminism. This new application of *The Beauty Myth* identifies harmful and inequitable practices within the FemTech ecosystem. Through such identification, it is possible for FemTech to reject these harmful practices and enact positive change by breaking the cycle of exploitation and oppression of women and marginalised genders that is so inherent within self- and personal care capitalism and within neoliberal feminism. It is important that the industry is focused on building intersectional inclusion and equity to ensure that life-improving health solutions and technologies can reach those that need them most. In the chapters that follow, especially in Part II of this volume which details case studies of FemTech solutions, readers can use the beauty myth as a critical lens through which to think about ideas of advertising, economic marginalisation, and self-surveillance in relation to other technologies.

References

Abendroth, A.-K., Melzer, S., Kalev, A., & Tomaskovic-Devey, D. (2017). Women at work: Women's access to power and the gender earnings gap. *ILR Review, 70*(1), 190–222. https://doi.org/10.1177/0019793916668530

Abraham, A. (2019). *30 years on from The Beauty Myth we ask Naomi Wolf 'what's changed?'* Dazed Beauty. https://www.dazeddigital.com/beauty/article/45639/1/30-years-on-from-the-beauty-myth-we-ask-naomi-wolf-whats-changed

Banet-Weiser, S. (2018). *Empowered: Popular feminism and popular Misogyny*. Duke University Press.

Banet-Weiser, S., Gill, R., & Rottenberg, C. (2019). Postfeminism, popular feminism and neoliberal feminism? Sarah Banet-Weiser, Rosalind Gill and Catherine Rottenberg in conversation. *Feminist Theory, 21*(1), 3–24. https://doi.org/10.1177/1464700119842555

Banet-Weiser, S., & Portwood-Stacer, L. (2017). The traffic in feminism: An introduction to the commentary and criticism on popular feminism. *Feminist Media Studies, 17*(5), 884–888. https://doi.org/10.1080/1468077 7.2017.1350517

Bartky, S. L. (1997). Foucault, femininity, and the modernization of patriarchal power. In D. Tietjens Meyers (Ed.), *Feminist social thought: A reader* (pp. 93–111). Routledge. (Work originally published in: Diamond, I. (1988). *Feminism and Foucault: Reflections on resistance*. Northeastern University Press).

Bell, S., Garbarino, P., Hubbich, J., Ingrum, A. Koehnline, L., & Wolhandler, J. (1980). Reclaiming reproductive control: A feminist approach to fertility consciousness. *Science for the People, 12*(1), 6–9, 30–35. https://archive.scienceforthepeople.org/vol-12/v12n1/reclaiming-reproductive-control-a-feminist-approach-to-fertility-consciousness/

Bertrand, M., & Hallock, K. F. (2001). The gender gap in top corporate jobs. *ILR Review, 55*(1), 3–21. https://doi.org/10.1177/001979390105500101

Breen, R., & Prince Cooke, L. (2005). The persistence of the gendered division of domestic labour. *European Sociological Review, 21*(1), 43–57. https://www.jstor.org/stable/3559583

Brown, E. A. (2021b). The FemTech paradox: How workplace monitoring threatens women's equity. *Jurimetrics, 61*(3), 289–329. https://www.proquest.com/docview/2568314630

Brown, M. R. [@montanarosebrown1] (2021a, March 7). *My mood when I can use natural cycles instead of putting hormones in my body* [Image]. Instagram. https://www.instagram.com/p/CMHy038AtZt/

Brown, M. R. [@montanarosebrown1] (2022, January 9). *Still loving my hormone-free journey, I have really enjoyed getting to know my body with this menstrual cycle app @naturalcycles* [Image]. Instagram. https://www.instagram.com/p/CYgnc3YgPIr/

Budlender, D. (2004). *Why should we care about unpaid care work?* Unifem.

Chernin, K. (1981). *The obsession: Reflectins on the tyranny of slenderness*. Harper & Row.

Chernin, K. (1985). *The hungry self: Women, eating and identity*. Times Books.

Cohen, R., Newton-John, T., & Slater, A. (2021). The case for body positivity on social media: Perspectives on current advances and future directions. *Journal of Health Psychology, 26*(13), 2365–2373. https://doi.org/10.1177/1359105320912450

Crawford, R. (1980). Healthism and the medicalization of everyday life. *International Journal of Health Services, 10*(3), 365–338. https://doi.org/10.2190/3H2H-3XJN-3KAY-G9NY

Criado-Perez, C. (2020). *Invisible women: Exposing data bias in a world designed for men.* Vintage.

Damelin, N. B. (2019). *The beauty myth: Is Naomi Wolf's classic still relevant today?* That's what she said. https://twssmagazine.com/2019/04/24/the-beauty-myth-is-naomi-wolfs-classic-still-relevant-today/

Della Bianca, L. (2021). The cyclic self: Menstrual cycle tracking as body politics. *Catalyst: Feminism, Theory, Technoscience, 7*(1), 1–21. https://doi.org/10.28968/cftt.v7i1.34356

Elias, A. S., Gill, R., & Scharff, C. (2017). *Aesthetic labour: Rethinking beauty politics in neoliberalism.* Palgrave Macmillan.

Emergen Research. (2020). *Femtech market to reach USD 60.01 billion by 2027.* [Online]. Cision. https://www.prnewswire.co.uk/news-releases/femtech-market-to-reach-usd-60-01-billion-by-2027-cagr-of-15-6-emergen-research-899205870.html

Hochschild, A. R., & Machung, A. (1989). *The second shift: Working families and the revolution at home.* Viking.

Iskiev, M. (2022). *How each generation shops in 2023 [New data from our state of consumer trends report].* Hubspot. https://blog.hubspot.com/marketing/how-each-generation-shops-differently

Lupton, D. (2016). The diverse domains of quantified selves: Self-tracking modes and dataveillance. *Economy and Society, 45*(1), 101–122. https://doi.org/10.1080/03085147.2016.1143726

Malone, N. (2017, March 20). Sexual-harassment claims against a 'She-E.O.' Thinx boss Miki Agrawal wanted to break taboos about the female body. According to some employees, she went too far. *The Cut.* https://www.thecut.com/2017/03/thinx-employee-accuses-miki-agrawal-of-sexual-harassment.html

Modibodi. (2020, September 16). *Modibodi | The New Way to Period* [Video]. YouTube. https://www.youtube.com/watch?v=qSnZSaWhtJs

Modibodi. (2022). *Support—How do you know when the product is at end of life?* https://support.modibodi.com/en-US/how-do-you-know-when-the-product-is-at-end-of-life-74123

Modibodi. (2023). *Shop—Moderate-heavy absorbency.* https://www.modibodi.co.uk/collections/moderate-heavy-absorbency

Mooncup. (2023). *Mooncup savings calculator.* https://www.mooncup.co.uk/menstrual-cup-savings-calculator/

Natural Cycles. (2023a). *Home page.* https://www.naturalcycles.com/

Natural Cycles. (2023b). *How does natural cycles work?* https://www.naturalcycles.com/how-does-natural-cycles-work

Orbach, S. (2005). *Fat is an advertising issue.* Campaign. https://www.campaignlive.co.uk/article/fat-advertising-issue/481078

Orgad, S., & Gill, R. (2022). *Confidence culture.* Duke University Press.

Periodpants.org. (2023). *Axe the period pants tax.* https://periodpants.org/

Progyny. (2023a). *Home page.* https://progyny.com/

Progyny. (2023b). *Is Progyny right for your company?* https://progyny.com/for-employers/for-your-company/

Riley, S., Evans, A., & Robson, M. (2022). *Postfeminism and body image.* Routledge.

Rodgers, R. F., Wertheim, E. H., Paxton, S. J., Tylka, T. L., & Harriger, J. A. (2022). #Bopo: Enhancing body image through body positive social media—Evidence to date and research directions. *Body Image, 41,* 367–374. https://doi.org/10.1016/j.bodyim.2022.03.008

Rostvik, C. M. (2022). *Cash flow: The businesses of menstruation.* UCL Press.

Rottenberg, C. (2018). *The rise of neoliberal feminism.* Oxford University Press.

Schoemaker, C. (2004). A critical appraisal of the anorexia statistics in *The Beauty Myth*: Introducing Wolf's overdo and lie factor (WOLF). *Eating Disorders, 12*(2), 97–102. https://doi.org/10.1080/10640260490444619

Smialek, D., & Zulawinska, J. (2023). *Period products cost calculator.* Omni Calculator. https://www.omnicalculator.com/everyday-life/period-products-cost

Stubb, C., Nyström, A.-G., & Colliander, J. (2019). Influencer marketing: The impact of disclosing sponsorship compensation justification on sponsored content effectiveness. *Journal of Communication Management, 23*(2), 109–122. https://doi.org/10.1108/JCOM-11-2018-0119

Thinx. (2023a). *Shop—Moderate flow.* https://www.thinx.com/thinx/collections/shop-all-period-underwear?absorbency=moderate

Thinx. (2023b). *How Thinx work.* https://www.thinx.com/thinx/how-they-work

Vitality Health. (2023). *Get rewarded for living a healthy life*. https://www.vitality.co.uk/rewards/healthy-living/

Wolf, N. (1991). *The beauty myth.* Vintage. (Original work published 1990 by Chatto and Windus)

Wolf, N. (2011). *A wrinkle in time: Twenty years after 'The Beauty Myth,' Naomi Wolf addresses The Aging Myth*. The Washington Post. https://www.washingtonpost.com/lifestyle/magazine/a-wrinkle-in-time-twenty-years-after-the-beauty-myth-naomi-wolf-addresses-the-aging-myth/2011/05/11/AGiEhvCH_story.html

WUKA. (2023a). *Period underwear for a medium flow*. https://wuka.co.uk/collections/medium-flow

WUKA. (2023b). *How period pants work*. https://wuka.co.uk/pages/how-period-pants-work

WUKA. (2023c). *Giving back*. https://wuka.co.uk/pages/giving-back

Zhao, H. (2018). Facebook and Microsoft are attracting top talent thanks to this cutting edge benefit [Video]. *CNBC*. https://www.cnbc.com/2018/12/07/progyny-is-working-to-expand-access-to-fertility-benefits.html

4

Fertile Becoming: Reproductive Temporalities with/in Tracking Technologies

Lara Reime, Marisa Cohn, and Vasiliki Tsaknaki

Introduction

If only we had known earlier…

This was a common phrase we encountered during our research on reproductive technologies and how they enable sense-making about fertility and reproductive potentials through data. *If only we had known earlier, we would have started earlier. If only we had known earlier, we would have frozen sperm (or eggs). If only we had known earlier, our future would look different as we could have acted accordingly.* These recurrent 'if only' narratives are just one example of how people who are concerned with infertility negotiate their present in relation to the past. They reveal what Barad (2010) refers to as lingering thoughts of the past and possible futures of what might yet be/have been.

In this chapter, we explore the multiple entangled temporalities of navigating fertility that we encountered in our research on menstruation

L. Reime (✉) • M. Cohn • V. Tsaknaki
IT University of Copenhagen, Copenhagen, Denmark
e-mail: lata@itu.dk; mcoh@itu.dk; vats@itu.dk

and fertility tracking applications (MFTAs) and how their users share and make sense of intimate bodily data tracked by these devices. In examining such apps and how people discuss their use in online forums, we observed many complex temporal relations such as rethinking and reencountering the past, managing expectations related to diagnosis and predictions in the present, and desires for the future. We are interested in understanding how such temporalities become structured through everyday engagements with technologies. We particularly investigate MFTAs and how they shape rhythms and relations to time and bodies. This includes how they embed particular biopolitical structures of reproduction through the ways they visually and narratively represent time, such as menstrual cycles, to the user; how they orient the user temporally in relation to their lived bodily experience of fertility and reproduction over time; and also, how users negotiate time through collective sense-making regarding data about their bodies within an ecology of apps and technologies aimed to assist with reproduction.

MFTAs make up a large part of the FemTech market with currently around 300 apps (both iOS and Android) available and the number is continuously increasing. Such apps prompt users to track their bodily sensations, activities, and practices. Through rendering this information into quantifiable data (Lupton, 2015a), they provide predictions on future beginnings of menstrual bleeding and fertile phases.

We scrutinize which particular temporalities are embedded into current MFTAs through how they represent, organize, and narrate time for the user. For example, they tend to capture data related to the present 'where am I in this cycle?' and display data related to the future—'when am I ovulating?'. We argue that the temporality of reproduction in these apps is reduced to linear, progressive narratives, as we will show through concrete examples. Overall, bodily experiences of the present (e.g. menstrual bleeding and ovulation) become translated into data archives of the *past* that serve as basis for action in the *present* (e.g. intercourse) to produce an anticipated *future* (becoming pregnant).

We ask how people navigate within the limitations and normativities of these apps, to understand how the complexity of reproductive temporalities often exceeds what these apps can represent. We find that people make sense of their data and the linear as well as progressive notions of time with others through in-app or online forums. We therefore examine extended discussions around reproductive self-tracking data in online forums where people share their tracking data and experiences with MFTAs more broadly or create alternative practices of data sharing. We analyze discussions of people encountering these apps from intersecting, and non-fixed relations to reproductive health, for example from infertile, queer, or non-binary positions. Such narratives reveal how reproductive temporalities are not only experienced in the present but also over the long durée and via retrospection.

Thus, this chapter offers an entry point into understanding the role MFTAs play in the narration of reproductive temporalities. At this point we briefly want to clarify our understanding of *reproductive time* and *temporality*. Reproductive time attends to moments where reproduction is biologically possible, i.e. ovulation and fertile years. Whereas temporality encompasses phenomenological modes focused on lived experiences of time (Freeman, 2010). In other words, with temporalities we refer to the lived and embodied experiences of reproductive time and the entanglements of past and future that form actions in the present. Temporality further entails social constructions of reproductive time, for example, through narratives of good time in one's life to become a parent. Thus, temporality, as opposed to time, is defined by multiplicity, entanglements, and relations.

To understand how temporalities are embedded in MFTAs and to map the interactions such self-tracking applications afford, we analyze data obtained from the walkthrough method (Light et al., 2018) and autoethnographic engagements with the MFTAs Drip, Clue, and Tilly.[1] The walkthrough method was employed to attentively and meticulously walk through an app's interface to unpack the social and cultural understandings of reproduction and reproductive bodies embedded in those. A1 expanded the 2nd phase (everyday use) of the walkthrough method with a longer autoethnographic engagement over a period of six months. Here, the author engaged daily with the tracking prompts of the three different MFTAs, taking screenshots, and writing down reflection notes when deemed necessary (see also Reime et al., 2023). To understand how people navigate reproductive temporalities and complexities, we also built on data conducted through digital ethnography in three online spaces on Reddit where infertility is being discussed.[2] Through these multiple data sources, we explore how time and temporalities are being understood and narrated in MFTAs and how these understandings bring

---

[1] Clue is one of the most used apps on the market for fertility and menstruation tracking, with a total of 12 million active users. Clue therefore builds part of the 'status quo' that some newer apps, like Drip, are positioning themselves against. Clue allows users to track bodily symptoms (e.g., bleeding, pain), activities (e.g., intercourse, exercise), emotions, as well as means of birth control (pills, IUD). The data is then analyzed and visualized by the app to predict future fertile windows and menstrual bleeding. Drip is a rather new app (first available for download since 2022), open source, and embodies ideals of inviting users to be in control of their data. Additionally, it is developed by women, and its creators communicate explicitly that this app departs from current MFTAs, by having addressed and improved particular aspects, such as transparency, data privacy, and bodily sensemaking. In Drip, users are actively encouraged to explore their bodies through touch, as the consistency of the cervical mucus is one of the markers Drip uses to make fertility predictions. Tilly is specifically targeted on tracking when in fertility treatment, which adds a different dimension and medicalization to menstruation and fertility tracking. Apart from tracking bodily sensations (e.g., cramps, bleeding, temperature), emotions (e.g., happy, calm), and activities (e.g., intercourse, exercise), Tilly also offers the possibility to track one's fertility protocol and medication. Tilly is conceptually developed by two women who have gone through fertility treatment themselves—a 'stressful journey' that they now want to support others with through data-driven personalization (see also Reime et al., 2023).

[2] We understand these as vulnerable spaces, despite their online availability. We have used quotes that are paraphrased in a way that they should not be traced easily. To further ensure anonymity, we refrain from naming the exact subreddits we are investigating. We are exploring three different forums which are freely accessible on Reddit, whereas one is addressing fertility more broadly, the second one is specifically geared towards aspects of queer reproduction, and the third one is used for picture sharing and comparison of fertility-related tests.

reproductive bodies into being.[3] Not only do lived experiences of reproductive temporality exceed these reductive temporalities presented by MFTAs, but the apps and their temporal frames are now part of the entangled experience of reproductive health.

MFTAs, while focused only on data collection and prediction, reshape and reconfigure experiences of reproduction. In that, they join other reproductive technologies, such as ultrasound or in vitro fertilization, taken up in prior critical Feminist STS work (e.g. Franklin, 2022) and are also entering the space of the socio-material making of reproduction. Recent technological advancement within reproductive health promises 'pregnancy for everyone' as the 'broken reproductive body' can (partly) be fixed through processes of assisted reproduction or IVF (Welsh, 2019). Prior 'infertile' bodies (either medically or socially) now have the possibility to become fertile and pregnant (Mamo, 2007; Welsh, 2019). Within this technoscientific development (some), queer bodies become fertility patients, not (or not only) because of their physical conditions but because of their sexuality (Mamo, 2007). Consequently, such technologies are entangled into broader cultural structures, carrying the potential to challenge heteronormative ideas of parenthood and family, while at the same time running the risk of reproducing such structures by reinforcing normativities of reproduction (ibid). These technologies are also part of complex temporal narratives of reproduction, as they (potentially) extend reproductive time by prolonging 'biological clocks' (Bach, 2022; Kroløkke, 2021; Wahlberg & Gammeltoft, 2017). Through egg or sperm freezing at a young age, reproductive futures are being secured, to realize one's reproductive potential, once the 'timing' is right, independent from bodily temporalities. Reproductive temporalities are thereby

---

[3] To situate our work and the ways we have surfaced the following analytical contributions, we find it important to spend some words on our own positionality. Each of us identifies as a woman, who, to different degrees, have been engaged with our own menstruating bodies and their fertile potential. One author has navigated infertility and participated as a subject of medical research on infertility as well as participating in data sharing among LBGTQ* groups related to fertility, while the other two authors previously tried to make sense of their fertile potential in order to avoid pregnancy. Therefore, our lived experiences in this regard are varied.

disconnected from bodily temporalities of aging and decreasing reproductive potential.

However, not only assisted reproduction and IVF are redefining reproductive time and temporalities; MFTAs are also suggesting timelines to act upon reproductive potentials through rendering intimate data archives into objective data outputs in forms of notifications and representations of 'fertile windows'. MFTAs, through such suggestive timings, shape what is 'good timing' for reproduction both at a moment in a particular cycle as well as throughout one's life course. They shape experiences of time through the habits of logging and calculation and people managing their expectations of such calculations. All in all, these apps and the data collecting and sharing they enable become tied up in processes of becoming (in)fertile, we argue.

In what follows, we first situate our work within existing research and theories on reproductive temporalities and self-tracking. We further hone into the processes of becoming fertile through and with technologies, particularly MFTAs. We attend to the temporal norms that are reinforced through MFTAs and how they become part of reproductive sense-making ecologies. Our research shows that people experience fertility through a complex entanglement of data tracking and sharing where MFTAs and their modes of embedding time are taken up by users to critically engage with their possibilities and limitations by employing an array of fertility sense-making practices.

Reproductive Temporalities

Theoretically, we anchor this chapter in feminist, crip, and queer theories of time and temporality. Donna Haraway's (2016) work, for instance, offers us vocabulary to talk about different temporalities as *ongoing pasts, thick presents*, and *still possible futures* pointing to the mutual entanglement of different temporal frames. In her words, 'there is nothing in times of beginnings that insists on wiping out what has come before, or, indeed, wiping out what comes after. Kainos ["new" in the Greek] can be full of inheritances, of remembering, and full of comings, of nurturing what might still be' (Haraway, 2016, p. 2). With ongoing pasts, Haraway refers to how our own pasts, but also worldly pasts, are still shaping our presents and the futures we can have. Thick presents capture the multiplicity of experiences of the present, which are always shaped by the past and the future. Still possible futures are nurturing what might still be, imagining futures not only for us but the world that comes after us and how that affects our being in the present.

This entanglement of temporal frames becomes crucial in understanding how reproductive time is being made, understood, and imagined, as we will point to throughout our analysis. In that, time is not only linear and forward oriented but always also entangled in the past: 'in our now lays the future [...] we're always coming into ourselves entangled in the past' (Gammeltoft, 2013). In her research of pregnancy in Vietnam, Gammeltoft (2013) highlights how past experiences of war and chemical pollution impact present approaches and concerns to reproduction. Here, pregnant bodies carry past traumas that might affect the future of their unborn child. Recent work also shows how not only a pregnant future is being negotiated but also how the future of the child is being imagined and how that becomes impacted by current issues of, i.e. climate change (see e.g. Lautrup, 2022). Further research argues that a pregnant person is already understood as 'a mother embarked on a life trajectory of mothering' (Browne, 2022), thereby not only entailing gendered ideas of pregnancy and parenthood but also pointing towards a 'future temporal horizon with pregnancy framed as a one-way passage to birth (when are you due?) and a forward time of teleological progress and being-toward' (Browne, 2022). Reproductive time becomes the means towards this future horizon of becoming a parent.

We further draw on the concept of *crip time* (Kafer, 2013) which allows us to view (reproductive) time as individual and multiple. In 'Feminist, Queer, Crip', Alison Kafer (2013) brings forward understandings of crip bodily temporalities as always already out of rhythm. Kafer (ibid.) argues that socially, time is seen as productive, and bodies that cannot reach a certain threshold of productivity are seen out of sync or, rather, experience their lived experience of time as out of sync with the world around them. In a similar vein, Freeman's (2010) notion of *chrononormativity* makes sense of the relationships between norms and time and builds on the 'use of time to organize individual human bodies towards maximum productivity'.

More specifically, Luciano's (2007) notion of *chronobiopolitics* tries to make sense of how lifespans become organized through 'teleological schemes […] such as marriage, accumulation of health and wealth for the future, reproduction, childrearing, and death and its attendant rituals' (Luciano, 2007 in Freeman, 2010, p. 4). In other words, chronobiopolitics moves beyond individual temporalities towards understanding how entire populations are managed through such schemes, synchronizing and relating bodies not only with each other but bigger temporal and social schemes, and rituals. For example, Martin's (2001) work shows how ideas of reproductive time, i.e. when a body is able to reproduce, is deeply entangled in gendered and social narratives of reproduction. Her work also highlights how narratives of reproduction are closely tied to ideas of citizenship and how such narratives cast the female body as a machine-like reproductive body 'producing' children (ibid). Thus, reproductive 'efficiency' takes on new meaning when it now becomes entangled in everyday practices of datafying reproductive bodies. In such teleological schemes, some bodies are always already outside of these normative temporalities through their positions in the world. This helps us to understand how MFTAs are remaking or reproducing such schemas and how the feeling body becomes an alternate collection of time (Luciano, 2007).

We draw on these theories of time and reproductive temporalities to frame questions for our analysis such as: How do people navigate their temporal schemes and make sense of them in relation to lived bodily experiences? How are crip and queer temporalities of being out of synch mediated by these apps? What are the 'thick' presents of becoming fertile? This allows us to surface moments where temporalities become visible, structured, and entangled, as well as to bring forward understandings of reproductive time which exceed biological terms, but rather asks how people make sense of their own reproductive time and temporality in becoming fertile.

Before moving into the analysis, we want to briefly situate practices of self-tracking within current research on MFTAs. Work in this field suggests that these apps are mainly designed for fertile, reproductive—willing and—able cis women in heterosexual relationships (Epstein et al., 2017; Lupton, 2015a), thereby neglecting the reality that not all women and not only women menstruate and excluding those who do not equate menstruating with being female (Homewood, 2018). Thus, critical and feminist scholarship argues that such technologies reproduce what it means to be sexed and gendered, as they are a product of entanglements with social structures, practices, and norms around reproduction (Cifor & Garcia, 2019; Homewood, 2018; Roberts et al., 2019). Other critiques from contemporary feminist research show how most reproductive health technologies still equate women's health with reproductive health, neglecting intersectional standpoints of women and gender as non-fixed categories (Keyes et al., 2020). Further critique attends to how those systems create issues of surveillance and data sovereignty (Mehrnezhad & Almeida, 2021). But research also points to their empowering potential of creating more self-knowledge and awareness (Andelsman, 2021; Homewood et al., 2020). For example, Hamper's (2020, 2022) work shows how women in the UK use MFTAs to make sense of their fertile window by learning about their bodies through tracking data. Further, Lupton's work (Lupton, 2015a, 2015b) offers a broad research scope on various socially entangled practices of self-tracking, bodies, and data. Specifically, her work on reproductive self-tracking points to the reconfigurations of bodies, as data is not only extracted from bodies but also shapes these bodies in return (Lupton, 2019). We build on this work by offering a critical engagement with normative temporal frames reinforced through engagements with MFTAs and an analysis of how reproductive bodies navigate these spaces.

Making and Understanding Temporalities Within MFTAs

The following analysis exemplifies different entangled modes of making and understanding time within reproductive sense-making. We move from analytical points of how we see temporality imagined within tracking applications towards practices through which these temporalities are

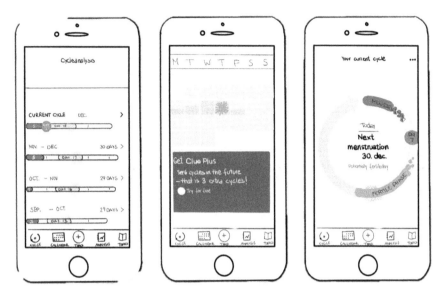

Figs. 4.1–4.3 Cycleanalysis, Calendar view, and Current Cycle

being made-sense-of through community practices. We present the first examples through data conducted from the walkthrough method and autoethnographic engagements, while the latter point is exemplified by community chats in reddit forums. We begin by presenting findings specifically on temporalities within MFTAs. Here, we surface how time is being represented and configured through such apps. Further, we look into which temporalities users become oriented towards, how datafied relations are built in the present towards the past and future, and how such apps are embedded in broader social schemas (chronobiopolitics) of reproduction.

The apps represent the reproductive journey as temporal linear and cyclical. For example, Clue uses three different representations of cyclic time. The visualization in 'Cycle history' (Fig. 4.1) views cycles in comparison, it individualizes each cycle—they have a distinct start and end. The calendar overview (Fig. 4.2) puts the reproductive cycle in connection with time around it (meaning days and dates). Figure 4.3 is probably the most used visualization for reproductive time, starting with the first day of menstruation, prediction of the fertile phase and locating one's current position on this cyclic trajectory that ends with the first day of menstruation and at the same time starts all over again. The idea of cyclic time stabilizes forward movement, promises renewal rather than rapture (Freeman, 2010). What all visualizations have in common is that they highlight and center fertile time (ovulation).

Apart from different modes of visualizing and representing time, they also afford the building of datafied relations to pasts and possible futures. Through fertility tracking in the present, data is being created that builds a 'digital archive of the body', which is then being used to calculate and predict fertile times. Thereby, MFTAs engage with different temporalities of the reproductive body (tracking data in the present to build an archive [past] that can predict future ovulations). 'The future' becomes the commodity of the app. The user shares their present and their past and the app predicts the future in return. In Clue, for example, the non-premium user only gets 3 months of prediction, whereas a longer prediction horizon of 6 months is available for users paying a monthly fee. If one has a 'regular' cycle, the difference between knowing 3 or 6 months in advance seems minor, as one could easily do the calculations oneself. Where it might be more meaningful for people with irregular cycles to make sense of their future reproductive times, as it might be harder to predict oneself, the apps fail to do these predictions, as they can only calculate with regularity. Thereby these apps are geared towards an ableist understanding of bodies and their regularity which makes them predictable.

Not only is the future being withheld from the non-premium user, so too is the analysis of their past. For example, Clue has A1's tracking data since January 2019 (more than 3 years of, more or less, consistent tracking data), but because A1 has not created an account, Clue does not give her any analysis on her past cycle data, other than providing the dates. This creates an imbalance, where the user loses their data sovereignty (Prainsack, 2019). The app now has more insights on the user than the user themself and is not sharing these insights with the user. By reading through the privacy statement of Clue and Tilly, we learn that both apps potentially share anonymized data with researchers for the purpose to 'create more knowledge around reproduction to help people with fertility issues' (Clue, 2022; Tilly, 2022). This help, however, does not directly reach the user, as they are not aware of the analysis that is being done about them based on their data. Creating a meaningful archive is also only possible by tracking consistently, which most people either do not do or where the apps do not allow for tracking, as they are only geared towards a certain life situation (getting pregnant/avoiding to) but do not encompass a more holistic view of reproductive life (Kumar et al., 2020), thus not allowing for consistent tracking throughout the life course. The user becomes part of an unknown future, a future where infertility supposedly can be better understood.

MFTAs orient[4] the user towards different temporalities such as rhythms, rituals, and durations, in multiple ways. Through notifications, the researched MFTAs structure daily engagements by sending reminders to track data, measure temperature, and even give suggestions for good timing of intercourse based on the data inputs. For example, 'mornings' become such a temporal orientation, as this is the moment where temperature measurements should take place. Though mornings should be understood as the time when bodies are waking up, not necessarily the temporal frame of morning (i.e. sunrise to noon). Through framings of 'mornings' rather than for example wake-up time, some bodies are already out of sync, as different work- and lifestyles allow for different moments of 'mornings'.

The researched MFTAs do not only structure users' time and engagement but also prompt them to 'make time' for taking self-care actions. For instance, Tilly has dedicated a whole section on self-care, including guides for meditation and yoga, as well as online courses regarding mental health, such as a 6-weeks course on dealing with miscarriage. While this might be helpful for some, it also assumes that users have time and can make time for taking care of themselves through meditation and have the capacity to become fertility experts of their own body by taking the courses they offer and engaging in tracking practices as well as community exchanges. Thus, tracking technologies 'bind' us (Freeman, 2010)

---

[4]To ask about orientation is to consider, how we arrive to the app as a designed object, what kind of attending to it requires of us and our body, and how it directs us along the 'well trodden paths'. 'Lines are both created by being followed and are followed by being created. The lines that direct us, as lines of thought as well as lines of motion, are in this way performative: they depend upon the repetition of norms and conventions, of routes and paths taken, but are also created as an effect of this repetition' (Ahmed, 2006, p. 16). This allows us to ask about what an app 'affords' in terms of how it orients the user to particular temporal experiences such as the menstrual cycle.

into specifically patterned lives, intimately linked to national narratives and timelines of reproduction (when is the right time and space to reproduce). That is to say, MFTAs do not only build on normative temporalities in the sense of cyclic temporalities (e.g. how long is a cycle, which day ovulation happens) but also on social temporalities of when it is socially acceptable to become pregnant. This becomes visible as the researched MFTAs are mainly addressing heterosexual couples in their late 20's early 30's. In the community space of Tilly, for example, most stories from people that are trying to conceive are from people in heterosexual relationships in their 30's. For example, one story recalls the experience of how a couple started to try to conceive when they were in their early 30's. After a few 'natural' tries, they took a consultation with a doctor who diagnosed the woman with fertility issues. She started treatment and eventually gave up trying, as she was getting too old. Throughout her narrative, we see the spell of the past lingering: 'if only I had known earlier, I might have had a chance'.

The past does not only become important on an individual level. As a campaign from the Copenhagen Municipality shows, potentially reproductive bodies are geared to take action in the present to ensure their ability to have children in the future (Copenhagen Municipality, 2015). This campaign illustrates that, in contemporary western societies, especially in bigger cities, people tend to have children at a later age, thus acknowledging, if not enforcing, a temporal shift in the chronobiopolitics of reproduction. Reproduction at a later age might lead to fertility issues as suggested by the campaign: 'your chance at becoming a mother is double as high when you are 25 than 35', or '40% have a low sperm quality. It can take time to become a father'. Such narratives not only reinforce gendered reproductive bodies but also fertile bodies; in other words, a younger body is more fertile than an older one. To battle a dwindling birthing rate, this Danish campaign suggests, for example, egg-freezing at a young age in order to ensure a reproductive future. Despite this campaign being critiqued for their involvement in citizens' reproduction, it thus points to entangled temporal relations. Rather than time being linear, it is nurturing of a future of what might still be, remembering a past where chances have been missed and ongoing presents infused with multiple temporalities and materialities (Haraway, 2016).

Collective Practices of Becoming Fertile

So far, we have shown, through data collected via the walkthrough method, the ways that MFTAs embed and represent temporality and temporal norms, not accounting for complex and individual temporalities. We now shift to these complexities of lived experiences of reproductive temporalities. In this section, we focus on the ways people make sense of these multiple and assembled temporalities in MFTAs in relation to their own experiences. We explore online forums, as we see these spaces as sites where people come to fill gaps encountered through the mismatch of lived experiences and engagement with the apps and reproductive health more generally. Here is also where alternative ways to share tracked data together beyond what the apps can offer are being developed and engaged with. Thus, these spaces also exemplify practices of knowledge and data exchange with others in similar situations. We are interested in understanding how people navigate these apps when they do not conform to their lived experiences. We look particularly at forums where people discuss queer experiences with fertility and experiences with infertility (these are also intersecting as we will discuss). We focus on how these forums are used to share experiences with the apps or reflect together on data tracking collection and analysis.

Generally, these online forums are spaces where information is being shared to make sense of one's own body and data. People share data regarding their reproductive experiences to varying degrees. Some have details such as diagnosis, age, gender, relationship status, miscarriages, and more in their 'flair' (a little information box behind their usernames, e.g. username1 [38F | Unexplained | Single | 1MC]). Some users actively seek help by posing questions while others provide help through sharing their own experiences or opinions, while another set of users might find it helpful to read discussions without actively engaging in them. Questions users ask relate to sharing frustrations and other emotions, but also to making sense of symptoms, cyclic stages, IVF treatment processes, pregnancy tests, or of doctors' advice. Users frequently share their diagnosis and the treatment doctors suggested, apparently trying to verify with the community if this is the 'correct' process. In that, time becomes an important normative horizon that can be oriented towards (e.g. duration of treatment). Within community chats for people in fertility treatment, normativities are a source for hope in that people tend to relate their own experience to someone else in the same situation. This becomes visible as people often answer with phrases like 'when I was at this stage', 'it looked the same for me', or 'I had the same diagnosis and treatment, and this happened to me'. Normativities of time are being used to make sense of one's situation. Where should I be at this stage of my pregnancy or at this stage of my IVF treatment? What did others do? How many tries did others have? What is normal?

These conversations could already be understood as data-sharing practices, where users share intimate information about their treatment, relationships, and diagnosis. But we also encounter examples where data sharing is approached in a more organized manner through, for instance, a spreadsheet. Whereas the forum entries are tied to experiences, emotions, and worries, the spreadsheet offers a collection of 'purer' data. Here, users can enter information including their reddit username, infertility diagnosis, age (at egg retrieval), cycle date, treatment protocol, the number of eggs retrieved, medication taken, whether sperm or egg donor were used, the costs, and much more.

Contrary to earlier examples, where MFTAs built data archives of users' data and share them with researcher beyond their control, this example can be understood as a bottom-up practice of creating a database that is accessible for everyone—a crowd-sourced resource from the community to the community people are engaged in. Such data sheets also fill another role, namely making sense of one's body in relation to others. The spreadsheet can be filtered in/excluding certain diagnosis or treatments. Consequently, users can find other users with similar parameters such as age, diagnosis, treatment, and from this information make assumptions about their own body, such as the amount of IVF procedures they will most likely need. What becomes visible when looking at the forum and the spreadsheet is that most users are in heterosexual relationships, and thus focus primarily on the female body for tracking and intervention. In that, social infertility is not specifically included though also not excluded, as the forum guidelines make clear that everyone concerned with infertility is welcome in the forum. However, there are different temporalities and relations at stake, depending on medical or social infertility (or an intersection of both), as we elaborate further.

Temporal and Bodily Pluralities

Medically, heterosexual couples are understood as infertile after one year of trying (having unprotected sex during the ovulation period), unless any affecting illness is known prior to that. Queer temporalities differ, as there is never a 'trying' period. From the beginning, queer bodies are entangled in multiple structures such as medical examinations, law, technology, hormones, and data. During this process, not only identities as parents become negotiated but also gender identities are being negotiated, gained, and lost. For example, Dahl's (2018) work illustrates how gay identities are being reshaped through pregnancy and parenthood, but also through national, in this case Swedish, narratives of reproduction. Focused on reproductive technologies and queer bodies, Mamo (2007) shows how wombs that have been previously outside of reproductive time are through technological and legal advancement embraced into this space: 'Becoming fertile, a process that involves a desire to reproduce through pregnancy, is a rather queer phenomenon; it is profoundly shaped by effects of and access to fertility medicine itself' (van Balen & Inhorn, 2002).

In the forums, we see people discussing their plans of becoming fertile in advance before even starting any treatment. For example, one user started planning treatment four years in advance, as processes such as sperm donor quarantine result in a longer temporal frame for conception. In response to this thread, most users share that they planned at least one year before they started trying to conceive. This includes finding a doctor, finding a donor, maybe even doing transitions, reducing/increasing hormones before the 'actual' trying can start. 'Queer Conception: The Complete Fertility Guide for Queer & Trans Parents-to-be' (Kali, 2022) is a book most frequently discussed and shared as an invaluable source for starting the journey. Here the 'pre-starting process', which includes making decisions and creating a timeline is the first chapter. This indicates how important planning is being understood and how the present is being planned towards the future. Knowing the exact time of ovulation becomes even more relevant in this process as not only the desire to get pregnant is involved but also different stakeholders (doctors, donors) and infrastructures, as well as financial resources (depending on location), and extended emotional labor.

Once a body has entered AR or IVF, their temporalities become more vulnerable due to repeated delays and disruptions. Users share their concerns with missing the 'perfect cycle' due to sickness or doctor office opening hours. 'What would have been if we would have been able to use this cycle?'—is a question we frequently encounter in the forums. The stories of several users show, for example, how they are affected by the COVID-19 pandemic, not only in terms of closing/opening hours of doctor offices but—in the longer perspective—shortages on sperm donations and resulting waiting lists. Answers to these posts are trying to see the positive, that they now have one more month of tracked data, which will make it easier for them in the future to determine 'good timing'. Other advice suggests zooming in and out of life, thinking about the decades of life staging. Instead of being upset about this moment, zooming out to realize that there is a whole 'family making decade' (20-40), so one month will not affect this. Another suggestion is to group cycles in 3-months blocks, which should help to minimize the disappointment of one failed cycle, making each cycle in itself less vulnerable.

Significantly, none of this can be represented in how MFTAs are currently designed. There is no possibility to think of/group cycles differently, as the apps offer a cycle-to-cycle thinking and set of representations. There is no such representation of a 'pre' phase, though apps might be mainly useful in the 'pre' phase, where users are learning about their bodies, and 'becoming fertile' in order to be 'ready' once they actually start trying. Moreover, the MFTAs we explored do not allow for adding insemination—only intercourse. Even though Tilly is an app developed for people concerned with infertility, the treatment categories only include treatment start date, egg retrieval, embryo transfer, follicle check, pregnancy test, ovulation injection, start of stimulation, appointment but not specifically insemination. This potentially indicates that most MFTAs are specifically designed for a certain part of the reproductive process. In this case, the 'becoming fertile' phase, adding medication and treatments, but once insemination happened it seems to transgress into a 'pregnant' body who cannot be tracked through this app anymore.

Ecologies of Becoming Fertile

Through research into MFTAs and online communities, we explored how temporalities of reproductive bodies are represented, configured, and navigated. We pointed towards complex temporalities of (in)fertile becoming. We now shift towards discussing the ecologies of reproductive bodies and how they come to matter through MFTAs and social narratives of reproduction.

MFTAs and other means of digital tracking have a linear understanding of reproductive time in the sense that they cannot deal with disruption of the linear forward movement towards pregnancy which ultimately results in the birth of a child. Thereby, MFTAs cater towards an ableist view of reproductive bodies. That is, through sufficient self-knowledge and observation, bodies can be moved, or progressed, into fertility. Reproductive time becomes the means towards this future horizon of becoming a parent, anticipating the right moment to establish this horizon by tracking and making sense of data. Miscarriages, abortions, and illness, however, destabilize the linearity and one-way nature of it. Pregnancy might end without becoming a parent. Miscarriages, for example, cannot be understood through most tracking applications, as there is no option of tracking pregnancy or miscarriage in the researched MFTAs. Once the body becomes pregnant, tracking through these apps is not possible anymore. This leaves a lack of possibilities for tracking the multiplicity of imaginary, sexualized, gendered, and technologically augmented bodies (Kroker, 2012). Even in a merit of apps that are specifically geared towards pregnancy tracking, pregnancy loss cannot be accounted for (Andalibi, 2021). This means that users need to delete their app to avoid the continuation of visualization of their lost pregnancy and to stop receiving notifications on the progress of growth. In the few cases where it is possible to add the loss, previous pregnancy data just becomes deleted, rather than offering a possibility to acknowledge and engage with the loss (Andalibi, 2021). Andalibi (2021) suggests that this reflects the cultural and social ecologies these apps are part of, namely ecologies in which miscarriages become individualized and tabooed rather than actively engaged with.

MFTAs are further part of shaping cultural and sociotechnical understandings of reproduction and bodies, for example, by embedding teleological schemas (Luciano, 2007) of reproduction. Thus, bringing reproductive bodies into matter through, for example, narrating when the right time to have children is not only in a particular cycle but at which stage in life. Expectations on how reproductive bodies should be acted upon and materialized are tied to cultural ideas about 'time and progression' (Franklin, 2022). When is it the right time to become a parent? What stage or life situation is best? Temporalities of reproductive bodies do not only bring norms into being in terms of which moments in one's life reproductive potential should be acted upon; it also brings into being very normative ideas of reproductive cycles that everyday life becomes acted upon and structured around. MFTAs thereby introduce a more normative and formalized temporal frame to reproductive bodies (Hamper, 2020).

In Barad's terms, coming into matter is a 'condensation of dispersed and multiple beings- times, where the future and past are diffracted into now, into each moment'. (Barad, 2015). Following that thought, reproductive bodies come into matter through MFTAs, where the past (bodily archive) and the future (becoming pregnant) are diffracted into actions in the now. Reproductive technologies are bringing reproductive bodies into being and altering reproductive temporalities. Tracking applications do not make people more or less fertile. But they create anticipation and visualize fertile moments, thereby making fertile bodies that can be acted upon. They are also remaking what a reproductive body is and moving bodies towards a reproductive future. Through collecting data in the present, predictions about future fertile potential are being made and anticipated by the user, affecting actions in the present (e.g. diet, sex, and doctor visits). Through MFTAs, these futures are visualized and acted upon, as bodies are becoming known as reproductive (Hamper, 2022).

In our exploration of the relationships between bodies, apps, data, and reproduction, we understand MFTAs not as singular way of making sense of fertility but as used together with other technologies, such as tests, thermometers, online forums, and analog notes. MFTAs are thereby part of an ecology of technologies that are used to make sense of one's fertility. Thus, reproductive bodies are complexly entangled in technologies, self-knowledge, and reproductive labour (Hamper, 2022). Within these entanglements of temporalities and technologies, we see reproductive bodies becoming fertile.

For example, through broader 'FemTech' developments, possible futures become intertwined with medical practices, in which reproductive bodies become spaces for constant repairs (Welsh, 2019). Infertile bodies are only temporarily 'broken' as, through technological intervention, everybody can get pregnant (Welsh, 2019)—in theory. In practice, however, some bodies will never become pregnant, partly by their own choice, but also due to the social and local situation they are moving within. Do they have access to healthcare? To inclusive healthcare? And in some cases, even technological advancement cannot make up for the historical medical neglect of the (female) reproductive organs that still leads to misconceptions and treatment errors. That is to say, the past lingers in the reproductive body in multiple ways. Not only our own past, and the decisions that we have made throughout our life course that might make it harder or easier for us to become fertile, but also decisions of the past that were not ours. The body inherits how reproduction has been studied in the past, especially how the uterus has been *understudied* in the past still affects the knowledge we (do not) have today. Fertility tracking gears us towards a hopeful future by contributing with our data in the present, to make future research more attuned and inclusive to the needs of diverse bodies and reproductive scenarios, and filling this historical research gap. However, we should remain cautious of the harm designs that are based on normative and under-researched understandings of embodied reproductive temporalities might do, even with the good intent of filling knowledge gaps.

Conclusion

This chapter has shown how specific FemTech developments, such as MFTAs, are entangled in a broader ecology of fertility sense-making. Empirically, we have engaged with the three tracking applications: Clue, Tilly, and Drip, as well as online forums in which users are making sense of their data and experiences together. We have shown how MFTAs represent and organize reproductive time, how they build datafied relations to pasts and futures, and how users become oriented towards temporalities that are embedded within broader social and cultural narratives of reproduction. We have further explored how people engage in collective practices to make sense of their fertile potential and find ways of 'queering' their temporalities.

Based on these explorations, we propose that future MFTAs should be designed with a more holistic purpose in mind: inclusive and accounting for a plurality of bodies, experiences, and temporalities. But as Barad (2015) pointed out: it is not about making 'trans or queer into universal features [...]. The point is to make plain the undoing of universality'. In other words, the question might not be about embracing other marginalized groups into these tracking spaces, but the mere idea that reproductive bodies can universally be tracked, categorized, and predicted is to be debated. However, we also want to take seriously users' need for objective sense-making about their reproductive bodies. We therefore propose that inclusive design might not completely abandon normative representations of temporalities but engage with them through intersectional and multiple perspectives. Thus, allowing to make sense of reproductive temporalities as entangled and non-linear.

References

Ahmed, S. (2006). *Queer phenomenology: Orientations, objects, others*. Duke University Press.

Andalibi, N. (2021). Symbolic annihilation through design: Pregnancy loss in pregnancy-related mobile apps. *New Media & Society, 23*(3), 613–631. https://doi.org/10.1177/1461444820984473

Andelsman, V. (2021). Materializing: Period-tracking with apps and the (re) constitution of menstrual cycles. *MedieKultur: Journal of Media and Communication Research, 37*(71), 054–072. https://doi.org/10.7146/mediekultur.v37i71.122621

Bach, A. S. (2022). The affective temporalities of ovarian tissue freezing: Hopes, fears, and the folding of embodied time in medical fertility preservation. In R. M. Shaw (Ed.), *Reproductive citizenship: Technologies, rights and relationships* (Health, Technology and Society) (pp. 51–73). Springer Nature. https://doi.org/10.1007/978-981-16-9451-6_3

Barad, K. (2010). Quantum entanglements and hauntological relations of inheritance: Dis/continuities, spacetime enfoldings, and justice-to-come. *Derrida Today, 3*(2), 240–268. https://doi.org/10.3366/drt.2010.0206

Barad, K. (2015). TransMaterialities: Trans*/matter/realities and queer political imaginings. *GLQ: A Journal of Lesbian and Gay Studies, 21*(2–3), 387–422. https://doi.org/10.1215/10642684-2843239

Browne, V. (2022). A pregnant pause: Pregnancy, miscarriage, and suspended time. *Hypatia, 37*(2), 447–468. https://doi.org/10.1017/hyp.2022.5

Cifor, M., & Garcia, P. (2019). Gendered by design: A duoethnographic study of personal fitness tracking systems. *ACM Transactions on Social Computing, 2*(4), 22.

Clue. (2022). Privacy policy. https://helloclue.com/privacy

Copenhagen Municipality. (2015). Ny kampagne: Få børn allerede mens du læser. DR. Retrieved October 5, 2015, from https://www.dr.dk/levnu/parforhold/ny-kampagne-faa-boern-allerede-mens-du- laeser

Dahl, U. (2018). Becoming fertile in the land of organic milk: Lesbian and queer reproductions of femininity and motherhood in Sweden. *Sexualities, 21*(7), 1021–1038. https://doi.org/10.1177/1363460717718509

Epstein, D. A., Lee, N. B., Kang, J. H., Agapie, E., Schroeder, J., Pina, L. R., Fogarty, J., Kientz, J. A., & Munson, S. (2017). Examining menstrual tracking to inform the design of personal informatics tools. In *Proceedings of the 2017 CHI conference on human factors in computing systems – CHI '17* (pp. 6876–6888). ACM Press. https://doi.org/10/cfbv

Forlano, L. (2017). Data Rituals in Intimate Infrastructures: Crip Time and the Disabled Cyborg Body as an Epistemic Site of Feminist Science Catalyst. *Feminism Theory Technoscience, 3*(2), 1–28. https://doi.org/10.28968/cftt.v3i2.28843

Franklin, S. (2022). *Embodied progress: A cultural account of assisted conception* (2nd ed.). Routledge. https://doi.org/10.4324/9781003284499

Freeman, E. (2010). *Time binds: Queer temporalities, queer histories.* Duke University Press. https://doi.org/10.2307/j.ctv1198v7z

Gammeltoft, T. M. (2013). Potentiality and human temporality: Haunting futures in Vietnamese pregnancy care. *Current Anthropology, 54*(S7), S159–S171. https://doi.org/10.1086/670389

Hamper, J. (2020). 'Catching Ovulation': Exploring women's use of fertility tracking apps as a reproductive technology. *Body & Society, 26*(3), 3–30. https://doi.org/10.1177/1357034X19898259

Hamper, J. (2022). Getting the timing right: Fertility apps and the temporalities of trying to conceive. In V. Boydell & K. Dow (Eds.), *Technologies of reproduction across the lifecourse* (Emerald Studies in Reproduction, Culture and Society) (pp. 149–162). Emerald Publishing Limited. https://doi.org/10.1108/978-1-80071-733-620221013

Haraway, D. (2016). *Manifestly Haraway. Posthumanities 37.* University of Minnesota Press.

Homewood, S. (2018). Designing for the changing body: A feminist exploration of self-tracking technologies. In *Extended abstracts of the 2018 CHI conference on human factors in computing systems, 1–4. CHI EA '18.* Association for Computing Machinery. https://doi.org/10.1145/3170427.3173031

Homewood, S., Karlsson, A., & Vallgårda, A. (2020). Removal as a method: A fourth wave HCI approach to understanding the experience of self-tracking. In *Proceedings of the 2020 ACM designing interactive systems conference, 1779–91.* Association for Computing Machinery. https://doi.org/10.1145/3357236.3395425

Kafer, A. (2013). *Feminist, queer, crip.* Indiana University Press. http://www.jstor.org/stable/j.ctt16gz79x.5

Kali, K. L. (2022). *Queer conception: The complete fertility guide for queer and trans parents-to-be.* Sasquatch Books.

Keyes, O., Peil, B., Williams, R. M., & Spiel, K. (2020). Reimagining (Women's) health: HCI, gender and essentialised embodiment. *ACM Transactions on Computer-Human Interaction, 27*(4), 1–42. https://doi.org/10.1145/3404218

Kroker, A. (2012). *Body drift: Butler, Hayles, Haraway. Posthumanities 22.* University of Minnesota Press.

Kroløkke, C. (2021). For whom does the clock tick?: Male repro-temporality in fertility campaigns, scientific literature, and commercial accounts. *Anthropology & Aging, 42*(1), 81–96. https://doi.org/10.5195/aa.2021.257

Kumar, N., Karusala, N., Ismail, A., & Tuli, A. (2020). Taking the long, holistic, and intersectional view to women's wellbeing. *ACM Transactions on Computer-Human Interaction, 27*(4), 23. 1–23:32. https://doi.org/10.1145/3397159

Lautrup, A. (2022). *Generation Carbon. Loss, goodness and youth climate activism in Norway's oil capital.* IT University of Copenhagen. https://en.itu.dk/-/media/EN/Research/PhD-Programme/PhD-defences/2022/PhD-Thesis-Temporary-Version-Andy-Lautrup-pdf.pdf

Light, B., Burgess, J., & Duguay, S. (2018). The walkthrough method: An approach to the study of apps. *New Media & Society, 20*(3), 881–900. https://doi.org/10.1177/1461444816675438

Luciano, D. (2007). *Arranging grief: Sacred time and the body in nineteenth-century America.* NYU Press.

Lupton, D. (2015b). "Mastering Your Fertility": The digitised reproductive citizen. SSRN Scholarly Paper 2679402. Social Science Research Network. https://papers.ssrn.com/abstract=2679402

Lupton, D. (2015a). Quantified sex: A critical analysis of sexual and reproductive self-tracking using apps. *Culture, Health & Sexuality, 17*(4), 440–453. https://doi.org/10.1080/13691058.2014.920528

Lupton, D. (2019). Toward a more-than-human analysis of digital health: Inspirations from feminist new materialism. *Qualitative Health Research, 29*(14), 1998–2009. https://doi.org/10.1177/1049732319833368

Mamo, L. (2007). Queering reproduction: Achieving pregnancy in the age of technoscience. https://doi.org/10.1215/9780822390220

Martin, E. (2001). *The woman in the body: A cultural analysis of reproduction: With a new introduction* (2001 ed.). Beacon Press.

Mehrnezhad, M., & Almeida, T. (2021). Caring for intimate data in fertility technologies. In *Proceedings of the 2021 CHI conference on human factors in computing systems* (pp. 1–11). ACM. https://doi.org/10.1145/3411764.3445132

Prainsack, B. (2019). Logged out: Ownership, exclusion and public value in the digital data and information commons. *Big Data & Society, 6*(1), 2053951719829773. https://doi.org/10.1177/2053951719829773

Roberts, C., Mackenzie, A., Mort, M., Atkinson, T., Kragh-Furbo, M., & Wilkinson, J. (2019). Fertility biosensing. In *Living data* (1st ed., pp. 33–66). Making Sense of Health Bio-Sensing. Bristol University Press. https://www.jstor.org/stable/j.ctvkwnqg0.7

Reime, L., Tsaknaki, V., & Cohn, M. 2023. Walking Through Normativities of Reproductive Bodies: A Method for Critical Analysis of Tracking Applications.

In *Proceedings of the 2023 CHI Conference on Human Factors in Computing Systems* (CHI '23). Association for Computing Machinery, New York, NY, USA. Article 658, 1–15. https://doi.org/10.1145/3544548.3581450

Tilly. (2022). Privacy policy. Tilly. 2022. https://mytilly.co/privacy-policy

van Balen, F., & Inhorn, M. C. (2002). Introduction: Interpreting Infertility: A View from the Social Sciences. In F. van Balen & M. C. Inhorn (Eds.), *Infertility around the Globe: New Thinking on Childlessness, Gender, and Reproductive Technologies* (pp. 3–32). University of California Press. http://www.jstor.org/stable/10.1525/j.ctt1ppfk5.3

Wahlberg, A., & Gammeltoft, T. M. (2017). *Selective Reproduction in the 21st Century.* Springer International Publishing AG. http://ebookcentral.proquest.com/lib/kbdk/detail.action?docID=4947292

Welsh, T. (2019). Broken pregnancies: Assisted reproductive technology and temporality. In *Phenomenology of the broken body*. Routledge.

Part II

FemTech at the Margins

5

One Size (Doesn't) Fit All: A Closer Look at FemTech Apps and Datafied Reproductive Body Projects in India

Paro Mishra, Ravinder Kaur, and Shambhawi Vikram

Introduction

The contemporary times are witnessing adoption of digital technologies for health wearables, implantables, sensors, mobile and web applications (popularly known as apps) and imaging/screening devices at a warp speed. These digital health technologies operate at a diverse scale, ranging from macro-level medical research, public health infrastructures, clinical health care to more micro-level practices of self-care and wellness. With an increase in multistakeholderism and technological innovation such products are increasingly centralised and connected through Artificial Intelligence. In this paper, we focus on a small but highly popular

P. Mishra (✉)
Indraprastha Institute of Information Technology, New Delhi, India
e-mail: paro.mishra@iiitd.ac.in

R. Kaur
Indian Institute of Technology, New Delhi, India

S. Vikram
Jawaharlal Nehru University, New Delhi, India

segment of FemTech apps for women's reproductive health tracking in India. The mobile health apps (m-Health apps) market has been expanding in India since 2016 and is estimated to be INR 337.89 billion industry by 2026 (Healthcare Apps Market in India Report, 2021). Within the wider health app market, FemTech apps catering to women's reproductive health is an important subcategory. The Australian network FemTech Collective describes FemTech as 'a category of software, diagnostics, products, and services that include fertility solutions, period-tracking apps, pregnancy and nursing care, women's sexual wellness, and reproductive system health care' (2021). FemTech has often been hailed for its emancipatory potential and its 'expansive focus and emphasis on addressing health inequities and tackling stigmatized conditions' (Sandhu et al., 2020). This is based on the recognition of long-standing gender bias in medicine (Dusenbery, 2018; Hamberg, 2008; Perez, 2019) and underserved health needs of women (Jafree, 2020). Within this context, such biomedical digital technologies are seen as addressing a gender gap (Zhao et al., 2016) and potentially transforming the relations between self, body and technologies (Wajcman, 2000).

India is now home to 5 percent of the world's total FemTech companies (Finology, 2022) and is the largest player in the South Asia region. In addition, it has also been a lucrative and expanding market for FemTech products and services emerging in developed parts of the world. The shift to women's reproductive health management through the digital is not driven by technology alone but is to be located in the Indian state's strong interest in digitisation of all services, including healthcare, which has been underway over the last several decades. Digital technology and data-driven approaches to health information systems have long been offered as solutions to unequal and exclusionary access to maternal and reproductive healthcare in the country (Rathi & Tandon, 2019). Mishra and Suresh (2021) note that initiatives like the Health Management Information System (2008), Mother and Child Tracking System (2011) and Reproductive and Child Health Portal (2018) were designed for delivery of pregnancy services and immunisation services. However, what is new about contemporary reproductive digital management is the rapid entry of private players and corporations into this domain, facilitated by what Mazzucato (2016) refers to as the 'entrepreneurial state' and state's incentivisation of startup culture in recent times. This startup culture has created fertile grounds for entry of new entrepreneurial ventures and private healthtech startups in the country and women's reproductive health startups too are riding on this wave. With programs and seed funding opportunities like *Make in India* (2014), Startup India Scheme (2016), *Atma Nirbhar* App Innovation Challenge (2020), Atal Innovation Mission (2016), Startup India Seed Fund (2021), eBiz portal (2013) and other myriad practices like innovators conclaves, hackathons and design research, the entrepreneurial community is expected to reimagine 'life as a latent opportunity and the masses not as an exploited or disadvantaged class to feed but as potential "users"—customers who could be managed and mined for value at the same time' (Irani, 2019, p. 8). It is within this wider political and economic climate that proliferation of FemTech has to be situated. Given this context, it is not surprising that several Indian FemTech apps have received seed funding from government bodies, one won the Indian Government's *Atma Nirbhar* App Innovation Challenge of 2020 and others boasted of being associated with the National Institute for Transforming India (NITI) Aayog.[1] Some FemTech apps have entered into public–private partnerships, advertising free trials and services at public health clinics in smaller towns and rural areas of the country. These trends reflect a legitimisation of FemTech by state endorsement and the symbiotic relationship between FemTech entrepreneurs and the state. It is also indicative of a larger shift towards privately owned healthcare services and neoliberal model of state playing a more facilitatory role for private players. Situating itself against this backdrop of rapid proliferation of FemTech in India backed by the Indian state, this paper we examine the growing adoption of reproductive health management apps in India by users for self-tracking menstruation, fertility, pregnancy/foetal development and menopause.

Critical studies on health tracking are skewed in favour of what has been called WEIRD demographics: Western, Educated, Industrialised, Rich and Democratic, and there is a paucity of similar research in diverse locales and cultural contexts (Epstein et al., 2017). In India particularly,

---

[1] A public policy think tank (replacing an older 'Planning Commission') of the Government of India.

not only do patriarchy and gender equations (Ravindran, 1992) shape questions of access to healthcare, but women's reproductive health has long been a culturally tabooed topic, often not discussed openly or worse, stigmatised. Further, Indian 'women' is a heterogeneous category in itself, highly diversified across class, caste, social capital, digital access/literacy and regional and linguistic categories. This locational complexity makes such a study necessary and revelatory—allowing us a better understanding of: what are the motivating factors, strategies and constraints shaping adoption and usage of FemTech apps; how are its benefits and harms distributed and to whom and what kinds of inequities and marginalizations might it produce?

Studies on FemTech applications have largely used a critical data studies approach to examine the impact and challenges of data and its power in society underpinning relations of inequality in data capitalism (Iliadis & Russo, 2016) focussing on extractive data regimes of the global north (Chami et al., 2021). Recent critical studies in the Indian context have highlighted a risky regime of surveillance that users are embedded in, once logged into FemTech, so to speak, which is sustained and exacerbated by the non-existent status of data protection architecture in the country (Rathi & Tandon, 2019; Mishra & Suresh, 2021). For this study, however, we focus on the incentives for users and the potential benefits and pitfalls of tracking, quantifying and managing reproductive health through the apps. This study is informed by a critical data perspective which involves in-depth examination of where and how the 'individual emerges in algorithmic cultures' (Dalton et al., 2016, p. 1). The theoretical perspective informing our method has been to empirically interrogate the everyday experience of big data (Lupton, 2016; Ruckenstein & Schüll, 2017), with a focus on the individual. Kitchin and Lauriault (2014) and Burns and Thatcher (2015) refer to it as 'small data' perspective, which seeks to bring out a detailed description of people's everyday data practices and to study the mutuality between contemporary technical innovation and social structures. Using this approach we seek to understand datafication of reproductive health in everyday life in the Indian context, through FemTech apps, and their appropriation and heterogeneous effects on end users (Fiore-Gartland & Neff, 2015) in the Indian context.

We argue that app-based management of reproductive health gives rise to what we call 'datafied body projects', drawing on Shilling's (2003) work. Shilling (2003) argued that the body in the postmodern era is best conceptualised as an unfinished biological and social phenomenon and marked by an increasing propensity of individuals to view their bodies as projects/entities which need to be worked upon. The body thus is no longer a 'given' biological entity but something at the forefront of messy boundaries and intersections of nature and technology. We demonstrate similarly how FemTech apps fuel datafied body projects driven by continuous streams of user generated data and algorithms which nudge users to undertake specific activities and to have a bearing on their understanding and experience of the reproductive body and shape its functioning and in the process shapes identities. But predicated on standard rhythms and routines of reproductive biological processes, such apps often end up marginalising and/or erasing specificities of diverse reproductive bodies and their needs. Thus, even as digital health data generated via FemTech apps opens up possibilities that may be emancipative/empowering, this data also has negative elements that merit scrutiny. Further, Shilling (1993) argues that body projects vary across social lines and are not without inequities and questions of gender, class, ethnicities and global inequalities that shape body projects. Similarly, we show how datafied reproductive body projects facilitated via FemTech apps is not an all-encompassing intervention. Their design and content have been built with the idea of catering to socio-economically privileged sections and thus leaving out a vast majority out of its fold. Ultimately, we suggest that although these tracking apps offer potential benefits of convenience and self-awareness in the context wherein women's ability to take control of their reproductive decisions and access healthcare is limited, it does so at the cost of invisibilizing entire populations, reproducing social inequalities and promoting a narrow standard of the fertile, fecund, female body excluding the subjective complexities of the lived everyday reproductive realities.

Methods and Data

Our study takes up four primary modes of engagement with the field in order to understand how 'datafied body projects' are produced via FemTech applications in India. First, we conducted 'platform analysis' of Indian FemTech apps (apps that were designed and owned by Indian companies) on Google Play store and Apple store corresponding to various stages of the reproductive cycle—such as menstruation, fertility/pregnancy and menopause. Our searches revealed a long list but we excluded the following apps from our analysis: blogging apps, apps developed for medical practitioners and apps that were games. This gave us a total of 41 apps. At the second level, we excluded apps that had less than 10 K downloads. Based on this exclusion, 12 apps were eliminated from analyses, and we finally identified 29 apps for content analysis. For this we created dummy accounts on the application to study the interface, design and features of the application, borrowing from the 'ethnographic walkabout method' (Light et al., 2018), to make visible the discursive foundations of the app imaginary and the system of actors at play. The shortlisted apps reflected a combination of these four features, borrowing from Tripp et al.'s (2014) classification: Informative and primarily educational (96.55%); Interactive, such as those that have live sessions with experts or host fitness classes (75.86%); Tools—apps that provide features to assess and track health parameters (48.27%) and Social media focused that provide features for writing blogs or connecting with other users (20.68%). The interface of all the apps was available in English, but 41.37% apps were available in other Indian vernaculars (one app could accommodate 14 Indian languages). Our platform analyses also revealed that that most of the companies are based out of Bengaluru, with Mumbai and Hyderabad housing a small minority. The app founders primarily have a background in engineering or management and the initial prototypes of many apps were developed at a 'startup incubation' of the country's premier technical education institutions. These founders have experience with diverse industries, sometimes unrelated to healthcare and wellness, such as hospitality, textiles and e-commerce.

Second, mass scale surveys via google forms in English and Hindi were rolled out through social media pages—Twitter, LinkedIn and Facebook—and posters with QR codes to the survey form were pasted around Delhi-NCR in conducive public spots. Further we reached out to several prominent social media health influencers who are also certified medical professionals to share our survey with their followers. Two of them agreed to our request and this helped us reach out to a large population group. This survey was filled by 1004 respondents but 977 met the eligibility criteria and the analysis is based on this number.

Third, qualitative data was collected through interviews drawing on Gusterson's (1997) conceptualisation of 'polymorphous engagement'. Semi-structured interviews, online and offline, were conducted with the primary users (22) of these apps. Further, as we wanted to explore the wider political economy within which appification of reproductive health is proliferating, other critical players in the FemTech landscape were also interviewed: medical professionals (6), FemTech founders/CEO's (6), health activists (1), coders (1), tech policy expert (1) and venture capitalists (2). Finally, the interviews are supplemented by ethnographic observations made in health innovation/startups events and conferences where the authors participated and in innovation and incubation hubs in Delhi. Table 5.1 gives an overview of our surveyed and interviewed user demographic.

As evident from the table above, FemTech app users are largely urban, highly educated, predominantly in the age group of 18–35 years and using apps for a variety of reasons—the most common being period tracking followed by pregnancy and fertility tracking. The data on usage shows that most users have been using apps for fairly long and thus sticking to the practice of tracking even as they may not be tracking all the biomarkers the app asks for. The five most common health data points inputted by the user include period flow, flow dates, premenstrual syndrome/mood, sexual history and fluid consistency in that order. Finally, most of the respondents in this study were using or had used a mix of FemTech apps—third party downloadable international (such as *Flow, Clue and In the Flow*) and Indian apps (such as *Maya, Niine, Mind&Mom and BabyChakra*) and also apps in-built in smartphones (*Apple Health,*

Table 5.1 User demographics from survey and interviews

Category	User survey data (977)	User interview data (22)
Age	5.7% <18 yrs; 90% between 18 and 35 yrs; 4% >35 yrs	1%<18 yrs; 95.8% between 18 and 35 yrs; 2% -36–45 yrs; 1.2% >45 yrs
Gender	Female: 98.77%; others: 1.33%	Female: 100%
Education	82% graduates and above	88% graduates and above
Location	Urban-92%; Rural-8%	Urban-96%; Rural-4%
Duration of app usage	39% (>3 years); 40% (1–3 years); others (<1 year)	72.7% (>3 years); 18.18% (1–3 years); others (<1 year)
Marital and sexual activity status	Married-28%; unmarried, sexually active-40%; unmarried, not sexually active-32%	Married-31.81%; unmarried and sexually active-54.54%; unmarried, not sexually active-13.65%
Tracking	Periods (82.7%); pregnancy/foetal development (7.2%); fertility (2.6%); baby growth (6.4%); menopause (1.1%)	Periods (72.78%); Pregnancy/Foetal Development (13.63%); Fertility (9.09%); Baby Growth (4.5%); Menopause (0)

Xiaomi Mi Calendar Tracker, etc.). Although inbuilt and foreign apps remain popular, there is also an expanding market for Indian FemTech apps. The next section elaborates on the appeal of datafied reproductive body from the user perspective.

Appeal of Datafied Body Projects

Insights into the reasons, motivations, benefits and practices of self-tracking reproductive health through FemTech apps was revealed in great detail through open-ended interviews. For the users, self-tracking apps eased the process of remembering and digital record keeping offering greater 'convenience' over other traditional methods (calendars, journals) which were 'cumbersome' and 'non-discrete'. Our respondents were fairly heterogeneous in terms of why they started tracking in the first place and often gave overlapping responses. Several stated that they wanted to 'give it a try' after hearing about it from their peers or social media. Others started using them 'just for fun' or 'out of curiosity' with this new technology. In a few cases, the respondents were asked by doctors to keep a track of their menstrual cycle if they were undergoing some reproductive health issue. Despite different reasons that prompted their use, most of the respondents found the apps 'quite helpful' and thus decided to continue with their usage. For example, women who were trying to conceive turned to menstruation or ovulation tracker apps for tracking their 'fertile window' or 'phase when [conception] chances are high' while pregnant women used apps to see 'week-by-week foetal growth' and associated developments. Those with 'irregular periods' (often a result of Polycystic Ovarian Syndrome (PCOS)) used the apps to overcome the 'difficulty of remembering last period dates'. However, others, whose menstrual cycles were fairly regular, used apps to 'just keep a record' of it to make sure 'everything is ok'. For instance, R23 who works as strategy and operations consultant at Google shared,

> My periods have been more or less regular. So it was just more like, you know, more like trying it out to see if the pattern was predictable, because sometimes it'd be like, maybe a day off here and there. It's just [that] I wanted to have more predictability about my periods. That was pretty much it…there was no other goal…the goal ideally would have been to just keep an eye on my period.

Heightened Awareness and Self-optimisation

The most frequent benefits our respondents cited pertained to awareness and understanding of corporeal processes. They referred to becoming 'more aware', 'getting a better picture' and 'better understanding' of how menstruation, fertility or pregnancy works. This increased awareness or understanding was expressed in myriad ways depending on the process being tracked. R8 who is currently pregnant with her second child, compares her first pregnancy journey with second one and shared how the app helped her 'know what dates [she] should try' for conception,

> 'I had difficulties in getting pregnant even with my first pregnancy and in the present one as well, so I had to go to the doctor for hormonal injections and medicines, and all of that, and after 4–5 months of that, I conceived. [In] this app there are two modes: one is 'trying to conceive' and one is

'pregnant'. I used it in the 'trying to conceive' mode before becoming pregnant. This app really helped me to know what dates I should try and you know have sex for conception so that helped and I am using it in the pregnancy mode right now'.

R23 shared how her understanding of menstrual cycle has shifted from the four-five days one bleeds to a more comprehensive understanding of the various phases of the cycle,

'So earlier, it was just like the period dates. With the app now it's more like, okay, I know,, I'm in the luteal phase or follicular phase, or I'm entering ovulation, whatever. I think I find that engagement more frequent and more useful. So I would say it's just like a full view as opposed to just the period dates right now and same for my symptoms as well.. I understand what corresponds to what phase'

Apps thus helped establish and maintain awareness of the reproductive process and our respondents drew satisfaction out of this greater awareness. Feminist scholarship on the relationship between data and body has argued how data is viewed as an extension of the human form, and control over the former is often experienced as control over the latter (Patella-Rey, 2018). In such a context, the distinction between physical and datafied body becomes amorphous due to the extent to which data is used to determine and control our bodily experiences (Van der Ploeg, 2012). To our respondents these datafied body projects felt 'more real' and objective markers of bodily processes as they provided information in 'nice graphs', 'neat diagrams' and 'charts displaying patterns over time', even as they problematically may produce 'biomedical bodily alienation' (Hendl & Jansky, 2022) by reducing space for the users to comprehend their own bodily processes. For our users, despite its associated problems, the awareness generated through self-tracking, offered possibilities of greater control over reproductive processes in a context like India where reproductive health is often shrouded in mystery and tabooed as the next section detail.

Reducing Uncertainties and Risk?

The awareness and satisfaction expressed by our respondents were typically tied to 'feeling more in control' or 'being in charge of oneself' and the bodily processes being 'more predictable'. They spoke about how reproductive tracking and self-monitoring became a way of dealing with 'uncertainty' and 'risks'. These risks and uncertainties pertained to management of reproductive processes—menstruation and fertility—both in their everydayness as well as in connection to future reproductive trajectories. Thus, app users spoke about using period trackers for 'being period ready' (having required menstrual supplies with one at the time needed), 'not scheduling important work/leisure/travel during periods' highlighting how safe management of periods has emerged as a necessity for urban, educated, upwardly mobile young women, which is the primary demographic using FemTech applications in India. R20, 31 years of age and a college lecturer, shared how by using the app:

> 'you could plan your clothes, carry menstrual hygiene supplies accordingly, and make your life much easier'

Similarly, R15, 24 years, based in Bangalore, who works as a development professional and whose work includes regular fieldwork, shared:

> 'I like to be at home for the first two days of my period and I absolutely hate travelling because of public transport and public toilets. I think the app is useful as I can plan my fieldwork around that'.

This safe management of periods is situated within the context of menstruating, leaking bodies being stigmatised (Ali & Rizvi, 2010) as lacking 'control' (Chrisler, 2011) and requiring self-policing and self-silencing (Ussher, 2006). In addition to menstruation management, we found Femetech apps being used for conception planning. R2, for instance, is married and currently based in Kolkata for pursuing PhD while her husband is employed in another city. Now keen to have a baby she has been using an ovulation tracking app and shared,

'When we got interested in having a child, I actually talked him into this [app] and he found it very useful and this way we can plan our intimate activity. We are busy with a tight schedule and are planning our life around conception'

For R23 and her partner, 'planning life around conception' while being in a long-distance marriage meant making sure that one of them travels to be with the other during peak fertility (as suggested by the app) days so that chances of conception are higher even as they juggle their 'busy' schedules. FemTech apps are thus adopted to respond to anxieties, aspirations and compulsions arising out of work and intimate life.

FemTech apps were also popular for the very same reasons of reducing risk and uncertainties among those who were avoiding conception and wanted safe management of fertility and thus 'not risk getting pregnant'. It should be noted that 40 percent of our survey respondents and 54.5 percent of interview respondents reported being unmarried and sexually active and given the stigma around premarital sex and pregnancy (Ganatra & Hirve, 2002; Jejeebhoy et al., 2010) in India, safe management of fertility was a heightened concern amongst this group of FemTech users. R17, a masters student based in Kolkata shared, shared, how she used a period tracker to know when she is not ovulating so that she could avoid getting pregnant as her partner refused to use a protection and would not entertain any conversations on that matter,

'I had a relationship in which it was something that was not even a topic of question anymore. I knew for a fact that was something that scared me completely. I would say that I am not comfortable in this so at that time I used to check whether it's okay, just to know if unprotected sex is going to be a problem right now, because it shows you the days you're ovulating, etc. So yeah, the app helped me a lot'.

Even as R17 confessed that she was in an unequal relationship where she 'didn't have a voice' and 'it was bad for [her] mental health' she thought the app was helpful in avoiding an unwanted pregnancy. This, as the paper discusses later, can be deeply problematic. Finally, management of risk and uncertainty via self-tracking is not only oriented to 'avoiding pregnancy' among young women but also to imaginations of desirable 'reproductive futures'. For example, R16, a 23 year old who has recently completed her Masters degree, shared how self-tracking periods and knowing they are 'normal' avoids unnecessary stress which later may have a bearing on her ability to procreate,

> 'I think post tracking, definitely like it has helped me remember a lot more I think…you know I am very panicky, and I have seen the kind of negative impact it puts on so many ways on your bodies, later on, you have a problem with having a baby. This just sort of seems right. And I think we want to be in control, in that sense. Like my mother's more panicky about this in that sense so she too keeps asking when did I get my last periods. Maybe in this sense [the app] just sort of gives comfort that everything is happening regularly you know'.

As is evident from these narratives, self-management of the reproduction through digital tracking practices promotes an entrepreneurial self-cultivation in very intimate areas of life (Ford et al., 2021). The respondent's narratives of using FemTech apps for bodily self-management, exercising procreative choices, and risk avoidance seem like furthering women's empowerment as they take ownership of their health but not without costs. Corbin (2020, p. 20), for instance, argues that FemTech devices often are 'more concerned with manipulating women's fears and insecurities about their bodies for the sake of profit' rather than really facilitating their agency and self-determination. Even as FemTech enabled datafied body projects are perceived by the users as mitigating risks of various sorts as discussed above, knowingly or unknowingly self-tracking behaviour also involves trading one set of risks for several others discussed in the later part of this chapter. Thus, in the section that follows we illustrate how FemTech apps in India reproduce dominant social inequalities rather than ameliorating them.

FemTech Apps Reproducing Dominant Social Inequalities

In this section, we illustrate how the rhetoric of empowerment evoked by FemTech and narratives of heightened awareness, self-optimisation, and greater control put forth by FemTech users can also distract us from the problems raised by these ordinary forms of biomedicalised self-quantification. One of these relates to questions of inequality and stratified access to healthcare in general and reproductive health in particular. While the emergence of FemTech in India does make possible some form of resistance to dominant Western narratives around digital health, FemTech apps in India continue to address a certain small segment of the Indian population while overlooking questions of accessibility, inclusion and affordability. Shilling (1993) argues that body projects vary across social lines and are not without inequities and questions of gender, class, ethnicities, global inequalities that shape body projects. Following a similar trajectory, this section reveals how datafied reproductive body projects facilitated via FemTech apps is not an all-encompassing intervention. The very design, language and content of FemTech apps caters only to socio-economically privileged sections leaving a vast majority out of its fold. Further, the apps also cause violent erasures of lived experiences of those who do not conform to the normative reproductive ideals. The section illustrates how FemTech in India is imprinted by and reinforces dominant social inequalities—some of which overlap with findings documented in other parts of the world while others being novel and specific to the cultural context in which the Indian FemTech ecosystem is based.

Reflection of Gendered Underpinnings

FemTech apps, more often than not further heteronormative, patriarchal ideals. This is evident in the design, content and imagery used in the apps. About 58.62% of the apps reviewed as part of this research had gendered imagery and 51.73% used gendered language. The interface of most of the apps (Healofy, Ava, Veera Health, Infano, Cicle, Period Calendar, etc.) was often pink loaded with flowers, hearts, stars, bees or butterfly stickers. Pregnancy and parenting app iMumz, for instance, always uses images of flowers on pregnant bellies as part of its app imagery. Period tracking, pregnancy and fertility apps invariably are loaded with imagery of thin, tall, able-bodied women with long hair catering to a cis-heterosexual male gaze. They are also not inclusive in their language, often using words like 'girl', 'women', etc. in their description assuming the user identifies as a woman. The incumbent alienation on account of explicit, normative gendering was clearly reflected in our survey respondents and interview narratives. Only a mere 23.07% of survey respondents identifying as LGBTQIA+ continued using self-tracking apps like Flow and Clue, the others choosing to discontinue or to not use the platform. Our respondents shared how non-female identified menstruators 'do not find the app accommodative of their gender identities' (R10, 32) and one survey respondent shared how the app does not work for menstruating persons undergoing hormonal replacement therapies. Similarly another female respondent in a homosexual relationship shared 'the app keeps telling me about my fertile window and when chances of conception are high even as I am a lesbian, there is no room for customization and it just assumes things' (R1, 37). When sexual and reproductive health behaviours and body functions are quantified, indicators and concepts of health risk become extremely exclusionary by creating homogenised models of the body. The intended user is heterosexual, fertile, biologically female, and FemTech thus others the experiences of women who do not fit the norm, alienating marginalised groups who are non-heteronormative women. By discriminating against these groups, FemTech creates 'digital micro-aggressions' (Corbin, 2020). Not just LGBTQIA+ but people with disabilities, aged populations, were largely outside the app's conceptualisation of who the intended user is. Pregnancy and parenting apps were also explicitly gendered. The language often assumed the user was a woman. One app upon logging asks with images, '*Are you "Mummy" or "Papa'?*'. Another application provided the following customisation options to choose from as soon as the user logged in: '*I carry a single baby(My bun in the oven);' 'Expecting Twin (It's a double treat)'; 'Assisted Pregnancy(I have superpowers)' and 'Single Mom! (I am an Iron Lady)'*. Our app analysis revealed that only 36% parenting apps provide a feature for a male/father as the user. The names of many of the apps reflected a play on the following words—healthy, mother/mom, her, baby, nine months. This (gendered) parent is imagined as female, reiterating hetero-patriarchal norms where the mother carries the primary burden of parenting.

Reflections of Class Imaginaries

In addition to reinforcing normative conceptions of sex and gender, our survey also revealed that FemTech users are a primarily urban, educated, relatively younger and technologically adept demographic. As smartphone and internet connectivity are prerequisites for these apps, those who do not possess these attributes—the poor, uneducated, living in underdeveloped areas—are automatically excluded from the reach of these apps. In India, where access to technology is both gendered and stratified (Doron & Jeffery, 2013), only 33.3% of women have used the internet (NFHS 5, 2020) making FemTech app usage a remote reality for the majority. The fact that FemTech apps only cater to the upper and middle classes is also reflected in the fact that while most of the apps made a basic version accessible to users upon free download, making it seem like they are more equitable, about 82.75% apps also had paid premium packages with monthly and yearly subscription charges for users allowing for an upgrade in features and services. Such features and services are of two kinds. One, they provide paid users an opportunity to liaison with institutions and individuals in the healthcare domain by either empanelling local hospitals, maternity and nursing homes and facilitate consultations with licensed experts like gynaecologists, endocrinologists, therapists, fitness and wellness coaches and nutritionists, etc. Second, nearly all applications had dedicated e-commerce sections and in-app purchase features, which are often built on the B2B model and the apps often send routine notifications to users to buy their products. These may include menstrual hygiene products, nutritional supplements, maternity and baby products, skincare and wellness products, etc. Some apps like Baby Chakra have now come up with their own line up bath, body and wellness products for mothers and infants. In pregnancy apps particularly, there is an emphasis on shopping for the right products, differentiated as per the pregnancy trimester and through the growing years of the child, accommodating up to the age of six, even. It is clear that the applications are designed keeping a user/consumer who can afford to pay for monthly or annual upgrades and maintain a certain lifestyle encoded in the kind of parenting ideals being promoted. Lupton (2016, p. 7) rightly notes in the case of FemTech apps in the global north that 'these discourses of ideal parenthood rest on middle-class, neoliberal assumptions about the individual's capacity and responsibility for educating themselves and acting upon information, positioning parenthood as autonomous and privatised'. FemTech apps are thus selling a lifestyle that rests on not just planned parenthood but also ideal parenting, which is pegged to indicators of purchasing power and a perfect consumer citizen who is upper or upper middle class. In a country where about 11% of pregnant women are unreached by a skilled birth attendant still, and only 1.9 and 0.9 per cent of the population has access to cervical cancer screening and breast examination (NFHS-5, 2020), there are looming gaps yet to be addressed. Self-management through FemTech apps, then, does not fill that void, further reinforcing the criticality of public health programs, services and infrastructures.

Reflections of Religious Undertones

While the gendered and classed assumptions underpinning FemTech apps have been highlighted in several past studies (Ford et al., 2021; Thomas & Lupton, 2016), we found Indian FemTech apps to be ideologically aligned in other specific ways. Some exclusively were organised around religious principles and promoting Hindu ideals, sometimes outrightly evident in their names like *Bal Sanskar* app, promoted as 'good parenting app' providing 'parents with the right perspective in raising their children as ideal citizens'. Available in four languages, English, Hindi, Marathi and Kannada, the app description says it is a guide to 'imbue good moral values (*sanskars*)' in children and 'sow the seeds of *dharmik* (religious) behaviour'. Several others provide counselling and education on vedic practices of *Garbh Samvad* (communicating with foetus in the womb) and *Garbh Sanskaar* (educating an unborn child) aimed at social, physical, spiritual and mental well-being of the unborn child. The apps stress how expectant mothers should listen to vedic *mantras* (hymns) as per Hindu religious beliefs including *mantras* like *Gayatri Mantra, Ram Raksha Stotra* and sanskrit shlokas and only eat *Satvik* (pure, vegetarian food as per ayurvedic recommendations) food 'to cleanse and purify the body'. These apps claim to have positive outcomes for foetal brain development promoting a certain kind of techno-spiritual engagement. About 48.3% apps had some of these features, promoting certain Hindu ideals through the application. A related but different example can be seen in the context of period-tracking app Femm which was criticized for being funded by anti-abortion and anti-gay Catholic groups in the U.S. that actively discouraged women from using hormonal birth control on highlyunscientific grounds that natural ways are more effective (Glenza, 2019). These reflect how rather than enabling participatory scientific health, the apps can also promote non-scientific ways and behaviour. For instance, one particular Indian app suggested that a foetus can get 'infected' if mothers' vaginal area is 'not kept clean' and thus recommended '*yoni dhupan* or fumigation of the perineal area with mediated herb fumes' once a week. These examples clearly reflect how technological advancements may not necessarily mean progressive consciousness and non-scientific ideas infiltrate into technospecs which sometimes can produce detrimental outcomes for the user.

Reflections on Normative Femininity and the Fecund/Fertile Body

Even as the underlying idea behind FemTech is to create a safe space for women to access sexual and reproductive health information, this space, at best, caters to only few while leaving out many others. Those women who do not adhere to conceptions of normative femininity find themselves obscured through the app. These include women who do not menstruate, menstruate irregularly, cannot conceive or have miscarried/lost a pregnancy. User narratives reflected the possible negative consequences of over-reliance on pattern prediction and the pressures experienced at having to self-quantify within the parameters of the application. This was especially stressful for two sets of users. One group included those grappling with adjacent health conditions such as endometriosis, PCOS, etc. Either the app was unable to account for the delays in their period cycle or helped mask the severity and symptoms of underlying chronic illnesses. One of our interviewees reported that she delayed approaching a doctor because the app continued to predict her period cycle effectively even as her menstrual cycle length fell way outside what is medically deemed to be the 'normal' period cycle length. In another case, a respondent's chronic endometriosis symptoms of extreme discomfort and pain were masked by the false comfort of a 'regular' period pattern which delayed medical consultation and was only diagnosed when it took the shape of a life threatening peptic ulcer. A false sense of normalcy sustained by the application points to the underlying totalising impulse of datafication that erases the subjective lived experiences of users. Violent erasures of lived experience were also witnessed in the case of pregnant women using pregnancy tracking apps to monitor foetal growth but who eventually miscarried, forming the second group. Our respondents using a diverse set of pregnancy tracking apps reported how their application's interface has no option to digitally record lost pregnancy/miscarriage. Their apps continued to send them notifications about baby size, organ development routinely causing distress to several users. Notifications in the form of text messages and repeated reminders were common even after uninstalling the apps. The algorithms of period tracking apps are unable to accommodate phases of no menstrual flow for months (during pregnancy) followed by sudden re-emergence of periods (following miscarriage) making their predictions go haywire. One of our respondents who recently experienced a miscarriage showed us how her app is signalling a 14-day window as the likely next period dates. She remarked,

> 'What sense do I make of this? This is almost a 2 week window and how does it at all tell me anything about my periods except a wild guess that it may be close to 15th. I just feel the app does not understand how women's bodies post miscarriage works and it is frustrating'.

Another way in which the fecund/fertile body is held as normative is reflected in the way in which the language of the apps is always geared towards a successful pregnancy. Thus, 'fertile window' is more commonly highlighted over 'safe days' and pregnancy is always viewed as a celebrated event evading any discussion about how to navigate unplanned/accidental pregnancies. Just as pregnancy testing kits adverts always assume a pregnancy to be 'good news', in a similar way FemTech apps adopt a pronatalist approach towards reproduction and the lifecycle support for women users who do not meet these normative reproductive expectations ends abruptly within the FemTech imaginary. Alfawzan et al. (2022) too note that, globally, most FemTech apps are overly focused on fertility, ovulation or menstrual cycle and pregnancy, further leaving no space for questions of menopause, sexual wellness, sexual pleasure, etc.—a gap we see in the Indian FemTech landscape as well. So, even as mobile applications are marketed as tools for control and better knowledge of one's body, there was in-built erasure of diverse body types, health issues, experiences and more. Thus, FemTech reassociates women in medicine with their biological reproductive functions, overlooking the wide variety of health conditions women may experience (Galea & Farretti, 2018).

Datafied Body Insecurities

Beset with exclusion and inequalities, FemTech emerges as a narrow solution to the needs and experiences of users, but also alarmingly implicates the set of users it does actively cater to into a paradigm of risk. T risks associated with datafied body projects are at two levels: the macro and the micro. The macro set of risks pertains to big data use for what Zuboff (2015) calls surveillance capitalism. When applied to health data it involves extraction, sharing, sale and commodification of sensitive and intimate personal information of users as big data within a global architecture of computer mediation (Lupton, 2016; Neff, 2013) often operating outside state jurisdictions (Martínez-Pérez et al., 2015). Indian apps on installation ask for detailed personal identifiers, including name, gender, age, number, email address, location and social media amongst others. However, the Terms of Services were often vaguely defined. About 34.48% of the apps did not have an outright policy disclaimer, many would assume user consent to terms and conditions as soon as the user input name and number. A select few (such as *Infano* and *Veera Health*) stated that user data would only be shared with third parties in cases of a legal obligation. Most openly stated that user data could be shared with third parties. One such disclaimer puts the burden on the user squarely, carrying the caveat: '*no information on the internet is 100% secure*'. Many Indian apps failed to provide links to the data policy and terms of services to the users despite requiring them to share intimate details. Discreet practices which evade the knowledge of the user were found in policy documents where many apps mentioned the collection of information about a non-registered user, for instance 'if a registered user provides the app/platform with their information to facilitative services'. This puts the user at risk of non-consensual targeted advertising and profiling in the database without ever having availed the services of the platform. Only about 37.93% of the apps sought permission to track activities across other companies' apps. About 68.96% of Indian apps did not have the option for a user to delete a profile, once it was created on their database. A few apps mentioned that they continued tracking the browsing history of the user prior and post the usage of the application. In our own experience of using the apps and then logging out or deleting the profile, we found that we continued to receive notifications over email or WhatsApp or SMSes with reminders or a new package deal or discount coupons. The Personal Data Protection Bill (2022) in India is still under deliberation, having been withdrawn previously on several occasions and given the vacuum created by absence of legislative checks, FemTech app users personal data is susceptible to large-scale privacy and security breaches.

We found that a majority of our survey and interview respondents were aware of the possibility of a data breach and that their data was being shared with third parties—about 54.35% said they were aware that data can be shared with third parties. Yet, 70.31% of the survey respondents said they did not know if their data was encrypted and most users reported that they had not read the Terms of Services of the apps. We noted a certain ambivalence in user narratives pointing to a normalisation of surveillance that has occurred recently. A kind of consent fatigue (Jain & Kovacs, 2021) could be noted where users feel they can either not fully decipher a lengthy Terms of Services section or that there was no option to challenge or modify their manner of usage of the app. As such they remain implicated in a power asymmetry that does not allow them any other option but to consent. Many said that privacy violation is the terms you must accept to become a datafied subject in contemporary times; a part of the bargain. R13 (F, 32 years) speaks of receiving targeted ads,

> *'If you are using google maps, you are using Google Pay, then your location is always available. It is kind of pointless to resist it'.*

Some chose to protect data by not providing to the app certain kinds of personal identifiers and access to social media platforms. R6 (F, 29 years), a PhD scholar studying the relationship between feminism and technology, shared

> *'Like I said, I only logged into my email, not with many other social media platforms, so in that sense, I feel that I have protected my personal data to a great extent'.*

When this is extended to parenting apps, where the unborn foetus and the child through the ages of infancy is also implicated in a surveillance paradigm for future targeting and prediction, called 'babyveillance' (Barassi, 2017), the normalisation alerts us to a privacy paradox (Shklovski et al., 2014). Users must either submit to data precarity or find ways of constantly balancing which and what data to input. Datafication then becomes a process of constant negotiation for the user with the conventions and paradigms that app developers create and the industry sustains.

The other set of risks to Femetch app users pertains to small data. For example, the fact that young, unmarried, sexually active women are highly dependent on the app to know their safe sex days is concerning for several reasons: One, the efficacy of FemTech applications as an alternative to birth control is questionable (Duane et al., 2016). Second, FemTech tracking app algorithms are predicated on standard rhythms and routines of reproductive biological processes; they often end up marginalising and/or erasing specificities of diverse reproductive bodies and their needs. Worsfold et al. (2021) in their analysis of menstrual tracking apps found that apps predict a long fertile window of seven days for all women even as the fertile window is not a fixed length for all women or all cycles as it is dependent on oestrogen hormone rise. This, on the one hand, puts a question on their contraceptive reliability; on the other hand, it can also lead to mistime intercourse for those trying to conceive resulting in failure. Third, some tracking apps may rely on fertility awareness-based methods (FABM) to determine pregnancy likelihood at a certain point in the cycle gauged through complex combinations of the body. Most of our respondents did not understand these complexities and often selectively entered information on the app depending on what they understood as more 'private', 'very intimate' or 'too personal'. Thus while menstrual dates, flow and mood was mostly recorded, users hesitated entering sexual activity and contraception use. This was particularly critical for unmarried women living jointly with family members and who did not want this information to be accessed by family members resulting in familial surveillance over their sexual and reproductive journeys. Further, our respondents also reported logging in basal body temperature and cervical mucus quality 'cumbersome' and 'confusing'. Studies on voluntary health self-tracking reveal how continuous datafication is often punctuated in multiple ways by user agency and resistance to datafication (Couldry & Powell, 2014; Rapp, 2016; Esmonde, 2020). Some studies show that users actively seek to strike a balance between the parameters of self-quantification when it crosses a certain line of excess (Noji et al., 2021). Given these omissions, it is not unlikely that this may affect app algorithms and impact its predictions. For those depending on apps as a contraceptive technique the risks can be egregious. Fourth, consciously or unconsciously the app reinforces the onus of 'reproductive management' and gendered burden of conception avoidance on women while not contributing to greater awareness and structural change in any way. Finally, these individual acts of 'self-management' of reproductive health through FemTech apps shrinks space for questions of access to non-judgemental reproductive healthcare, contraceptives, sex-education and societal awareness which are much needed conversations in India.

Conclusion

In India, digital interventions into reproductive health are proliferating, with FemTech apps for menstruation, fertility, pregnancy/foetal development and menopause self-tracking and management as their most popular articulation. Backed by an entrepreneurial state and a booming startup culture in India, several app-based FemTech companies are promising to offer easily accessible, adaptable addendum to users' lives that promises self-optimisation through self-monitoring; the entrenchment of ideals of 'healthism' (Lupton, 2018). Through a multi-pronged enquiry involving both qualitative and qualitative data, the chapter reveals who the main adoptees of FemTech apps are in the Indian landscape and how these users are actively pursuing datafied body projects through reproductive self-tracking and management. The minutiae of shifts and transformations that create the datafied, reproductive body project has been achieved through the imperative of self-quantification. The app has relative power to shape behaviour as the users themselves produce 'serviceable truths' (Jasanoff 2015, as cited in Bianca, 2021) and often take what the app provides as objective, factual truth in the form of digital data.

Our study reveals that FemTech users in India are primarily from an 'urban, young, highly educated, middle and upper class, upwardly mobile' bracket who use tracking apps to navigate complex reproductive journeys while managing busy lives, work schedules and travel plans and fell the apps offer them better 'control' over uncertainties and risks. The digital nature of healthcare support provided via FemTech apps is unable to accommodate those on the margins—socioeconomically marginalised women, rural populations and those for whom access to digital technologies and digital literacy is a yet unrealised goal. However, beyond these inequalities which inscribe the FemTech app landscape in India, the limits of datafication of sexual and reproductive health emerge in sometimes detrimental outcomes for the end users, not only in terms of the threat of intimate data breaches but also by not accounting for those end users whose reproductive journeys do not adhere to the normative, fecund, fertile ideal. Under quantification, health standards become extremely narrow and create a homogenised model of the body. The app algorithms, while making predictions with a certain accuracy, are often unable to accommodate any lived experience deviating from the norm resulting in erasures of certain categories of persons as well as their health conditions. By revealing these complexities, this chapter has shifted the dominant way of looking at data in terms of the traces it leaves, making populations/conditions 'visible' to reveal how we need to be attentive to the ways in which data also invisiblizes people; how it obliterates them, their lived realities and diverse bodily experiences.

Without underestimating the potential of these technologies, it needs to be reiterated that in absence of a structural, social and progressive change in women's healthcare, these technologies may further only cause self-monitoring for automation of oneself and others. With further expansion across the country, it is yet to be seen how FemTech technologies adapt to the challenges of women's sexual and reproductive health needs in non-urban centres. Towards this, better accountability from the industry, attention to biases and effective regulatory practices by state bodies would be paramount.

References

Alfawzan, N., Christen, M., Spitale, G., & Biller-Andorno, N. (2022). Privacy, data sharing, and data security policies of Women's mHealth apps: Scoping review and content analysis. *JMIR mHealth and uHealth, 10*(5). https://doi.org/https://doi.org/10.2196/33735

Ali, T. S., & Rizvi, N. S. (2010). Menstrual knowledge and practices of female adolescents in urban Karachi, Pakistan. *Journal of Adolescence.* https://www.academia.edu/58704602/Menstrual_knowledge_and_practices_of_female_adolescents_in_urban_Karachi_Pakistan

Barassi, V. (2017). BabyVeillance? Expecting parents, online surveillance and the cultural specificity of pregnancy apps. *Social Media & Society.* https://doi.org/10.1177/2056305117707188

Burns, R., & Thatcher, J. (2015) Guest Editorial: What's so big about Big Data? Finding the spaces and perils of big data. *GeoJournal, 80*(4), 445–448. https://doi.org/10.1007/s10708-014-9600-8

Chami, N., Bharati, R. V., Mittal, A., & Aggarwal, A. (2021). Data subjects in the FemTech matrix: A feminist political economy analysis of the global Menstruapps market. *IT for Change*. https://itforchange.net/sites/default/files/1620/FDJ-Issue-Paper-6-Data-Subjects-In-the-FemTech-Matrix-IT-for-Change.pdf

Chrisler, J. C. (2011). Leaks, lumps, and lines: Stigma and Women's bodies. *Psychology of Women Quarterly, 35*(2), 202–214. https://doi.org/10.1177/0361684310397698

Corbin, B. (2020). Digital micro-aggressions and discrimination: FemTech and the 'othering' of women. *Nova Law Review, 44*, 1–27. https://ssrn.com/abstract=3630435

Couldry, N., & Powell, A. (2014). Big data from the bottom up. *Sage Journals*. https://doi.org/10.1177/2053951714539

Dalton, C. M., Taylor, L., & Thatcher, J. (2016). Critical data studies: A dialog on data and space. *Big Data & Society, 3*(1). https://doi.org/10.1177/2053951716648346

Doron, A., & Jeffery, R. (2013). *Cell phone nation: How Mobile phones have revolutionized business, politics & ordinary life in India*. Harvard University Press.

Duane, M., Contreras, A., Jensen, E. T., & White, A. (2016). The performance of fertility awareness-based method apps marketed to avoid pregnancy. *The. Journal of the American Board of Family Medicine, 29*(4), 508–511. https://www.jabfm.org/content/29/4/508

Dusenbery, M. (2018). Doing harm: The truth about how bad medicine and lazy science leave women dismissed, misdiagnosed, and sick. *HarperOne*.

Epstein, D., Lee, N., Kang, J., Agapie, E., Schroeder, J., Pina, L., Fogarty, J., Kientz, J., & Munson, S. D. A. (2017). Examining menstrual tracking to inform the design of personal informatics tools. *Proceedings of the SIGCHI Conference on Human Factors in Computing Systems. CHI Conference 2017.* 6876–6888. https://doi.org/10.1145/3025453.3025635.

Esmonde, K. (2020). There's only so much data you can handle in your life: Accommodating and resisting self-surveillance in women's running and fitness tracking practices. *Qualitative Research in Sport, Exercise and Health, 12*(1), 76–90. https://doi.org/10.1080/2159676X.2019.1617188

Fiore-Gartland, B., & Neff, G. (2015). Communication, mediation, and the expectations of data: Data valences across health and wellness communities. *International Journal of Communication*, [S.l.], v. 9. https://ijoc.org/index.php/ijoc/article/view/2830

Ford, A., de Togni, G., & Miller, L. (2021). Hormonal health: Period tracking apps, wellness, and self-Management in the era of surveillance capitalism. *Engaging Science, Technology, and Society.* https://doi.org/10.17351/ests2021.655

Galea, M., & Farretti, T. M. (2018). Improving pharmacological treatment in brain and mental health disorders: The need for gender and sex analyses. *Frontiers in Neurology, 50,* 1–2. https://doi.org/10.1016/j.yfrne.2018.06.007

Ganatra, B., & Hirve, S. (2002). Induced abortions among adolescent women in rural Maharashtra, India. *Reproductive Health Matters, 10*(19), 76–85. https://doi.org/10.1016/S0968-8080(02)00016-2

Glenza, J. (2019, May 30). Revealed: Women's Fertility app is funded by anti-abortion campaigners. *The Guardian.* https://www.theguardian.com/world/2019/may/30/revealed-womens-fertility-app-is-funded-by-anti-abortion-campaigners

Gusterson, H. (1997). Studying up revisited. *Political and Legal Anthropology Review, 20*(1), 114–119. http://www.jstor.org/stable/24497989

Hamberg, K. (2008). Gender bias in medicine. *Women's Health*, 237–243. https://doi.org/10.2217/17455057.4.3.237

Hendl, T., & Jansky, B. (2022). Tales of self-empowerment through digital health technologies: A closer look at 'Femtech'. *Review of Social Economy, Taylor & Francis Journals, 80*(1), 29–57. https://doi.org/10.1080/00346764.2021.2018027

Henrich, J., Heine, S. J., & Norenzayan, A. (2010). The weirdest people in the world? *The Behavioral and Brain Sciences, 33*(2–3), 61–135. https://doi.org/10.1017/S0140525X0999152X

Iliadis, A., & Russo, F. (2016). Critical data studies: An introduction. *Big Data & Society., 3.* https://doi.org/10.1177/2053951716674238

Irani, L. (2019). *Chasing innovation: Making entrepreneurial citizens in modern India.* Princeton University Press. https://doi.org/10.23943/princeton/9780691175140.003.0001

Jafree, S. R. (Ed.). (2020). *The sociology of south Asian Women's health.* Springer.

Jain, T., & Kovacs, A. (2021). Informed consent – Said who? A Feminist perspective on principles of Consent in the age of Embodied Data. *Internet Democracy Project.* https://internetdemocracy.in/policy/informed-consent-said-who-a-feminist-perspective-on-principles-of-consent-in-the-age-of-embodied-data-a-policy-brief

Jejeebhoy, S. J., Kalyanwala, S., Zavier, A. J., Kumar, R., & Jha, N. (2010). Experience seeking abortion among unmarried young women in Bihar and

Jharkhand, India: Delays and disadvantages. *Reproductive Health Matters, 18*(35), 163–174. https://doi.org/10.1016/S0968-8080(10)35504-2

Kitchin, R., & Lauriault, T. (2014). Towards critical data studies: Charting and unpacking data assemblages and their work. https://www.researchgate.net/publication/267867447_Towards_critical_data_studies_Charting_and_unpacking_data_assemblages_and_their_work

Light, B., Burgess, J., & Duguay, S. (2018). The walkthrough method: An approach to the study of apps. *New Media & Society, 20*(3), 881–900. https://doi.org/10.1177/1461444816675438

Lupton, D. (2016). *The quantified self: A sociology of self-tracking* (1st ed.). Polity Press. http://au.wiley.com/WileyCDA/WileyTitle/productCd-1509500634.html

Lupton, D. (2018). Digital health: Critical and cross disciplinary perspectives. Routledge.

Martínez-Pérez, B., de la Torre-Díez, I., & López-Coronado, M. (2015). Privacy and security in mobile health apps: A review and recommendations. *Journal of Medical Systems, 39*(1), 181. https://doi.org/10.1007/s10916-014-0181-3

Mazzucato, M. (2016). Innovation, the state and patient capital. *The Political Quarterly*. https://doi.org/10.1111/1467-923X.12235

Mishra, P., & Suresh, Y. (2021). Datafied body projects in India: FemTech and the rise of reproductive surveillance in the digital era. *Asian Journal of Women's Studies, 27*(4), 597–606. https://doi.org/10.1080/12259276.2021.2002010

Neff, G. (2013). Why big data won't cure us. *Big Data, 1*(3), 117–123. https://doi.org/10.1089/big.2013.0029

Noji, E., Kappler, K., & Vormbusch, U. (2021). Situating conventions of health: Transformations, inaccuracies, and the limits of measuring in the field of self-tracking. *Historical Social Research / Historische Sozialforschung, 46*(1), 261–284. https://www.jstor.org/stable/10.2307/27000005

Patella-Rey, P. J. (2018). Beyond privacy: Bodily integrity as an alternative framework for understanding Non-Consensual Pornography. *Information, Communication & Society, 21*(5), 786–791. https://doi.org/10.1080/1369118X.2018.1428653

Perez, C. (2019). Invisible women: Exposing data bias in a world designed for men. *Chatto*. https://doi.org/10.1111/1475-4932.12620

Rapp, R. (2016). Big data, small kids: Medico-scientific, familial and advocacy visions of human brains. *BioSocieties, 11*, 296–316. https://doi.org/10.1057/biosoc.2015.33

Rathi, A., & Tandon, A. (2019, February 9). Data infrastructures and inequities: Why does reproductive health surveillance in india need our urgent attention? *Economic & Political Weekly, 54*(6). https://www.epw.in/engage/article/data-infrastructures-inequities-why-does-reproductive-health-surveillance-india-need-urgent-attention

Ravindran, S. T. K. (1992). Engendering health. *UNDP Seminar, 396*, 21–25. https://www.undp.org/content/dam/india/docs/engendering_health.pdf

Ruckenstein, M., & Schüll, N. D. (2017). The datafication of health. *Annual Review of Anthropology, 46*(1), 261–278. https://doi.org/10.1146/annurev-anthro-102116-041244

Sandhu, M., Gambon, E., & Stotz, C. (2020, March 8). FemTech is expansive – It's time to start treating it as such. *RockHealth.* https://rockhealth.com/FemTech-is-expansive-its-time-to-start-treating-it-as-such/

Shilling, C. (1993). *The body and social theory.* Sage Publications.

Shilling, C. (2003). *The body and social theory.* Sage Publications.

Shklovski, I., Mainwaring, S. D., Skúladóttir, H. H., & Borgthorsson, H. (2014). Leakiness and creepiness in app space: Perceptions of privacy and mobile app use. *CHI '14: Proceedings of the SIGCHI Conference on Human Factors in Computing Systems,* April 2014, pp. 2347–2356. https://doi.org/10.1145/2556288.2557421.

Thomas, G. M., & Lupton, D. (2016). Threats and thrills: Pregnancy apps, risk and consumption. *Health, Risk & Society, 17*(7–8), 495–509. https://doi.org/10.1080/13698575.2015.1127333

Tripp, N., Hainey, K., Liu, A., Poulton, A., Peek, M., Kim, J., & Nanan, R. (2014). An emerging model of maternity care: Smartphone, midwife, doctor? *Women and birth: journal of the Australian College of Midwives, 27*(1), 64–67. https://doi.org/10.1016/j.wombi.2013.11.001

Ussher, J. M. (2006). *Managing the monstrous feminine: Regulating the reproductive body.* Routledge/Taylor & Francis Group. https://doi.org/10.4324/9780203328422

Van der Ploeg, I. (2012). The body as data in the age of information. In Ball, K., Haggerty, K., & Lyon, D. (Eds.), *Routledge Handbook of Surveillance Studies* (pp. 176–185). https://doi.org/10.4324/9780203814949

Wajcman, J. (2000). Reflections on gender and technology studies: In what state is the art? *Social Studies of Science, 30*(3), 447–464. https://doi.org/10.1177/030631200030003005

Worsfold, L., Marriott, L., Johnson, S., & Harper, J. C. (2021). Period tracker applications: What menstrual cycle information are they giving women? *Women's Health.* https://doi.org/10.1177/17455065211049905

Zhao, N., Schmitt M. & Fisk, J. (2016). Zhao et al. reply. https://www.research-gate.net/publication/305318790_Zhao_et_al-2016-FEBS_Journal/citation/download

Zuboff, S. (2015). Big other: Surveillance Capitalism and the prospects of an Information Civilization. *Journal of Information Technology, 30,* 75–89. https://doi.org/10.1057/jit.2015.5

6

Providing Care When There Is No Cure: How FemTech Can Help Destigmatize Autoimmune Diseases

Georgia M. Roberts

In the 1950s, the medical community began using the term "autoimmune disease" to categorize a range of chronic disorders generated by the body's overactive immune response to perceived infection. By overproducing antinuclear antibodies (the biomarker of autoimmunity), the immune system turns against itself and attacks healthy cells, causing new disease.[1] Two-thirds of those diagnosed with autoimmune conditions are

---

[1] See *Origins and history of autoimmunity – A brief review.* Ahsan H. Origins and history of autoimmunity—A brief review. Rheumatology & Autoimmunity. 2023;3:9–14. https://doi.org/10.1002/rai2.12049. Ahsan writes, "it was not widely recognized, until the 1950s, that an immune response could be developed not only against "foreign" but also "self" antigens from the studies of chronic thyroiditis leading to the acceptance of autoimmune diseases. Paul Ehrlich coined the term "horror autotoxicus" to emphasize the pathogenesis of autoimmunity and how the immune system distinguishes "foreign" from "self." The process led to the concept of immune tolerance. The discoveries of allergy and anaphylaxis were the first signs that the immune system was capable of self-damage. The first autoantibodies were discovered in the 1940s, when antinuclear antibodies and rheumatoid factors were described as serum factors that could bind nuclear antigens and immunoglobulins, respectively."

G. M. Roberts (✉)
University of Washington, Bothell, WA, USA
e-mail: gmr2@uw.edu

born female, and in the last forty years, reported cases of more than eighty different autoimmune diseases have been steadily on the rise in the United States and around the world.[2] The thing they all share in common is that they cannot be cured.

Experts have long acknowledged the extraordinarily difficult task in diagnosing and understanding the multicausal factors contributing to both the onset and progression of autoimmune disease. Even the more common conditions like rheumatoid arthritis, lupus, and multiple sclerosis are not well understood. Both genetics and the environment play a role in individual susceptibility to autoimmune disease, with mounting evidence to suggest the latter may be more instrumental than previously thought. Scientists are now focused on understanding how ultra-processed foods, environmental pollution, and so-called "forever chemicals" can provoke inflammatory response, because once cells turn against the body, treatment options are limited.[3] Drugs therapies and biologics can be effective in easing symptoms in conditions like rheumatoid arthritis, eczema, and ulcerative colitis by suppressing the entire immune system or, as in the case of JAK (Janus family kinases) inhibitors, by targeting specific proteins involved in overactive cell growth.[4] Yet none of the present treatments are not curative. In almost all cases, drugs have to be taken indefinitely, or the disease returns.

Advancing technologies in Artificial Intelligence (AI) and machine learning offer hope in diagnosing and better understanding autoimmune conditions. For example, AI programs such as Tibot® can utilize patient-submitted photos to analyze and identify an array of dermatological conditions. Recent studies have shown near-perfect accuracy in recognizing

---

[2] Dinse, Gregg E et al. "Increasing Prevalence of Antinuclear Antibodies in the United States." *Arthritis & Rheumatology (Hoboken, N.J.)* vol. 72,6 (2020): 1026–1035. https://doi.org/10.1002/art.41214.

[3] See Carolyn Beans "How 'Forever Chemicals' Might Impair the Immune System" https://www.pnas.org/doi/10.1073/pnas.2105018118 Accessed April 4, 2023. See also K. Persellin "Study: PFAS Exposure Through Skin Causes Harm Similar to Ingestion" https://www.ewg.org/news-insights/news/study-pfas-exposure-through-skin-causes-harm-similar-ingestion Accessed April 4, 2023.

[4] The FDA recently announced it had approved JAK inhibitors to treat alopecia areata, an autoimmune-related form of hair loss. See F.D.A. Approves Alopecia Drug Found to Regrow Hair. https://www.nytimes.com/2022/06/13/health/alopecia-drug-approved-fda.html?searchResultPosition=1 Accessed March 27, 2023.

visible forms of diseases like alopecia areata, an autoimmune-related skin condition that causes hair loss, and is the primary focus of this essay.[5] Self-initiated detection can offer privacy and empower patients to seek out appropriate medical expertise. The collection and aggregation of data also presents a unique opportunity to make real breakthroughs in advancing treatment options.

Considering that nearly 80% of all people diagnosed with autoimmune disease are born female, it seems obvious that research and tech-related solutions can benefit from the growing market and scholarly interest in the field of FemTech. In a January 2022 interview at the FemTechnology Summit, Mette Dyhrberg, the founder of Mymee, (a "digital care program" that employs "health coaches" to assess a customer's self-reported activity and turn it into a personalized plan of action), pointed to the ways data might help women better understand and manage autoimmune conditions. According to their website, Mymee's design is based on Dyhrberg's personal experience of managing her own diagnosis of reportedly six different autoimmune conditions, including psoriatic arthritis and Sjögren's syndrome.[6] The company's approach is similar to other autoimmune-related apps on the market that focus primarily on self-surveillance and disease management.[7] They ask clients to track food and activities, helping them identify and eliminate inflammation-causing foods. The coaches encourage lifestyle changes that draw on more general forms of perceived wisdom such as getting proper exercise, eating a balanced diet, and reducing stress.

---

[5] See Patil, Anant, Sharmia Patil, DheerajN Rao, Faisal Basar, and Salim Bate. "Assessment of Tibot® Artificial Intelligence Application in Prediction of Diagnosis in Dermatological Conditions: Results of a Single Centre Study." *Indian Dermatology Online Journal* 11, no. 6 (2020): 910. https://doi.org/10.4103/idoj.idoj_61_20.

[6] See https://www.mymee.com/about-mymee Accessed April 3, 2023.

[7] From preliminary research, it looks like Mymee has supported both of the available studies on the effectiveness of the app and personal coaching. The first article is a proof-of-concept and lists Dyhrberg as one of the authors. The other is funded by Mymee. Both use populations of older adults living with lupus and chronic pain, respectively. They track water intake, exercise, food, etc. and have Meetings with coaches (to go over self-tracking data) which cost about one hundred dollars per session. See Kaul, Usha et al. "A mobile health + health coaching application for the management of chronic non-cancer pain in older adults: Results from a pilot randomized controlled study." Frontiers in pain research *(Lausanne, Switzerland)* vol. 3 921428. 25 Jul. 2022, https://doi.org/10.3389/fpain.2022.921428.

Perhaps the greatest value in using apps like Mymee is digitalizing the combination of food and symptom tracking with fee-based forms of accountability, yielding more consistent outcomes and generating an understanding of potential patterns. Nutritionists have been helping patients track food sensitivities and develop autoimmune diet protocols since at least the 1970s, and self-reporting can be especially helpful in managing conditions like type-one diabetes and celiac disease. But it's also important to understand that when it comes to living with an autoimmune disease, knowledge doesn't always equal power. Even though autoimmune-related apps have names like My Life, Manage My Pain, and Mymee (my me) doesn't mean they can provide a magical salve to restore the loss of control experienced through the unpredictability of living with autoimmune disease. Food-tracking and expensive vitamin supplements are not pathways to a cure. I'm not at all suggesting an absence of good intention, but rather that treatments geared toward women and autoimmune disease that rely on an unexamined faith in data and prioritize biopolitical self-management can work to further stigmatize women with autoimmune disease. I'm interested in the ways FemTech might help us redefine care beyond the individual and imagine more expansive approaches to living with autoimmune disease. For example, how can FemTech draw on important lessons from feminist theory to understand and treat autoimmunity within the sociohistorical and cultural matrixes of race, class and gender? As science moves us toward curative therapies (of which data plays an important role), how can we leverage the space of FemTech to help strengthen existing networks of care and build new coalitions toward more effective healthcare and inclusive policy? In short, how can technology help provide care when there is no cure?

"Alopecia is Trending!"

These questions were literally brought centerstage at the 94th Annual Academy Awards ceremony in the controversy surrounding actor Will Smith's physical assault of comedian Chris Rock for a joke made in reference to Jada Pinkett-Smith's baldness and alopecia areata. The night of the Oscars, I was home grading papers when my phone began to ping nonstop. Several friends and family members sent texts with the same question, "Did you see what just happened? 'Alopecia' is trending!" The sudden and overwhelming interest in learning about alopecia areata demonstrated what researchers and those of us living with the autoimmune condition already knew; there is a long way to go in educating the general public about what it means to live with an autoimmune disease.

The term alopecia is a wide-ranging, generic term for hair loss and can develop for a variety of reasons, including hormone levels and aging. Damage to the hair follicle from harsh chemicals and pulling can also lead to both temporary and permanent hair loss.[8] Alopecia areata, on the other hand, is classified an autoimmune-related skin disease that causes people to lose hair in smooth, round patches. It can affect any age (including babies in the womb) and affects all races and ethnic groups. The patchy form of alopecia areata is fairly common, and about 2% of the larger population experiences patchy hair loss in some form during their lifetime. More severe and less-common forms of alopecia areata are alopecia totalis (where a person loses all the hair on their head and reportedly Pinkett-Smith's diagnosis) and alopecia universalis (the most severe form and leaves the person completely hairless, including loss of eyelashes, eyebrows, and nose hair). Alopecia universalis is categorized as a rare disease, affecting less that 200,000 Americans. Unlike the majority of autoimmune conditions, which are invisible and often physically debilitating, alopecia areata is experienced largely as a stigmatized social condition. The constant management and unpredictability of social expectations, especially around gender identity, racialised standards of attractiveness, and for those who wear wigs—the fear of discovery, can pose serious social and mental health challenges.

Pinkett-Smith has been open in recent years about struggling with alopecia areata totalis, and after recently shaving her head on her show, *The Red Table Talk*, she attended the Academy Awards without a wig or head covering. People have speculated as to whether Rock knew Pinkett-Smith had alopecia areata, but either way, during his short monologue, Rock

---

[8] https://theconversation.com/amp/what-is-alopecia-its-no-laughing-matter-for-millions-of-black-american-women-180213.

turned to her and said "Jada – love ya. *G.I. Jane 2* – can't wait to see it." There was an immediate reaction from the crowd, a combination of bemusement and condemnation. As a woman diagnosed with alopecia universalis in my teens, I have lived nearly thirty years without hair and wasn't at all surprised by the old *GI Jane* reference. It's typical and quite ordinary, a reference drawn from a very limited number of pop culture-inspired insults aimed at bald women (the other two being Sinead O'Conner and Britney Spears). I've heard it a million times in passing. Yet to hear it on live TV and in public had a different effect.

As trite and outdated as the reference may have sounded to some, Rock's choice of comparison was far from harmless. If he meant nothing by it, why not compare Pinkett-Smith's shaved head to those of the Dora Milaje, the all-female military unit entrusted to protect the King of Wakanda in the more recent (and far more successful) movie, *Black Panther*? What was the point in referencing a twenty-five-year-old film about a woman who shaved her head while training to join the U.S. Navy SEALs? Whether intended or not, Rock's joke relied on a residual, yet still powerful cultural image not so easily removed from its original referent. As the first female recruit, Lieutenant Jordan O'Neil (*G.I. Jane*'s main character) challenges the heteropatriarchal forms of masculine power at the core of U.S. military power by her mere *presence* in the program. The pivotal scene where Lt. O'Neil (played by Demi Moore) sneaks into the barber shop to shave her head is meant to demonstrate her absolute commitment to complete the training. There is more to say about the scene and the film beyond the scope of this paper, but suffice it to say that Rock's reference to G.I. Jane was not harmless. It was performative and drew on a well-established cultural grammar used. As a bald, Black woman at the Oscars that night, Pinkett-Smith's presence already challenged Hollywood's historically white beauty standards, and Rock's invocation of G.I. Jane recast Pinkett-Smith's brave decision into a symbolic threat to American heteropatriarchy.

Stigma is about public shaming through calling attention to physical difference and finding a way to assign individual blame to the person. According to sociologist Erving Goffman, the word and concept of "stigma" comes from the Greeks and refers to "bodily signs designed to expose something unusual and bad about the moral status of the signifier.

The signs were cut or burnt into the body and advertised that the bearer was a slave, a criminal or a traitor—a blemished person, ritually polluted, to be avoided, especially in public places."[9] A stigma sets the person apart from society, and their physical difference "spoils" their identity and standing in the social sense. It was the audacity to be seen in public as she is (and not wear a wig) that made Pinkett-Smith a vulnerable target for Rock's humiliation, and his joke transformed the general perception of her as someone dealing with a health condition into someone who was making a deliberate "choice."

Across social media, people speculated that Will Smith's reaction to the joke demonstrated Pinkett-Smith's dominance in their relationship; her baldness simply showed up as the manifestation or surface-level proof that something was deeply wrong with her as a wife and mother. Rather than showing empathy, many people castigated Pinkett-Smith for previously speaking publicly (with Smith, on her show) about their previous separation and practicing non-monogamy in their marriage. Several widely circulated memes, such as the one below, went as far as to characterize her baldness as mental illness, listing it among her other alleged personality disorders (Fig. 6.1).

Not to belabor the point, but it's important to note that the larger narrative of what transpired at the Oscars has been cast as an unfortunate rupture between men, where one of them took it too far and resorted to violence. The initial interest in finding out about alopecia quickly morphed into an endless flurry of successive think-pieces about Black masculinity, the Smith's marriage dynamics, and respectability politics. Will Smith granted his first public interview to Trevor Noah in November of 2022, and Chris Rock waited until the week before the 2023 Oscars to give his public statement—in the form of the first-ever live-streamed Netflix show, and for a reported for a 20 million dollars. Neither Smith nor Rock mentioned Pinkett-Smith's autoimmune diagnosis, and their collective silence served as further proof that the public stigma would be hers to bear alone.

---

[9] Goffman, E. (1963). *Stigma: Notes on the management of spoiled identity.* New York: Simon & Schuster, 1–3.

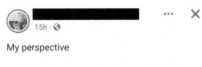

My perspective

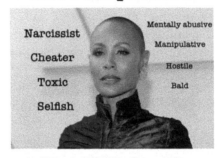

Fig. 6.1   Jada Pinkett-Smith meme

Pinkett-Smith's response to the incident, on the other hand, though not as publicized or commented-upon in mainstream press as the others, was instructive and extremely helpful for thinking more carefully about the main question animating this essay: how best can we use technology and FemTech as a space to address the medical and social concerns of people living with incurable autoimmune conditions like alopecia areata? Pinkett-Smith invited people of all ages diagnosed with alopecia areata to appear on the June 1, 2022 episode of her Facebook show, Red Table Talk, to share a wide-range of experiences with the various types of alopecia. She approached the topic from the awareness that Black women in the U.S. are disproportionately impacted by alopecia and the understanding that alopecia areata is an incurable autoimmune condition that affects all people and at all ages. She included doctors, advocates, spouses, and parents to talk about the ongoing challenges of caring for loved ones, and started the show by interviewing the mother of a 12-year-old girl from Indiana with alopecia totalis who died by suicide just a few short weeks before the Oscars. She spoke to Pinkett-Smith about the note her daughter left saying she could no longer endure the constant bullying at school. Overall, the show emphasized proper diagnosis, public education to reduce stigma, and connecting with others who share similar experiences.

Some might consider my focus on the Oscars incident and the stigma of hair loss as merely superficial or surface level when it comes to larger discussions about health outcomes associated with autoimmune disease. But that is exactly the point. The vast majority of autoimmune disorders affecting women are not always visible, with notable exceptions like vitiligo and psoriasis. More public figures and celebrities have stepped forward in recent years to disclose their struggles with autoimmune conditions, such as Christina Applegate and Selma Blair (multiple sclerosis) and Selena Gomez (Lupus), but many people speak up only when they begin to show outward signs of their condition, such as limited mobility and weight fluctuation due to medication. It's still unusual to see someone in the public eye with a visible autoimmune diseases like alopecia areata and vitiligo may not be physically debilitating in the same way as other autoimmune conditions, but they are much more than simply "cosmetic." The social stigma associated with physical difference can have devastating mental health impacts on people, with one recent study showing that newly diagnosed cases of with alopecia areata correspond to an almost 40% increase in new diagnosis of clinical depression.[10] Stigma can be exacerbated by social media and contemporary standards of beauty based on gender, age, race, class, and culture. Finding better ways to deal with the more surface-level aspects and *social reality* of living with autoimmune disorders can remind us that care must also move beyond self-surveillance and disease management and toward education and support.

FemTech has offered interventions and proposed solutions to destigmatize topics like menstrual health, reproductive care, and menopause. How might we leverage the category in ways that attend to both the medical and the social environments that patient outcomes in

---

[10] Abby E. Macbeth, Susan Holmes, Matthew Harries, Wing Sin Chiu, Christos Tziotzios, Simon de Lusignan, Andrew G. Messenger, Andrew R. Thompson, The associated burden of mental health conditions in alopecia areata: a population-based study in UK primary care, *British Journal of Dermatology*, Volume 187, Issue 1, 1 July 2022, Pages 73–81, https://doi.org/10.1111/bjd.21055.

autoimmune disease? As mentioned above, advancing AI technologies in the diagnosis and management of autoimmune disease can provide earlier and more discreet modes of diagnosis, connect people to medical information and advice, and outline potential management/treatment options. But FemTech can also play an essential part in supporting women and people with autoimmune diseases in more specific ways: (1) help to educate patients, providers, and the general public about autoimmune conditions, including how they may impact a person's experience at school, work, or in relationships, (2) create platforms to connect people with similar conditions in ways that assure maximum privacy, and (3) use data in ways that help researchers and patients better understand the relationship between reproductive health and autoimmune disease.

One of the most important aspects of providing better outcomes for people with autoimmune conditions is through public education, including educating doctors, insurance companies, employers, and the larger community.[11] A study conducted in 2021 surveyed over 2000 adult respondents in the U.S. to assess the relationship between social stigma and alopecia areata. Researchers used technology to create three versions of six people, eighteen images total, representing both women and men, and black and white. The participants were shown different versions of the same computer-generated image, each with varying forms of autoimmune-related hair loss. Over 80% of those surveyed expressed no knowledge of alopecia areata, and when shown the pictures before being told that the person had a medical condition, described people with

---

[11] JAMA Dermatology April 2021 volume 157 #4. Creadore A, Manjaly P, Li SJ, et al. Evaluation of Stigma Toward Individuals With Alopecia. *JAMA Dermatol.* 2021;157(4):392–398. Creadore and colleagues surveyed over 2000 adult respondents in the US to assess the average layperson's understanding and perception of alopecia areata, specifically alopecia totalis and universalis. They used technology to create three versions of six people, eighteen images total, representing both women and men, black and white people. The survey "presented each internet respondent with one randomly selected portrait to be used in answering a series of stigma-related questions from three domains: stereotypes, social distance, and disease-related myths; the third domain was presented only to respondents who believed that the individual pictured had a medical condition." About a third of respondents described photos of people with totalis and universalis as them as "unattractive" but among the group of people who were told or "who believed the individual pictured had a medical condition…there was decreased stigma including change in perceived masculinity or femininity." As Dr. Goh points out in her essay in the same volume, one of the "key takeaways from this study are that there is a public stigmatization about alopecia totalis the universalism and that seeing them as medical conditions may reduce stigma," 383–384.

totalis and universalis as "unattractive." On the other hand, attitudes were significantly less judgmental about physical appearances among participants "who believed the individual pictured had a medical condition", Commenting on the significance of the study in the same issue, dermatologist Dr. Carolyn Goh" recalls her personal experience of living with a alopecia totalis for the better part of four decades:

> I have been mistaken for male, asked numerous times if I am undergoing chemotherapy, and have even been taunted by those who incorrectly assumed I shaved my head. When wearing wigs as a child, I experienced bullying and lived in fear of the wig being misplaced or falling off my head. Similar experiences have been reported by others with alopecia. Their experiences epitomize the public stigma of alopecia and are not merely perceptions. In fact, the idea that the perceived stigma of an individual with alopecia is distinctive or should be differentiated from public or external stigmas should not be acceptable. Yet there is the need to provide evidence for external stigma for practical reasons, and this study by Creadore and colleagues establishes the pervasiveness of the stigmatization of alopecia.[12]

As Goh points out in the article, research and evidence that people are socially stigmatized by the condition can help patients advocate for more effective treatment options and insurance coverage for hair pieces and mental health care, "thus reducing stigma and financial burden for patients with alopecia."[13] One of the most common issues people face is insurance companies refusing to cover the cost of hair pieces because they are classified as cosmetic. Many of the same companies will cover the cost of wigs during temporary treatment for chemotherapy but not for someone with alopecia areata.

Social media has surfaced some of these inconsistencies and helped in lobbying for better coverage. FemTech can also help us build similar understanding and connections around Goh's point about gender-based bullying and misgendering. This is an extremely common occurrence for small children and teens with alopecia universalis and for people who do not wear wigs. Policies that target transgender and queer people also harm gender nonconforming people with alopecia. Transphobic bathroom laws and doubling down on definitions of gender presentation in binary terms like "feminine" and "masculine" also normalize discrimination against people with alopecia areata. There is an opportunity to develop more intersectional approaches that help educate patients and the public and foster connections between communities of people who are suffering in disproportionate ways.

I'd like to see FemTech become a space that listens to and learns from communities about what they want and need in terms of diagnosis, treatment options, educational resources, and community support. In the course of researching and writing this essay, I found several that are addressing the first two, but only a couple that came close to the others. The Global Autoimmune Institute has compiled a list of recommended apps that help patients remember medication, track food, monitor pain, or connect to mental health services. Some also offer disease-specific discussion boards. Although not autoimmune-specific, the most interesting among them is an app called Healp that allows people with the same medical conditions to connect with one another.[14] According to an interview with the Healp's founder, Elizabeth Tikoyan, the app's structure is similar to Tinder or Bumble, "allowing people to enter the database and swipe right or left, then start talking to people with similar conditions." Tikoyan said some members (mostly thirty-five and younger) join to ask each other questions about treatments, while "others use it for social questions, like how to talk to partners about their conditions."[15] On paper, this model comes very close to the role support groups have played for years. Meeting other people going through the same thing is a gamechanger, and as someone who has personally benefited from support groups for over two decades, I am most drawn to of this kind approach. However, the potential benefits in doing so online not currently outweigh the risks to privacy (I took the time to read the entire privacy statement). I've met hundreds of women with alopecia areata over the last 25 years whose family and friends knew little-to-nothing about their condition and/or have never seen them without a hairpiece.

---

[14] https://www.healp.co/how-it-works.

[15] https://technical.ly/diversity-equity-inclusion/healp-elizabeth-tikoyan.

A similar connection-focused mobile app called Ally (UK-based) proposed to connect women with alopecia to one another across the world.[16] Founded by a woman with alopecia areata, the project received a lot of initial press in the FemTech space in 2019, but no longer seems to be active. I'd like to see more projects like Healp and Ally that center and support the social needs of people with autoimmune disease. Speaking from the perspective of someone with three autoimmune conditions, I think the most useful projects would intervene at the nexus of culture, meaning they would find ways to disrupt or complicate commercial narratives that implicitly link anxiety, vitamin supplementation, and "hair growth journeys." They would be honest about the lack of scientific understanding when it comes to autoimmune disease. They'd prioritize privacy when connecting people to resources and to each other, and encourage deeper conversations about how social stigma emerges in relationship to race, class, gender, and sexuality. They would expand what we mean when we talk about environmental triggers and find ways to balance individualized disease management with community-wide organizing efforts for less-polluted food sources and more inclusive social spaces. The most successful interventions will be feminist, collaborative and draw on the decades-long experience of people who have been showing up for one another since the days before the internet or the non-profit patient foundation, when treatment meant a handful of people in a coffee shop trying to understand what an autoimmune disease was, and finding ways to provide care when there is no cure.

---

[16] https://www.forbes.com/sites/nicholasfearn/2019/07/04/how-one-entrepreneur-is-creating-a-global-online-community-for-people-with-alopecia/?sh=719ed73e15d1.

7

The Insta-Trainer: A Study of How Instagram Is Used as a Biopedagogical Tool for Health and Wellbeing Among Young Women in Qatar

Sara Al Derham

Introduction

This chapter introduces the concept of the "Insta-Trainer," its functionality as a gendered technology of power, and the impact such phenomena have on young content consumers in Qatar. The original study focuses on Instagram as a platform, but this chapter will also touch upon Insta-Trainers and their representation on TikTok in order to demonstrate the pertinency of the concept across multiple social media platforms.

In doing so, I maintain that, if the scope of feminine technologies (FemTech) includes software, hardware, as well as worn devices, medical implants, communication technologies and artificial intelligence, then included within the remit of FemTech must also be consideration for social media platforms. Moreover, the relationship between women's health technologies and social media is growing increasingly close with platforms such as Facebook and Instagram being used not only to market

S. Al Derham (✉)
Newcastle University, Newcastle upon Tyne, UK
e-mail: S.A.A.Alderham2@newcastle.ac.uk

products, but to manage a consumer base and serve as a medium for the sharing of health data accumulated by other FemTech applications.

I define "Insta-Trainers" as a concept of instantly training the self via the use of digital platforms. In detail, it is a concept that represents content gathered from various content creators including individuals, businesses, and organisations[1] within a hypermedia[2] space under one umbrella, as a multiservice assemblage. Their activity is designed to operate hand in hand with the algorithmic functions of the platform as a neoliberal self-training and self-managing tool. In other words, Insta-Training, then, works to discipline the (female) body using social media as the delivery mechanism for self-tracking and improvement.

Through intensive qualitative data collection—consisting of (1) an interactive survey designed with open-ended questions, completed by 41 women from Qatar ranging between 18 and 30 years, and (2) 10 semi-structured interviews from the same pool—I have confirmed that the young Qatari women from my study heavily rely on Insta-Trainer content to learn about and manage their overall health. It was also revealed that they do so particularly for the purpose of achieving a feminine, normalized, and productive sense of self through performing self-discipling practices. A noteworthy finding was the heavy reliance on Insta-Trainers originating from the West rather than from the Middle East, which has had a clear impact on the participants' relationship with diet habits, their relationship with cultural food, and even the language in which they consume digital media.

For this chapter, I aim to discuss one out of the three themes that I have extracted from my datasets using Braun and Clarke's thematic methods. I focus on how young women from Qatar benefit from Insta-Trainers through meta-texts that I have termed "curated digital manuals". I define these manuals as visual collages that are either assembled by users through directly interacting with and meticulously bookmarking content created by Insta-Trainers in organised and labelled folders, or the result of

---

[1] This includes private, public, and governmental institutes and organisations.

[2] A hypermedia space, as defined by the Cambridge Dictionary, are "a combination of videos, images, sounds text, etc. that are connected together on a website, which you can click on in order to use them or to go to other related videos, websites, etc." or "an interactive system that allows users to navigate a network of linked *hypermedia* objects" (2023).

engagement with Insta-Trainer content, which feeds into the algorithm of the platform resulting into algorithmically curated collages of content in the form of the popular page or daily feed.

On Instagram, I have identified three types of curated digital manuals: (1) the pre-curated—created outside of the platform yet hyperlinked and marketed within; (2) the self-curated, bookmarked and curated by the users using the "Saved Folders" feature on Instagram; and finally (3) the algorithmically curated digital manual, generated by the algorithm based on user engagement and presented in the form of the "Daily Feed" and "Popular Page." These categories also apply to TikTok as well.

Indeed, the platform TikTok was cited by six out of the ten (60%) of the women interviewed for this study. It is worth briefly mentioning that TikTok has a function similar Instagram's "Saved Folders," called "Collections." In the same way the "Explore Page" and "Feed" on Instagram function, TikTok's version, which is the "For You Page," acts as an analogue. The purpose of highlighting TikTok's features is purely in an effort to point out that such bio-pedagogical functionalities and ethical practices extend outside of Instagram and can be found on other social networking platforms, which is an area for further research. Further, examining the digital curation of "healthism," which works alongside other forms of digital health software and hardware, demonstrates the extent to which discourses of self-management operate across devices *and* platforms.

In what follows, I offer some background context on the relationship between heath management and social media and provide a close analysis of an Insta-Trainer profile and how it functions under the definition presented above. I then turn to the phenomena of digitally curated manuals and how they function as biopedagogical tools. The example that I plan to present is of a fitness influencer who fits into the description of an Insta-Trainer as per the definition mentioned above. However, it is important to reiterate that Insta-Trainers include private, public, and governmental organisations as well and are not limited to individuals or influencers. However, this chapter will not address this example to remain within the scope of the volume.

Finally, before concluding the chapter, I will briefly discuss the lessons learned from heavy interaction with Insta-Trainer content during the first wave of the Covid-19 lockdown in a section titled, "The Qatari post-pandemic conscious user." I will present this chapter through discussing the experiences shared from the interviewees of this study. The relevance of the section is due to the fact that the majority of data was collected in the midst of lockdown, which led me to two of the most important findings: the first is that there exists a clear shift in the way users traditionally interacted with Insta-Trainers compared to after the pandemic. The second is the existence of a user-disjuncture, where the participants claim that they do not trust content created by Insta-Trainers, yet they subscribe and increasingly follow and purchase their content and products.

Looking at Insta-Trainers through the lens of Qatari women's experiences with social media provides a rich contribution to the field of FemTech research by considering the unique relationship between gender, culture, race, and class, and reveals the deep complexity of gender, health, and technology in Qatar and the Middle East. The Qatari society, like other Gulf countries, tend to be a private and discreet community with cultural norms and traditional values that are rooted in Islamic beliefs. Despite this and contrary to the popular belief that portrayed Arab women as passive and silent, women have always played an active role in the making and shaping of society, particularly in Qatar (Diaconoff, 2009; Al-Fassi, 2012; Nasser, 2012; Sonbol, 2012). Ultimately, I argue that examining such complexities is vital in understanding how aspects of FemTech is playing a significant yet discreet neoliberal globalised role in shaping cultural identities and health-related behaviours in traditionally private tribal populations.

Background

A health report conducted by Northwestern University in Qatar has found that young users in Qatar heavily rely on digital platforms when interacting with health-related information (Schoenbach et al., 2017). Based on an interactive dataset from a seven-nation survey on media use within the Middle East, women from Qatar were found to be among the most active users of social media platforms, particularly Instagram 71%

with around 51% checking the platform at least once a day (Dennis et al., 2018).

A follow-up survey also concluded that "Instagram is more popular among younger respondents," which has been the case within the findings since the project had launched in 2013 (Dennis et al., 2013, 2014, 2018). In regard to TikTok, studies published by the platform itself has reported that Qatar was among the top five countries, at fifth place, in terms of platform penetration worldwide in 2022—it is important to note that the other top three countries were reported to be neighbouring Gulf countries, ranging between 87.9 and 95.4% in penetration (Statista, 2022). These number show heavy exposure to TikTok content within the Gulf countries, which provides a rich area for further research of social media usage, and on women within a region that is already underrepresented (Al-Fassi, 2012; Sonbol, 2012).

In terms of social media usage among the participants in my study, the interviewees reported spending an average of four hours a day on Instagram alone. This is approximately 16% of their entire day specifically spent on Instagram, and not including other social media platforms. It is important to note that while my study focuses on Instagram that all the ten interviewees have referenced TikTok usage when discussing interactions, engagements, and the health impact of Instagram. Through the semi-structured conversations, I discovered that the interviewees view Insta-Training functionalities on Instagram and TikTok as one. Again, this further confirms that the concept of the Insta-Trainer and their functions apply to other social media platforms, and that the concept itself can be used as a tool for further research in this area, particularly in further investigations into the relationship between social media and digital health.

Further, the numbers and facts above indicate two very important factors, the first is that young women in Qatar use social media extensively as part of their daily routine. They do not only spend most of their day online as passive users but are actively interacting and then enacting the messages and information in the content. In the case of the participants in my study, this has proven to directly impact their health in ways that are both productive and problematic. For example, one participant claimed that she, "got the results that she paid" for from an Insta-Trainer's booklet on exercise and nutrition, whereas another claimed that fitness content from Insta-Trainers were the main cause of a 27-day stay in hospital. Other studies on Instagram usage among young users have found similar results in relation to users' wellbeing, fitness, and nutrition habits—they confirm a change in attitude, mindset and routine due to content found and consumed on Instagram and other social media platforms (Talbot et al., 2017; Ambwani et al., 2019; Camacho-Miñano et al., 2019; DiBisceglie & Arigo, 2019; Rodney, 2019).

The second factor is that Instagram is indeed used as a bio-pedagogical tool that users benefit from to learn how to maintain both their physical and mental wellbeing. Other responses revealed the extent to which users desired to be thinner, to lose weight, to stop feeling guilty about eating, to feel good about themselves, and to be healthy. Significantly, these goals have been described by participants as achievable through either learning from influencers' journeys, subscribing to health profiles, and/or purchasing products and services from highly curated and cleverly hidden advertisements (Habibi et al., 2014; Abidin, 2016; Liu et al., 2018). Moreover, the content created by Insta-Trainers is often commercially driven and alludes to the notion that certain degrees of health and wellness cannot be obtained without the consumption of such products, services, and paid advice (Pilgrim & Bohnet-Joschko, 2019; Reinikainen et al., 2020; Sokolova & Kefi, 2020).

Important to note is that Insta-Trainers who are female social media influencers exist within an extremely gendered profession that consists of "(mostly) uncompensated, independent work that is propelled by the much-venerated ideal of *getting paid to do what you love*" (Duffy, 2017, p. 4; Cirucci, 2017; Duffy & Hund, 2019). Despite this, it is evident that women themselves, to some degree, are indeed creators and contributors of features that build FemTech, or create the standardised ideals put forward by most feminine technologies. The constant need to be updated and keep up with current trends, while simultaneously self-regulating, curating, and manging both their content and bodies does indeed add pressure on Insta-Trainers and the consumers of their content. Furthermore, it adds complexity to a sub-genre of FemTech in which women act as entrepreneurs and influencers in ostensibly feminist ways, while at the same time promoting conventional versions of gender and beauty.

At its core, such practices promoted by Insta-Trainer align with the popular ideology that looking a certain type of way, thin, hairless and with no signs of aging, equate to being in good health and being considered as a virtuous bio-citizen as well as maintaining a normalised sense of femininity (Bartky, 1990; Gill, 2007; Heyes, 2007; Halse et al., 2009; Lupton, 2013; Camacho-Miñano et al., 2019; Sikka, 2023). Additionally, this frames personal health outcomes as a direct result of personal choices (Gordon, 2023). Such self-managing, self-surveillance and individualising mechanisms reflect a dominant theme across chapters in this volume, in which women's bodies in particular are subject to (self) scrutiny in the surface of surveillance capitalism.

All the above directly leads young Qatari women, who are already heavy users of social media, to physically and mentally self-moderate, and increasingly adds an extra layer of pressure and stress on their shoulders (Dennis et al., 2018). Arguably, this places the users' agency in crisis, as they have normalised and internalised self-surveillant practices, which have turned them into docile subjects continuously seeking to self-transform themselves through disciplinary actions (Foucault, 1978; Han, 2017). This is achieved, of course, with the help of Insta-Trainers and their biopedagogical functionality on social media platforms, one such function being the feature of the curated digital manuals.

Biopedagogical Relations Between Apps and Platforms: A Case Study

Denice Moberg's Instagram profile documents the lifestyle of a fitness influencer who meets the criteria of an Insta-Trainer and has a following of one million users as of April 2023. She was identified twice within the survey and once within the interviews, particularly among participants who mentioned "mom stuff" and "postpartum workouts" within their save folders on Instagram. Notably, I have found that the participants from my study heavily rely on Western Insta-Trainers to learn about health and wellness, another influencer who was mentioned multiple times was Kayla Itsines, who has a following of 16 million as of April 2023. One participant even proclaimed in the interview that she does not trust Middle Eastern Insta-Trainers and prefers learning about her health and body from Western profiles.

The data that I have collected does not directly justify the preference that young Qatari women have for Western Insta-Trainers, however I do believe that the algorithmic biases that favours White and Eurocentric features do play a role in terms of the content exposure of these content creators (Benjamin, 2019; Noble, 2018). Another plausible factor could be that the Western Insta-Trainers mentioned have followers within the millions, whereas the regional Insta-Trainers' followings usually range within the hundreds of thousands, such as Dr Hanadi Al Badir (@drhanadialbadir) at 170k followers and Naji Al Hammadi (@naji__alhammadi) with 106k followers.

Moreover, Moberg is also a brand ambassador for *GymShark*, a fitness apparel company and fitness and training application. As such, Moberg's account can also be considered as an Insta-Training profile, with shopping and training options both hyperlinked in her biography. This alone demonstrates how Insta-Trainer profiles operate as an assemblage and are interlinked across hypermedia and app-based spaces, in this case between Instagram and the *GymShark* training application. Her photo grid on Instagram represents content that is highly curated, sponsored and biopedagogical at its core. Here, I rely on the definition of biopedagogy brought forward by Camacho-Miñano et al. (2019), which includes "normalizing and regulating practices that provide individuals with the knowledge to understand themselves, change their behaviour and take action upon themselves and others to improve health." Worth noting here is that fitness content on social media is indeed considered biopedagogical content, whether they contain advice, product placements or services relating to fitness or health, which can be found on Moberg's profile (Wright, 2009).

Indeed, in addition to lifestyle content, Moberg's account includes an overwhelmingly repetitive collage of (1) recipes that are framed as quick and healthy meal preparation solutions targeted at busy mothers or fitness enthusiasts; (2) work-out montages of Moberg that offer tips and advice in the description, some of which include the word "SAVE," in an effort to encourage followers to save the videos as reference for later consumption; and (3) highly curated snippets of her life as a mother of two followed by advertisements for fitness related products, like *Barebells'* protein milkshake cleverly placed in the centre between her and her daughter during a fun day at the pool.

Denice Moberg's page is a good example of influencers utilising Insta-Trainer functions such as urging her followers to save her video in their "Saved Folders," which I identify as one of the curated digital manuals, a main feature of Insta-Training functionalities. The urgency to bookmark her content and the use of words such as, "get upper body strength" and "learn how to fix your [pelvis]" in the description implies a biopedagogical approach that offers a solution to a problem that could very well be non-existent, but at the same time building upon a narrative targeted at women that presents intensive labour a solution for healthier and stronger body.

The gestures made in the video,[3] which signal to the users to "do this and not this," frame the knowledge that is provided as the only method to achieve "better contact with your core." As a sidenote, the Insta-Trainer is wearing *GymShark* gear in the video and is filmed in a gym using barbell weights, which (1) indicates that the video is a sponsored video, and (2) indirectly implies that one needs certain products, accessories, and gear in order to perform certain functions to achieve good physical health.

Through this example, it is clear that self-surveillant, self-disciplinary and self-managing practices are being encouraged by the content creator to better improve oneself. It is presented and packaged to be achievable through the support of the Insta-Trainer's knowledge, services, and the products from brands that they represent, which are inaccessible to many, and promote an unrealistic standard health and beauty. Young women from Qatar who consume content by Insta-Trainers, such as Moberg and Itsines, have expressed benefiting in terms of losing weight, maintaining weight, or gaining muscles for strength. However, they also have excluded

---

[3] As of 28 April 2023, the video I am referring to was played 213,583 times. The number of likes is not visible, but the users who have liked the video are overwhelmingly female users. The post was originally uploaded on 18 April 2023.

cultural and regional food from their everyday diet, labelling them as "evil food," which have replaced it with Western inspired options tied to trendy diets, such as Mediterranean and Keto diets.

The Curated Digital Manuals

The curated digital manuals like traditional manuals, primarily those that focus on health and wellbeing, are pedagogical tools in nature. They present themselves as guidelines, references, and instructions on self-conduct, which are often rooted in self-disciplinary practices. In this study, all the 41 participants have confirmed that the content within the three types of digitally curated manuals encourage self-transformative and self-surveillant practices. It is important to reiterate that the biopedagogical nature of Insta-Training functionalities, the curated digital manual being a main feature, have been found to produce moderately productive and significantly problematic patterns among users within the study. This is entirely due to the fact that such practices are labour-intensive, exclusionary, unsustainable, and require a certain amount of privilege to enact.

The first out of the three types of digital manuals that I identify in my study are the pre-curated digital manuals, this is one that is originally created outside the platform by or for Insta-Trainers. They consist both of traditional manuals and technologically designed programmes, such as printable PDF booklets, mobile applications, and/or websites that are all heavily marketed on Instagram. Like historic and traditional manuals, they all share a similar narrative of self-transforming to a better and virtuous version of oneself. The pre-curated manuals are hyperlinked on the Insta-Trainers' profiles, and occasionally within the content or directly on the profiles of their partners and/or brand ambassadors (Habibi et al., 2014; Abidin, 2016; Sokolova & Kefi, 2020). In short, they are manuals that are either printable, technologically developed, and/or embedded as instructions within content that are created outside of Insta-Trainer platforms and are marketed within Instagram and other platforms, such as TikTok.

An example of the pre-curated manuals cited by the participants were those created by Kayla Itsines, the *Bikini Body Guide* booklet turned mobile application, *SWEAT*. The application is accessible through an annually or monthly subscription fee, as opposed to the booklet, which was a one-time purchase. Ghaya,[4] in the interview, has mentioned that she purchased the booklet and then upgraded to the application as soon as it launched. She has mentioned using the application at least two to three times a week. Other self-surveillant applications, which can be considered as a pre-curated digital manual and have also been identified by the participants are *MyFitnessPal* and *TrainingPeaks*, which they stated learning about through Instagram.

One example from the region, also mentioned extensively by participants of the study is Dr Hanadi Al-Badir's Instagram profile. She is a popular family doctor based in Kuwait, who tailors calorie-restricted diets based solely on customers' BMI. She markets her services as a diet that allows one to incorporate their cravings within the daily meal plan. Dr Al-Badir operates exclusively through Instagram and WhatsApp,[5] which is where she collects payment for her services and where shares the tailored diet manuals.

The second type of digital manual is the self-curated digital manuals, which are created by users bookmarking content in categorised folders. This is done through the built-in feature of the "Saved Folders" on Instagram and is "a way of keeping [the] posts you want to look at again" (Aguiar, 2019). The women in my study have indicated doing so in an attempt to organise the flood of information from their feed or the popular page. Interestingly, this does not only show that young users of social media are critical of the content they consume, but it also gives insight to how users navigate through a constant influx of information whilst rating those they deem as beneficial and important to save for future consumption.

Further, the top three saved folders or individually curated manuals as reported by the respondents of the survey were; (1) fitness content and products, such as work-out montages and fitness accessories reported by 68% of respondents; (2) food related, particularly diets trends and healthy recipes, such as keto friendly meals, Mediterranean diets or protein packed meal preparations reported by 50% of respondents; and finally (3) mental health, meditation and self-care was tied with content on

---

[4] All the names of the participants have been changed to protect identity of the participants.
[5] The way Dr Al-Badir operates as an Insta-Trainer is based on data collected between 2019 to 2021.

fashion and make-up reported by 35% of respondents. Interestingly, all the types of content reported were those that are inherently rooted in self-surveillant and self-disciplinary practices. These findings indicate that the young women from my study heavily rely on feminine technology to exert ethical practices that share the same ideology that aligns with the popular discourse on women and health, one that frames the female body as a site for constant work, transformation, and improvement (Amigot & Pujal, 2009; Bartky, 2020; Gill, 2007; Heyes, 2007).

The third type of digital manual is the algorithmically curated manuals, and this comes in the form of content displayed on the "Daily Feed" or the "Popular Page," generated by the algorithmic design of the platform. The way in which content is algorithmically curated within these pages are purely based on users' activity, engagement, and overall consumption patterns. Also, these algorithms control what the users see and do not see, which is problematic in the sense that "they reflect and reproduce existing inequities but that are promoted and perceived as more objective and progressive than the discriminatory systems of a previous era" (Noble, 2018; Benjamin, 2019, p. 5). Such oppressive systems directly affect cultural visibility on the online platforms through favouring certain types of features, skin-tones and body types while restricting visibility to others (ibid., 2018; Poell et al., 2021). It is worth mentioning that there have been instances of algorithmic resistance from the participants, such as labelling sponsored advertisements that may be of interest as "Hide Ad" or "Report Ad," in an attempt to mislead the algorithm.

Overall, this constant exposure to such content not only suggests constant transformative actions on the body and mind of young women in Qatar, but also suggests that social norms and traditions may indeed be impacted. This is directly reflected across all the datasets where the majority of respondents have listed Insta-Trainers who are white, thin and conventionally attractive. This also means that the content they consume is not in their native language (Arabic). One interviewee has expressed preference for non-Arab Insta-Trainers and prefers Western Insta-Trainers instead as they appear to be more trustworthy, qualified, and genuine when sharing health-related information.

Moreover, two interviewees, Naimah and Ola, have mentioned that they used to think of Middle Eastern and Qatari cuisine as "evil or bad food" that was unhealthy and fattening due to the fact that healthy recipes on social media were overwhelmingly Italian, French or Mediterranean. However, after critically engaging with, performing and applying the techniques learnt from Insta-Training content on "healthy food recipes." They both reported repurposing the skills they learnt to modify different dishes from the Middle Eastern cuisine in order to fit their health/diet requirements. In this example, we see a productive outcome to the biopedagogical content produced by Insta-Trainers in aiding users with newfound skills that has been used to further embrace their culture and traditions.

Indeed, as we can infer from the above, Insta-Trainer content does in fact enhances users' capacities and allows for the development of new skills. However, it can also feed back into "the crushing effects of normalization" (Rabinow, 1994; Heyes, 2007, p. 7). This is evident among the participants who have reached their health goals, they have reported constantly self-managing and monitoring their bodies, which confirms the ideology that their bodies are a site for constant work. There is a pattern that exists through enforcing the image of feminine body type as a stand in for good health, social acceptance, and self-achievement (Amigot & Pujal, 2009; Bartky, 2020; Sikka, 2023).

These biopedagogical practices that are encouraged through feminine technology, such as labour-intensive exercise, cosmetic surgery, and "weight-loss dieting has long been associated with the tyranny of slenderness and the enforcement … of an ideal body type that carries powerful symbolism of self-discipline, controlled appetites, and the circumscription of appropriate feminine behaviour and appearance" (Heyes, 2007, p. 63). In addition, these practices are a result of intensive digital labour and are cleverly packaged to women as costly yet essential products and services of which one cannot reach certain health goals without.

The Post-pandemic Conscious Qatari Users

The Covid-19 pandemic has created a profound and long-lasting toll on the physical and mental health of entire populations across the globe (Masciantonio et al., 2021; O'Connor et al., 2021; Knox et al., 2022). One of the most significant findings across studies on mental health and the Covid-19 pandemic is that mental health outcomes were worse for women as well as young adults who are typically within the age range of the women in my study (Swami, Todd, et al., 2021; O'Connor et al., 2021). Since the beginning of the outbreak, a large volume of fatphobic social media content emerged with a focus on weight loss and dieting with many of them containing weight-stigmatising attitudes (Lucibello et al., 2021; Swami, Horne, & Furnham, 2021; Swami, Todd, et al., 2021). Such content can easily be categorised as encouraging self-regulating and self-transformative targeted at young women, as confirmed by the participants of my study. In other words, the young Qatari women from my study have confirmed an influx of fatphobic and weight-stigmatising content on their feed and popular page during the first phase of the Covid-19 lockdown in Qatar, which indeed had a negative effect on their mental and physical wellbeing.

One interviewee, Faten, who struggles with "chronic illness, chronic fatigue, and depression," shared that many of the Insta-Trainers she followed during the early days of the pandemic have certainly shared fatphobic and sexist memes on their stories. The same accounts also posted content that indirectly shamed people who were not physically active or productive during the first phase of lockdown in Qatar. The same insight regarding the influx of content on productivity, in health, school, and career were shared by two other interviewees, Marwa and Naimah, who have all reported negative mental outcomes due to such content. These insights have been found in similar studies on social media and Covid-19 across the United Kingdom and Canada, which suggests an international trend (Lucibello et al., 2021; Swami, Horne, & Furnham, 2021). While Instagram did indeed play a significantly positive role in the enhancement of social support during lockdown, the visual-based application also increased instances of social comparison, which reportedly negatively affected physical and mental well-being (Masciantonio et al., 2021; Pittman & Reich, 2016; Wagner et al., 2020).

The content often created and circulated through Insta-Trainers and their followers were found to be rooted in a fear of "inevitable weight gains due to changes in eating, physical activity, and sedentary behaviours resultant from self-isolating" (Pearl, 2020, p. 1; Wagner et al., 2020; Lucibello et al., 2021). This fear was described by the interviewees of my study and has pushed them to purchase expensive workout equipment, perform intensive workouts at home with or without the proper gear, and follow calorie restricting diets which had negative outcomes on their health within the first phase of lockdown dated March 2020 to May 2020.

Tala, who spent the first phase of lockdown alone, mentioned that she relied on the self-curated digital manuals and often accessed them in the middle of work meetings on Zoom to perform the workouts that she had saved, which she described as a bonus in productivity, both career and health-wise. Also, she reported that she had also purchased a pre-curated manual from a popular dietician during that time, which restricted her to 1000 calories per day. She did this in fear of gaining weight due to the lack of the lack of movement during quarantine.

In a conversation with Faten, she shared that in the early days of the quarantine she, "felt guilty, I felt like I should be working-out... it was an insane amount of pressure." Shortly after following a few Insta-Trainers and copying their methods, she sustained an injury and was rushed to the emergency on multiple occasions and had spent a total of 27 days in the hospital within the span of one month. She stated that, "it was mainly because I have such a bad relationship with myself, with food, with exercise, you know? I was following all these accounts and just trying to keep up ... and after that happened it hit me ... I could have easily died."

This is when a shift appeared in Faten's attitude, precisely towards the type of Insta-Trainers she followed. She had realised that none of the Insta-Trainers she had followed were struggling with the same chronic illness that she struggles with, nor did they have any information on it. This led her to conduct further research on her condition, which in turn led her to the "the right" Insta-Trainers for her, which is when she learned how to reach her weight-loss goals while simultaneously maintaining her health and being in control of her illness. Important to note, is that Faten reported that she regularly uses the feature of the self-curated digital manuals, where she stores content on fitness and health.

While this example is a positive reflection of how users benefit from Insta-Trainers through learning new skills and health-related information, we must keep in mind that in order for this interviewee to benefit and reach her goals, she is still conditioned to self-regulate and manage her illness while doing so—adding stress and an additional layer of labour on her shoulders. Interestingly, Faten concluded the interview by stating that, "we were in quarantine, and we were consuming so much online content. … I just knew I had to do better for myself," and that she approaches such packaged content with conscious and caution. Despite her injury and multiple hospital admissions, she still believes that information from Insta-Trainers is generally reliable and trustworthy.

The same contradictory belief was found with other interviewees, including Marwa, Naimah, Tala, Ghaya, Sumaiyah, and Dalal, who either claim that they do not trust Insta-Trainers, yet confirm purchasing, subscribing to, and continue to follow their content, or say that they have had negative health-outcomes from Insta-Trainers but state that they do in fact trust the information that is shared by them. Another common belief found among the participants was that performing high-intensity fitness sessions and following regulated diets were the best way obtain positive emotional, social and health outcomes, even though the data reflects the contrary. These areas are precisely where I locate the user-disjuncture, which is mainly a clear disconnect or contradiction between what the participants have reported feeling and what they practice and/or the actual outcome of those practices.

Conclusion and Beyond

In my overall analysis, I have found that there is a clear optimistic approach by young women when interacting with feminine technology. There also exists a constant need to obtain and sustain both physical and mental wellbeing using FemTech through the aid of the various biopedagogical practices on social media. Within this ideology exists the notion that frames wellbeing as a personal responsibility through self-acquired knowledge from digital platforms. This is extremely problematic in nature, as not all health outcomes are a direct result of personal choice. Also, this ideology is one that links contemporary representations of good health, feminine bodily ideals, and wellness to Western standards of health and beauty (Gordon, 2020; Sikka, 2023; Streeter, 2023).

As a concept for further research, Insta-Training, or instantly training the self via the aid of social media, can be applied to areas other than health and wellness. Such areas may include but are not limited to the personal, career, and academic development of one's knowledge, ideologies, and practices on social media. The concept along with the various aspects opens the door to multiple research opportunities within the field of new media and internet studies. My study, in particular, has found that young women in Qatar are critically active when interacting with the features and functionalities that feminine technology provides.

Indeed, feminine technology has, to some degree, provided women in Qatar with opportunities to express and exercise their agency in multiple ways. Keeping in mind that women interacting with FemTech have also been found to be passive users in previous studies, whereas in reality, female users are undeniably critically active users of such technologies (Camacho-Miñano et al., 2019; Lupton, 2017; Rodney, 2019). Despite this agency, it is crucial to keep in mind that freedom is in fact still constricted through the use of such technologies and devices, whilst (and in the case of women in Qatar) a discreet process of the detachment from certain traditional and cultural societal elements takes place.

References

Abidin, C. (2016). Visibility labour: Engaging with Influencers' fashion brands and #OOTD advertorial campaigns on Instagram. *Media International Australia, 161*(1), 86–100.

Aguiar, R. (2019). *The ultimate glossary of Instagram terms | Kicksta*. [online] Kicksta Blog. Tips & Tricks to Get More Real Followers on Instagram. Retrieved 2023, from https://blog.kicksta.co/the-ultimate-glossary-of-instagram-terms/.

al-Fassi, H. A. (2012). Women in Eastern Arabia: Myth and representation. In *Gulf Women*. Bloomsbury.

Ambwani, S., Shippe, M., Gao, Z., & Austin, S. (2019). Is #cleaneating a healthy or harmful dietary strategy? Perceptions of clean eating and associations with disordered eating among young adults. *Journal of Eating Disorders, 7*(1).

Amigot, P., & Pujal, M. (2009). On power, freedom, and gender. *Theory & Psychology, 19*(5), 646–669. https://doi.org/10.1177/0959354309341925

Bartky, S. (1990). *Femininity and domination: Studies in the phenomenology of oppression*. Routledge.

Bartky, S. L. (2020). Foucault, femininity, and the modernization of patriarchal power. In *Feminist theory reader*. Routledge.

Benjamin, R. (2019). *Race after technology: Abolitionist Tools for the New Jim Code*. Polity.

Camacho-Miñano, M., MacIsaac, S., & Rich, E. (2019). Postfeminist biopedagogies of Instagram: Young women learning about bodies, health and fitness. *Sport, Education and Society, 24*(6), 651–664.

Cirucci, A. M. (2017). A new women's work: Digital interactions, gender, and social network sites. *International Journal of Communication, 12*(2018) https://doi.org/10.1932-8036/20180005

Clarke, V., & Braun, V. (2017). Thematic analysis. *The Journal of Positive Psychology.* [online] *12*(3): 297–298. https://doi.org/10.1080/17439760.2016.1262613

Dennis, E. E., Martin, J. D., & Hassan, F. (2018). Media use in the Middle East: A seven-nation survey. http://www.mideastmedia.org/2018

Dennis, E. E., Martin, J. D., & Wood, R. (2013). Media use in the Middle East: An eight-nation survey. http://menamediasurvey.northwestern.edu/

Dennis, E. E., Martin, J. D., & Wood, R. (2014). Entertainment media use in the Middle East: A six-nation survey. http://www.mideastmedia.org/2014

Diaconoff, S. (2009). *The myth of the silent woman*. University of Toronto Romance.

DiBisceglie, S., & Arigo, D. (2019). Perceptions of #fitspiration activity on Instagram: Patterns of use, response, and preferences among fitstagrammers and followers. *Journal of Health Psychology*, 1359105319871651.

Duffy, B., & Hund, E. (2019). Gendered visibility on social media: Navigating Instagram's authenticity bind. *International Journal of Communication, 13*(19).

Duffy, B. E. (2017). (Not) getting paid to do what you love. https://doi.org/10.12987/yale/9780300218176.001.0001

Foucault, M. (1978). *The history of sexuality*. Pantheon Books.

Gill, R. (2007). Postfeminist media culture: Elements of a sensibility. *European Journal of Cultural Studies, 10*(2), 147–166.

Gordon, A. (2023). *What we don't talk about when we talk about fat*. Beacon Press.

Habibi, M., Laroche, M., & Richard, M. (2014). The roles of brand community and community engagement in building brand trust on social media. *Computers in Human Behavior, 37*, 152–161.

Halse, C., Wright, J., & Harwood, V. (2009). *Bio-citizenship: Virtue discourses and the birth of the bio-citizen. Biopolitics and the "Obesity Epidemic": Governing bodies* (pp. 45–59). Routledge.

Han, B.-C. (2017). *Psychopolitics*. Verso Books.

Heyes, C. J. (2007). *Self transformations: Foucault, ethics, and normalized bodies*. Oxford University Press.

Knox, L., Karantzas, G. C., Romano, R., Feeney, J. A., & Simpson, J. A. (2022). One year on: What we have learned about the psychological effects of COVID-19 social restrictions: A meta-analysis. *Current Opinion in Psychology, 46*.

Liu, L., Lee, M., Liu, R., & Chen, J. (2018). Trust transfer in social media brand communities: The role of consumer engagement. *International Journal of Information Management, 41*, 1–13.

Lucibello, K. M., Vani, M., Koulanova, A., deJonge, M. L., Ashdown-Franks, G., & Sabiston, C. M.. (2021). #quarantine15: A content analysis of Instagram posts during COVID-19. *Body Image, 38*, 148–156, ISSN 1740-1445. https://doi.org/10.1016/j.bodyim.2021.04.002

Lupton, D. (2013). The digitally engaged patient: Self-monitoring and self-care in the digital health era. *Soc Theory Health, 11*, 256–270. https://doi.org/10.1057/sth.2013.10

Lupton, D. (2017). Digital media and body weight, shape, and size: An introduction and review. *Fat Studies, 6*(2), 119–134.

Masciantonio, A., Bourguignon, D., Bouchat, P., Balty, M., & Rime´, B. (2021). Don't put all social network sites in one basket: Facebook, Instagram, Twitter, TikTok, and their relations with well-being during the COVID-19 pandemic. *PLoS ONE, 16*(3), e0248384. https://doi.org/10.1371/journal.pone.0248384

Nasser, H. H. S. M. B. (2012). Forward. In *Gulf women*. Bloomsbury.

Noble, S. U. (2018). *Algorithms of oppression: How search engines reinforce racism*. New York University Press.

O'Connor, R. C., Wetherall, K., Cleare, S., McClelland, H., Melson, A. J., Niedzwiedz, C. L., O'Carroll, R. E., O'Connor, D. B., Platt, S., Scowcroft, E., Watson, B., Zortea, T., Ferguson, E., & Robb, K. A. (2021). Mental health and well-being during the COVID-19 pandemic: Longitudinal analyses of adults in the UK COVID-19 Mental Health & Wellbeing study. *The British Journal of Psychiatry*. Cambridge University Press, *218*(6), 326–333. https://doi.org/10.1192/bjp.2020.212

Pearl, R. L. (2020). Weight Stigma and the "Quarantine-15". *Obesity (Silver Spring, Md.), 28*(7), 1180–1181. https://doi.org/10.1002/oby.22850

Pilgrim, K., & Bohnet-Joschko, S. (2019). Selling health and happiness how influencers communicate on Instagram about dieting and exercise: Mixed methods research. *BMC Public Health, 19*(1).

Pittman, M., & Reich, B. (2016). Social media and loneliness: Why an Instagram picture may be worth more than a thousand Twitter words. *Computers in Human Behavior, 62*, 155–167.

Poell, T., Nieborg, D. B., & Duffy, B. E. (2021). *Platforms and cultural production*. Polity Press.

Rabinow, P. (1994). *The Foucault reader: An introduction to Foucault's thought*. Penguin.

Reinikainen, H., Munnukka, J., Maity, D., & Luoma-aho, V. (2020). 'You really are a great big sister' – Parasocial relationships, credibility, and the moderating role of audience comments in influencer marketing. *Journal of Marketing Management, 36*, 1–20.

Rodney, A. (2019). The rise of the blogspert: Biopedagogy, self-knowledge, and lay expertise on women's healthy living blogs. *Social Theory & Health*.

Schoenbach et al. (2017). NU-Q study explores health information and monitoring among youth. *Northwestern University Qatar*. Available at: https://www.qatar.northwestern.edu/news/articles/2017/12-Health-Comms.html.

Sikka, T. (2023). *Health apps, genetic diets and superfoods*. Bloomsbury Publishing.

Sokolova, K., & Kefi, H. (2020). Instagram and YouTube bloggers promote it, why should I buy? How credibility and parasocial interaction influence purchase intentions. *Journal of Retailing and Consumer Services, 53*, 101742.

Sonbol, A. (2012). *Gulf women*. Bloomsbury.

Statista. (2022). *TikTok penetration in selected countries and territories 2022*. [online]. https://www.statista.com/statistics/1299829/tiktok-penetration-worldwide-by-country/

Streeter, R. (2023). "Bargaining with the status quo": Reinforcing and expanding femininities in the #bodypositive movement. *Fat Studies, 12*(1), 120–134. https://doi.org/10.1080/21604851.2021.2006958

Swami, V., Horne, G., & Furnham, A. (2021). COVID-19-related stress and anxiety are associated with negative body image in adults from the United Kingdom, Personality and Individual Differences, *170*, 110426. ISSN 0191-8869. https://doi.org/10.1016/j.paid.2020.110426

Swami, V., Todd, J., Robinson, C., & Furnham, A. (2021). Self-compassion mediates the relationship between COVID-19-related stress and body image disturbance: Evidence from the United Kingdom under lockdown, Personality and Individual Differences, *183*, 111130. ISSN 0191-8869. https://doi.org/10.1016/j.paid.2021.111130

Talbot, C. V., Gavin, J., van Steen, T., et al. (2017). A content analysis of thinspiration, fitspiration, and bonespiration imagery on social media. *Journal of Eating Disorders, 5*, 40. https://doi.org/10.1186/s40337-017-0170-2

Wagner, D. N., Marcon, A. R., & Caulfield, T. (2020). "Immune Boosting" in the time of COVID: Selling immunity on Instagram. *Allergy Asthma Clin Immunol, 16*, 76. https://doi.org/10.1186/s13223-020-00474-6

Wright, J. (2009). Biopower, biopedagogies and the obesity epidemic. In J. Wright & V. Harwood (Eds.), *Biopolitics and the 'obesity epidemic': Governing bodies* (pp. 1–14). Routledge.

8

Hoop Dreams or Hoop Nightmares: Athletics, Fitness Tracking, and the Surveillance of the Black Body

Rachel D. Roberson

If your heart and your honest body can be controlled by the state, or controlled by community taboo, are you not then, and in that case, no more than a slave ruled by outside force.—June Jordan

Introduction

The state of intercollegiate athletics is one of the most polarizing topics in public higher education today. However, much of this dialogue spends little time addressing the socio-historical trajectory of the relationship between athletes and the institution of sport. This chapter provides a conceptual rendering of the barriers to agency and liberatory practices for Black female basketball players, by unpacking the use of wearable surveillance as a tool for reinforcing power stratification within intercollegiate athletics. Additionally, this chapter is strategically positioned to both

R. D. Roberson (✉)
University of California, Berkeley, CA, USA
e-mail: rachel_roberson@berkeley.edu

© The Author(s), under exclusive license to Springer Nature Singapore Pte Ltd. 2023 **167**
L. Balfour (ed.), *FemTech*, https://doi.org/10.1007/978-981-99-5605-0_8

deepen conceptual scholarship on FemTech Studies as well as add nuance to the question posed by Sara Diaz: "What role can technoscience play in the movements to achieve gender justice" (Diaz, 2020). Ultimately, this work adds to our understanding of the valuing and devaluing of Black female bodies within society at large, emphasizing our historical dehumanization through labor exploitation and domestication.

Defining Surveillance

Coaches, academic personnel, university leaders, and trainers maintain consistent, holistic monitoring of student-athletes that is tantamount to surveillance. Methods of surveillance range from the use of two-way mirrors within study hall rooms to optimize administrative monitoring to requiring teammates to surveille each other and deliver comprehensive dossiers on player etiquette and adherence to dress codes (Foster, 2003; Newhall & Buzuvis, 2008); however, the use of biometric technologies is on the rise. Implicit in most understandings of surveillance is the idea that certain people are being watched, often unknowingly, while participating in everyday activities. "Surveillance" is generally used to identify a systemic and focused manner of observing, or in the words of David Lyon, "any collection and processing of personal data, whether identifiable or not, for the purposes of influencing or managing those whose data have been garnered" (Lyon, 2007). Mann (2013) advanced modern surveillance studies by charting the veillance plane, which helps us visualize the relationship between surveillance tools and power. Specifically, the veillance plane illustrates eight variations of (sur)veillance and situates their net impact on the stratification of power (Fig. 8.1).

Figure 8.1 illustrates the eight variations of (sur)veillance, and while all eight forms of veillance are important and warrant further study the distinction necessary for understanding my framework are: veillance, surveillance, and sousveillance. Veillance stems from the French: to watch and serves as a neutral form of watching without gaining or losing power. Surveillance occurs when organizations observe power—the act of watching is done by an entity in a position of power. Sousveillance serves as an inversion of power, where the watched become aware of their surveillance

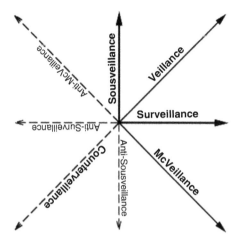

Fig. 8.1 The veillance plane depicts the relationship between the act of watching and power stratification

and utilize their understanding of systems of power to neutralize and disrupt (Mann, 2013). Browne (2015) builds upon Mann's theory by offering dark sousveillance, which is an explicitly racialized means of resisting surveillance within the imaginary. Browne posits, "dark sousveillance charts possibilities and coordinates modes of responding to, challenging, and confronting a surveillance that is almost all-encompassing (Browne, 2015). In the analysis section, I will offer a theorization of the ways in which dark sousveillance can be harnessed by Black student-athletes as a means of reclaiming their agency and bodily autonomy within a hyper-surveilled system operationalized through gendered tools of fitness tracking and other digital health technologies.

Review of Literature

Race and Gendered Frames of Labor Capital

This chapter is anchored by a comprehensive historiography of Black women's labor exploitation in the United States, supplemented by a range of theoretical threads. This historical understanding is imperative to my analysis of modern biometric technologies and frames the volume's ultimate question: *Who is FemTech for?* Spillers (1987) is foundational to this historiography, as she was one of the first scholars to frame the labor of Black women on slavery plantations, explicitly centering the role Black women's labor played within the plantation economy. Similarly, hooks (1981) maintained that in anticipation of the nuanced, i.e., physical, emotional, and sexual assault Black women were forced to endure within the plantation economy, their treatment on the Middle Passage was intended to prepare them via curated violence. Haley (2016) extended this history post emancipation, where carcerality emerged as a key to the relationship between Black women's labor capital and United States western expansion. Murray's foundational work, *Jane Crow,* positions the ways in which laws, policies, and practices were leveraged to maintain cheap access to Black women's labor primarily within but not limited to the Jim Crow South (Murray & Eastwood, 1965).

Despite the gruesome history of sexual abuse and assault from slavery to the present, and the limitation of Black women's labor market options, there are equally rich and important examples of resistance, refusal, and radical reimagining. By revisiting hooks through "the oppositional gaze," we can recognize that for as long as Black women have had their labor exploited within the United States, there have been robust acts of refusal and defiance. hooks described the various methods Black women used to both subtly and overtly resisted institutions and systems of exploitative labor (hooks, 2010). Finally, Patton-Davis applied a Black feminist lens to labor within public higher education (Cobham & Patton-Davis, 2015; Patton & Haynes, 2018; Patton, 2009; Davis, 2021). Her work explored the role of Black women's labor expectations within higher education—maintaining that this labor is multifaceted, quantifying emotional labor and naming the impact "battle labor" and institutional advocacy (Cobham & Patton-Davis, 2015). This scholarship is vital for offering a more comprehensive framework for cultural taxation and labor. For the purpose of this chapter, a Black feminist frame for labor capitalism not only shapes the ways in which Black women's basketball players are expected to provide multifaceted labor to the institution but also serve as compulsory test subjects for emerging biometric technologies.

Intersectionality

One of the ways in which the relationship between gendered tracking technologies and Black female labor can be theorized is through the concept of intersectionality. Intersectionality stems from the school of thought that various forms of oppression are connected, mutually constitutive, and that laws and institutions are ill equipped to acknowledge and remedy specific raced and gendered discrimination. This notion is most attributed to Black feminisms—where Patricia Hill Collins (2000) described the matrix of domination as "structural, disciplinary, hegemonic, and interpersonal domains of power reappear across quite different forms of oppression" (p. 306). To be clear, intersectionality is not a process of framing identities as playing cards where privilege in one area gets cancelled out by subjugation in another. At its core, intersectionality attempts to conceptualize the lived experiences of being marginalized within an already marginalized group, as well as that marginalization and privilege can exist within the same person. Intersectional feminism thus helps conceptualize how race, class, sexuality, and gender intersect in the proliferation of wearable surveillance and impact the lived experiences of women's basketball players. Crenshaw argues that without intersectionality, Black women are erased theoretically. The lack of intersectional analysis in sport has already perpetuated this erasure-based framing (Crenshaw, 1989).

Surveillance scholars have moved to racialize the field of surveillance studies (Fiske, 1998; Wiegman, 1995; Wood, 2016), calling attention to the need for a framework that evaluates the specific ways in which surveillance is used as a tool to control and regulate Black bodies. However, Simone Browne is among the only scholars (Dubrofsky & Amielle Magnet, 2015; Smith, 2015; Rifkin, 2011; Morgensen, 2011) to create a specific framework for an intersectional evaluation of surveillance; that is, the intersection of surveillance and dark sousveillance. To properly consider these interlocking systems of oppression coming to roost within the institution of sport, I apply intersectional surveillance to an analysis of FemTech tools that are becoming increasingly adopted into intercollegiate athletics. Browne builds upon Patricia Hill Collins's intersecting paradigms work to introduce intersecting surveillance, which Collins (2004a) defined as "the interdependent and interlocking ways that practices, performances, and policies regarding surveillance operate" (p. 9).

Browne employs intersectional surveillance to understand the lived experiences of Black people under surveillance throughout history, building upon the work of Collins (1998) and hooks (1989), specifically within the Jim Crow South. During the time of Jim Crow in the South, surveillance was used to ensure "Blacks would stay in their designated, subordinate places in white-controlled public and private spheres" (p. 20). Collins (1998) also notes that this time-period served as a "testing ground for surveillance as a form of control" within the labor-oriented market of domestic workers (p. 21). Browne too sees the connection between refining surveillance practices and the domestic worker structure of power: "Yet within these labor condition of hypervisibility, black domestic workers needed to assume a certain invisibility where, as bell hooks observes, 'reduced to the machinery of bodily physical labor, black people learned to appear before whites as though were zombies, cultivating the habit of casting the gaze downward so as not to appear uppity" (hooks, 1989; emphasis Browne, 2012). Even though the consequences were severe, hooks catalogs accounts of Black people defiantly staking claim in their humanity by daring to set an "oppositional gaze" toward Whites (hooks, 2010). In other words, "Black looks" or watching Whites during Jim Crow frames the eyes as the "technology of whiteness" (Fiske, 1998). Similarly, Mann refers to the eyes as one's body-borne camera, which can again be leveraged as tools of resistance or control.

This historical example presents one form of counter surveillance; under Mann's assessment, we could also code this resistance as a form of sousveillance because the action is meant to challenge and shift power stratification. The act of resistance directed toward existing power structures intended to signal "our movement from object to subject—the liberated voice" (hooks, 1989; emphasis Browne, 2012). This tool of veillance is fashioned as a "gesture of defiance that heals, that makes new life and new growth possible" (hooks, 1989; emphasis Browne, 2012). During this historical moment, Black people's use of sousveillance became a method for demanding a recognition of humanity. I raise this history not only to recognize that both surveillance and the resistance to it have a gendered and racialized legacy but also to draw attention to the ways in which technologies of power have always been the mechanism of such oppression. Now repacked in literal digital form, these new technologies of power remind us that acts of resistance that utilize sousveillance are just as necessary within the institution of sport today, as they were in the Jim Crow South.

Historical Studies of Surveillance

Much like the historiography of Black women's labor, a brief review of the history of surveillance studies demonstrates the necessary nuance for contemporary discussions of FemTech practices in sport. Bentham (1791) developed the concept of the Panopticon as a blueprint for surveillance meant to enable the few to consistently watch and therefore control the many. The most well-known proposed application for this design is within prisons. Bentham's design places a tower or opticon in the center of the facility with cells or rooms opening in-ward, toward the opticon, surround the tower. Some designs also include exterior mirrors so those incarcerated could not know for certain when they were being watched. The goal behind this design was for inmates to assume they were always being surveilled and in turn modify behavior accordingly in fear of retribution. In essence, Bentham's design enables the powerful few to condition the behavior of the masses through surveillance and fear of punishment. The behavior modification promised by this design was highly appealing to other areas of social service most notably schools (Bushnell, 2003; Tait, 2000; Webb et al., 2009). Bentham's paternalistic motivations rely heavily on the belief that it is the role of the powerful to save the masses from themselves.

Foucault is the foundational scholar to theorize the underlying power structures at play in the panoptic blueprint. Foucault (1979) named the inherent problem in building physical structures for the sole purpose of surveillance and control: "That of an architecture that is no longer built simply to be seen ... or to observe the external space, ... but to permit an internal, articulated and detailed control—to render visible those who are inside it; in more general terms, an architecture that would operate to transform individuals: to act on those it shelters, to provide a hold on their conduct, to carry the effects of power right to them, to make it possible to know them, to alter them" (p. 125). This sentiment sparks the Foucauldian tradition named panopticism. Panopticism can be defined as "an ensemble of mechanisms brought into play in all the clusters of procedures used by power," including the permanent surveillance of a group of individuals through a generalized set of procedures (Foucault & Gordon, 1980, p. 200). Mathieson countered panopticism's framing of the few surveilling the many by introducing the synopticon, where the many watch the few. Mathiesen (1997) applied this shift in framing to the viewing society consuming mass media. In the case of the institution of sport, both the framing of the panopticon and synopticon are necessary, and I will argue, occur simultaneously (Mathiesen, 1997). Boyne built upon Mathieson's work to assert that society has entered a state of post-panopticism, where we experience a reversal of panoptical polarity. Boyne asserted, like I do, that this shift works in conjunction with the panopticon. Although the surveilled are actively being the watcher, they are also conditioned to watch themselves (Boyne, 2000). This understanding of the various forms of surveillance helps better situate the role that institutions of power play in surveillance and its control over the body, mind, and spirit of the Black student athlete.

Panoptic discipline is thus reanimated through contemporary issues such as the impacts of surveillance for the Black student-athlete, particularly as those forms of surveillance are increasingly digitized. Foucault's notions of discipline and docility are indeed well reflected in discourses surrounding self-tracking technologies in both wearable and app form. These contemporary discussions, however, must also consider the ways in which Black bodies continue to be overly scrutinized are surveilled within this regime. Browne (2015), for instance, calls forth Sylvia Wynter's sociogeny or the sociogenic principle, paraphrased as "the organizational framework of our present human, and that fixes and frames blackness as an object of surveillance" (p. 29). This concept serves as a grounding principle in why Black bodies are surveilled and speaks to the lack of boundaries for the methods used to surveille Black bodies. In other words, if an object is being surveilled, there is no need for consent or a moral consideration of the potential dehumanization consequences. I argue that the sociogenic principle is being readily applied to the surveillance of Black student-athletes, wherein their ability to consent to the use of biometric technologies like microchipped sports bras is revoked and they maintain little to no tangible ownership over their bodies or data (Wynter, 2001; emphasis Browne, 2015). Fiske (1998) intentionally built upon Foucault's surveillance critiques, naming that many Foucauldian scholars apply a racialized lens to Foucault's panopticon critique, yet further holds that this was not Foucault's intent: "has been racialized in a manner that they did not foresee, today's seeing eye is white" (Fiske, 1998, p. 85). Fisk called this dichotomy racializing surveillance and claimed that because society is built upon White capital, actions taken by Black people are surveilled, then coded as criminal. This racialized coding leads directly to skewed punishment and the widening of the equity gap.

Intersectional Surveillance in Fitness Tracking Apps and Devices

I utilize Collins' intersectional framing to situate the exploitative use of biometric technologies to surveille Black female athletes. Collins (2002) used athletics to showcase the potential for race, class, gender, and sexuality uplift. Collins's use of the shifting perception of femininity (signals a shift toward the masculine) paved the way for her ultimate evaluation of Black female athletes and sexual orientation. Collins writes: "In essence, the same qualities that are uncritically celebrated for Black male athletes can become stumbling blocks for their Black female counterparts. Corporate profits depend on representations and images, and those of Black female athletes must be carefully managed in order to win endorsements and guarantee profitability" (Collins, 2002, pp. 135–136). Self-tracking technologies have a critical role to play in ensuring that this careful curation of marketable Black athletic identity is achieved. Moreover, Collins points to profitability through marketing strategies employed by the WNBA, which, to Collins, is meant to directly silence the supposed threat of lesbian domination. These strategies include hyper-sexualization of individual, hand-selected players, and showcasing motherhood and family.

Black female athletes are under constant scrutiny to perform and uphold White hegemonic expectations of femininity. Such expectations become compounded when Black athletes are compelled to use tracking technologies in which Whiteness and heterosexuality are usually the norm or baseline upon which performance is measured. That financial security and, conversely, the economic consequences of resistance are reasons through which individuals acquiesce to these forms of tracking begs the question of how Black female athletes can effectively push back on existing power structures within a system of surveillance. As such, I employ intersectional surveillance as a means of discerning how said structures and systems of control are present within the Black student-athlete's experience in order to deepen current understandings of the lived experiences of Black basketball players. It is my hope that this work will be used to identify opportunities for agency and bodily autonomy within a surveilled system perpetuated by tracking technologies, by challenging current student-athletes to defiantly *look back.*

Surveillance in Sport—Current Conversations

Sites of Surveillance wWithin Women's Basketball

In order to appropriately frame the use of biometric tools of surveillance within women's basketball, we center Cahn's seminal history of the institutionalization of women's basketball. Cahn (1994) situates women's basketball's institutionalization as a tool for regulation by first tracing the sport's history. Cahn's historical analysis helps to explain why women's basketball became a site for regulation. Coupling Cahn's foundation with feminist surveillance studies (Bell, 1992; Koskela, 2012; Senft, 2008), further shows why women's basketball became and continues to be a site for surveillance. Many feminist and colonial surveillance scholars communicate the expressed threat the female body poses to White heteropatriarchal frames of masculinity. These scholars take up the frame of power through gender normative behavior. At the crux of surveillance sits the positioning and reinforcement of power.

Basketball players at highly selective athletic programs also experience surveillance while navigating the larger campus community. In this context, hypervisibility occurs when student-athletes are simultaneously highlighted and isolated on campus, while also having their experiences erased and minimized. Browne (2012) unpacks the dynamics of hypervisibility for Black domestic workers, which is eerily similar to the experiences of student-athletes. She writes: "Yet within these labor conditions of hypervisibility, black domestic workers needed to assume a certain invisibility where, as bell hooks observes, 'reduced to the machinery of bodily physical labor, black people learned to appear before whites as though they were zombies, cultivating the habit of casting the gaze downward so as not to appear uppity." For basketball players, this often results in ostracization from the larger campus community. With experiences such as these on campus it not only begs the questions as to how student-athletes are meant to succeed within the classroom but also challenges the notion that they are intended to be members of the community at all.

Other scholars have deemed these occurrences as a byproduct of the hyper-athletic identity, specifically for Black students. In multiple studies, Black student-athletes are found to have a stronger and more salient athletic identity than their non-Black teammates. Bimper also contests that Black student-athletes often felt as though other members of the campus community only see them as athletes, resulting in an increased focus on sport.

Ethics of Biometric Technologies

In 2016, the Duke University men's basketball team began using sleep sensors for student-athletes. These sensors are placed under the beds of each player and are intended to measure their REM sleep nightly. The data are automatically sent to the coaching staff each morning. In addition to sleep sensors, many basketball teams have begun using microchipped workout layers that are using during every practice and workout gear: for men's basketball, the biometric technology is built into the compression layer, and for women's basketball and volleyball, the biometric technology is built into the sports bra. These devices collect an array of bodily data from the student-athlete, from the number of times they move their feet in a practice to their resting heart rate. Because student-athletes are required to waive their FERPA rights, and to a lesser extent their HIPPA rights, as a contingent to participating in intercollegiate athletics, the unfiltered Big Data is freely shared among the coaching staff, medical trainers, and the brand proctors of the wearable technology; that typically includes Nike, Under Amour, and Adidas. These surveillance tools are intended to intrude upon and actively shape the student-athlete's intimate life. The implicit *cost* of playing intercollegiate athletics—even with a *payment* of scholarships and fee remissions— requires the giving up of intimate data with no ownership and control over how it is used. The implication of this *cost* in a "post-Roe United States" is especially worrisome for women's athletics. For instance, there have been several instances where commercial wearable tech, using the same technoscience as the microchipped sport bra, served as early detections of pregnancy through the identification of irregularities in a woman's heartrate. Again, the women whose bodily data is freely shared with members of their coaching staff, medical personnel, the brad proctoring the tech, and now accessible by state agencies, do not have ready access to the happenings of their own bodies. In today's United States political landscape, it is not hyperbole to name that it is entirely likely and wholly worrisome that a woman who has become pregnant could have less information about their body than the state, let alone maintain autonomy over critical medical options for terminating an unwanted and/or unsafe pregnancy—an offense that is now an arrestable offense.

As the story above shows, one of the most salient applications of surveillance tools within the institution of sport is the use of biometrics and big data (Browne, 2012; Gandy, 2012; Hutchins, 2016; McKittrick, 2021). Hutchins (2016) cautioned against the uncritical embrace of Big Data in sport, contending, "a collective fascination with the digital sublime obscures the complex interaction between corporate power, digital data markets, history and culture, and contributes to inequalities that demand ongoing attention and critique" (Hutchins, 2016). While these biometric technologies are framed as performance enhancing tools, the consent of the student-athlete is not required for mandating and regulating use. In contrast, many professional athletes are looking toward biometric technologies to measure their athletic growth; however, unlike intercollegiate athletes, they possess bodily autonomy by maintaining the power to change devices or stop using the tools entirely if they so choose. Most importantly, they have primary ownership of the bodily data collected. This ownership was won during the bargaining negotiations in the summer of 2017. Specifically, in the summer of 2017, for the first time, the NBA Players' Association recently won the ability to bar the team's ownership from using biometric data in player contract negotiations, essentially leaving the ownership of the data to the player's discretion. Importantly, student-athletes, legally registered as amateurs, are unable to employ the same labor-oriented channels to voice and exercise their bodily autonomy with biometric and other technologies. As such, institutional regulation of athlete's bodies through biometric technology serves as a tool for reinforcing power stratification and access to uncompensated labor.

In many academic support spaces for student-athletes, biometric surveillance tools are used as means of control, monitor, and condition student behavior (Bimper & Harrison, 2011; Sailes, 1998; Van Rheenen, 2012). In practice, the use of technological tools to monitor and report on student-athlete off court behavior has reached the national stage. In 2020, the National Association of Academic Advisors for Athletics convened to introduce the uses of class-checking products: "ClassCheck" and "Spotter," which are intended to relay electronic messages directly to academic advisers and coaches when student-athletes are absent from class. These products are designed to utilize microchipped backpacks as well as smartphone GPS technology to track the student-athlete's physical location in relation to their class and workout schedules. These biometric technologies are marketed toward the multitude of athletic programs that already implement class monitoring of student-athletes— mostly through the physical surveilling of coaches and team managers. "ClassCheck" claims their product could save individual teams tens of thousands of dollars a year in personnel costs alone, seeing as many programs currently charge an assistant coach with physically checking that student-athletes are attending courses (Wolverton, 2015).

There are several intersections between physical punishment for the purpose of academically disciplining students. The tutoring space is most salient. Certain students, the highest percentage of whom are Black, are mandated to attend tutoring sessions. Tutors, who monitor these sessions, must draft reports following each session, thus cataloging the student's academic progress, grades, and other pertinent information as necessary. These reports are directly connected to the payment system for the tutor, meaning if they elect not to participate in this form of surveillance, they will not receive payment for their work. These reports are shared with learning specialists, academic advisors and coordinators, and the coach staff. Tutors are not required to share the report's contents with students. The "run list" is determined in part from this information. This physical punishment is intended to discipline the minds of the student-athletes, with the goal of changing the student-athlete's behavior. This surveillance tool can be traced directly back to Bentham's motivating philosophy for the panopticon.

Students who fail to comply with the regulation and control established by coaches and the support staff face a range of consequences. The run-list is the catalog of student-athletes who have broken the rules (whether it be a code of conduct violation or simply being unfocused during a workout). Student-athletes on the run-list must complete a set of physical exercises, intended to produce both physical and mental discipline. Examples of run-list exercises include running up every stair of the football stadium or sprinting the lines of an empty parking lot. Elevated forms of punishment carry more implicit, long-term consequences. If a player frequently resists the regulation of coaches and support staff, they risk being branded uncoachable. This scarlet letter for athletes can jeopardize the student-athlete's role on the team, potentially resulting in the loss of their athletic scholarship. For those student-athletes with the potential to play professionally, this drastic form of punishment can impact their career options and reputation.

Resistance

While the central purpose of this chapter is to document the exploitative intent and consequences of the use of biometric technologies within intercollegiate athletics, it is equally necessary to explore the ways in which biometric technologies can also serve as a tool of resistance in the right hands. Dark sousveillance could bridge the gap between sousveillance and the Black imaginary toward liberation for the Black female intercollegiate basketball player. Sousveillance utilizes the act of watching but as a tool for upending and dismantling the stratification of power, rather than reinforcing it. An example of this form of resistance is using cell phone cameras to capture police misconduct, brutality, and murder. To be clear, this form of resistance goes beyond circumventing the intended surveillance tool, such as refusing to wear a biometric tracker, i.e., anti-surveillance. At its core sousveillance allows for the intended subject of surveillance to defiantly cast their gaze or body-borne cameras (Mann, 2013) toward those in power and the root of their subjugation, which is what hooks (2010) deemed as an act of defiantly *looking back*. This reclamation of biometric technologies is made particularly difficult within intercollegiate athletics due to the limitations of amateurism. That being said, the invasive nature of the technologies offers a unique argument for increased bodily autonomy and agency for the student-athlete. In other words, leveraging technological tools like microchipped sports bras and sleep sensors to advocate for the creation of a collective bargaining process for student-athletes to directly negotiate the regulation of said tools and the ownership of the data they collect.

The intervention discussed above provided a tangible action item for actors within intercollegiate athletics and higher education, and there remains an abolitionist path forward for student-athletes. Dark sousveillance takes us into a space of the unknown: true Black liberation. Dark sousveillance boldly asks us to dream of a truly free Black female body, an existence we can now only dream of. Future work aims to look toward dark sousveillance as a finish line of sorts, allowing Black women to dream freely of basketball, the game they love, without the institution of sport and the state, both of which are structures that are built and persist because of the exploitation of their labor. While Sexton (2016) proclaims true Black liberation is an ideal so far removed from our current reality, we cannot rationally fathom its reimagining, dark sousveillance plants the liberatory seeds to aid our dreaming of radical transformation and the dismantling institutional power stratifications.

References

Bell, D. A. (1992). *Faces at the bottom of the well*. Basic Books.

Bentham, J. (1791). *Panopticon*. Printed for T. Payne.

Bimper, A. Y., & Harrison, L. (2011). Meet me at the crossroads: African American athletic and racial identity. *Quest, 63*(3), 275–288.

Boyne, R. (2000). Post-Panopticism. *Economy and Society, 29*(2), 285–307.

Browne, S. (2012). *Routledge handbook of surveillance studies* (pp. 72–81). NY. Routledge. Race and surveillance.

Browne, S. (2015). *Dark matters: On the surveillance of blackness*. Duke University Press.

Bushnell, M. (2003). Teachers in the schoolhouse panopticon: Complicity and resistance. *Education and Urban Society., 35*(3), 251–272.

Cahn, S. K. (1994). Sports talk: Oral history and its uses, problems, and possibilities for sport history. *The Journal of American History, 81*(2), 594–609.

Collins, P. H. (1998). It's all in the family: Intersections of gender, race, and nation. *Hypatia, 13*(3), 62–82.

Collins, P. H. (2000). Gender, black feminism, and black political economy. *The Annals of the American Academy of Political and Social Science, 568*(1), 41–53.

Collins, P. H. (2002). *Black feminist thought: Knowledge, consciousness and the politics of empowerment*. Routledge.

Collins, P. H. (2004a). *Black sexual politics: African Americans, gender, and the new racism*. Routledge.

Collins, P. H. (2004b). Black feminist thought in the matrix of domination. In C. Lemert (Ed.), *Social theory: The multicultural and classic readings* (pp. 535–546). Westview.

Crenshaw, K. (1989). Demarginalizing the intersection of race and sex: A black feminist critique of antidiscrimination doctrine, feminist theory and antiracist politics. *The University of Chicago Legal Forum, 1*, 139–167.

Davis, L. P. (2021). *Keynote-Dr*. Lori Patton Davis.

Diaz, S. (2020). Science, technology, and gender. In N. A. Naples (Ed.), *Companion to Women's and gender studies* (pp. 111–137). John Wiley & Sons.

Dubrofsky, R. E., & Amielle Magnet, S. (Eds.). (2015). *Feminist Surveillance Studies*. Duke University Press.

Fiske, J. (1998). Surveilling the City: Whiteness, the black man and democratic totalitarianism. *Theory, Culture and Society, 15*(2), 67–88.

Foster, K. (2003). Panopticonics: The control and surveillance of black female athletes in a collegiate athletic program. *Anthropology & Education Quarterly, 34*(3), 300–323. American Anthropological Association.

Foucault, M. (1979). *Discipline and punish: The birth of the prison*. Vintage.

Foucault, M., & Gordon, C. (1980). *Power/knowledge: Selected interviews and other writings, 1972–1977*. Pantheon Books.

Gandy, O. H., Jr. (2012). Statistical surveillance. *Routledge handbook of surveillance studies, 125.*

Haley, S. (2016). *No mercy here: Gender, punishment, and the making of Jim crow modernity.* UNC Press Books.

hooks, b. (1981). Ain't I a woman: Black women and feminism.

hooks, b. (1989). *Talking Back: Thinking feminist, thinking black.* South End Press.

hooks, b. (2010). *Teaching Critical Thinking: Practical Wisdom.* Routledge.

Hutchins, B. (2016). Tales of the digital sublime: Tracing the relationship between big data and professional sport. *Convergence: The International Journal of Research into New Media Technologies, 22*(5), 494–509.

Koskela, H. (2012). You shouldn't wear that body. The problematic of surveillance and gender. In *Routledge Handbook of surveillance studies*, edited by Kirstie B., Kevin H., and David L. (pp. 49–56).

Lyon, D. (2007). *Surveillance Studies: An Overview.* Polity Press.

Mann, S. (2013, June 27–29). Veillance and reciprocal transparency: Surveillance versus sousveillance, AR glass, lifelogging and wearable computing. In *IEEE International Symposium on Technology and Society (ISTAS)* (pp. 1–12).

Mathiesen, T. (1997). The viewer society: Michel Foucault's panopticon revisited. *Theoretical Criminology, 1*(2), 215–234.

McKittrick, K. (2021). *Dear science and other stories.* Duke University Press.

McNeely Cobham, B. A., & Patton, L. D. (2015). Self-will, power, and determination: A qualitative study of black women faculty and the role of self-efficacy. *NASPA Journal About Women in Higher Education, 8*(1), 29–46.

Morgensen, S. L. (2011). *Spaces between us: Queer settler colonialism and indigenous decolonization.* University of Minnesota Press.

Murray, P., & Eastwood, M. O. (1965). Jane crow and the law: Sex discrimination and title VII. *Geo. Wash. L. Rev., 34*, 232.

Newhall, K. E., & Buzuvis, E. E. (2008). (e)racing Jennifer Harris: Sexuality and race, law and discourse in Harris v. *Portland. Journal of Sport & Social Issues, 32*(4), 345–368.

Patton, L. D. (2009). My sister's keeper: A qualitative examination of significant mentoring relationships among African American women in graduate and professional schools. *Journal of Higher Education, 80*(5), 510–537.

Patton, L. D., & Haynes, C. (2018). Hidden in plain sight: The black women's blueprint for institutional transformation in higher education. *Teacher's College Record, 120*(14), 1–18.

Rifkin, J. (2011). *The third industrial revolution: How lateral power is transforming energy, the economy, and the world*. Macmillan.

Sailes, G. A. (1998). The African-American athlete: Social myths and stereotypes. In G. A. Sailes (Ed.), *African-Americans in sport: Contemporary themes* (pp. 183–198). Transaction.

Senft, T. M. (2008). *Camgirls: Celebrity and community in the age of social networks* (Vol. 4). Peter Lang.

Sexton, J. (2016). The social life of social death: On afro-pessimism and black optimism. In *Time, temporality and violence in international relations* (pp. 85–99). Routledge.

Smith, A. (2015). Not-seeing: State surveillance, settler colonialism, and gender violence. *Feminist Surveillance Studies*, 21–38.

Spillers, H. J. (1987). Mama's baby, papa's maybe: An American grammar book. *Diacritics, 17*(2), 65–81.

Tait, G. (2000). *From the panopticon to the playground: Disciplinary practices* (pp. 7–18). Social and cultural perspectives.

Van Rheenen, D. (2012). Exploitation in college sports: Race, revenue and educational reward. *International Review for the Sociology of Sport, 48*(5), 550–571.

Webb, T., Briscoe, F., & Mussman, M. (2009). Preparing teachers to resist the neoliberal panopticon. *Educational Foundation, 23*(3-4), 3–18.

Wiegman, R. (1995). *American anatomies*. Duke University Press.

Wolverton, B. (2015, June 17). Electronic checking on athletes in class sparks debate about their privacy. *The Chronicle of Higher Education*.

Wood, D. M. (2016). *Beyond the panopticon? Foucault and surveillance studies* (pp. 257–276). Routledge.

Wynter, S. (2001). Towards the sociogenic principle: Fanon, the puzzle of conscious experience of 'identity' and what It's like to be 'black. In A. Gomez-Moriana & M. Duran-Cogan (Eds.), *National Identities and sociopolitical changes in Latin America* (pp. 30–66). Routledge.

9

FemTech and Taboo Topics: Raaji as a Tool for Educating Women in Pakistan

Khawar Latif Khan and Farah Azhar

Introduction

Periods and menstruation fall on the list of words that are silenced in Pakistani households. "Are you feeling down?" One sister asks the other. A nod in response means she is on her period. In the month of Ramadan, even when the religion excuses them from fasting during their periods, women pretend to fast. The male members of the household should never know. Talking about menstruation is not an option. As a result, girls and boys grow up with little or no knowledge about this physiological process. So much so that many girls do not even learn about periods before menarche (Ali & Rizvi, 2010, p. 537). Indeed, according to a study

K. L. Khan (✉)
North Carolina State University, Raleigh, NC, USA
e-mail: kkhan3@ncsu.edu

F. Azhar
Minnesota State University, Mankato, MN, USA
e-mail: farah.azhar@mnsu.edu

© The Author(s), under exclusive license to Springer Nature Singapore Pte Ltd. 2023
L. Balfour (ed.), *FemTech*, https://doi.org/10.1007/978-981-99-5605-0_9

conducted by UNICEF, 49% of young Pakistani girls "had no knowledge of menstruation prior to their first period" (Hafeez-Ur-Rehman, 2017).

There are, then, several myths and misconceptions associated with menstruation and menstrual hygiene within the Pakistani context. Rizvi and Ali (2016) discuss some of these misconceptions, such as labeling menstruating girls as impure, keeping them away from newborns, and restricting social gatherings (pp. 51–54). The misconceptions and social stigma attached to menstruation lead to guilt and shame, thus impacting the lives of girls in numerous ways. For example, the inability to manage menstrual hygiene increases school absentees and results in poor academic performance (Singh et al., 2008, p. 394). Additionally, societal pressure and stigma lead to "episodes of anxiety and depression during or near the menstrual period" (Michael et al., 2020, p. 2). It is within these contexts, and cultures of silence, that digital tools are entering the discussion. Raaji, for example, is a chatbot developed by Aurat Raaj and is used to educate women about reproductive health and address myths and misconceptions regarding menstruation (Aurat Raaj, n.d).

This chapter explores the development of Raaji as a conversational agent transforming menstrual health and awareness. In what follows, we aim to highlight its current positionality and importance in Pakistan. In particular, the chapter discusses the extent to which Raaji serves as a modern and inclusive tool, standing in opposition to "master" narratives in order to pave the way for women's access to information in a patriarchal society (Lorde, 1984). We use Gibson's (1979) theory of affordances and its application to the design of physical and digital designs (Norman, 2013) to identify and analyze the key aspects of Raaji. The affordances, in this case, refer to the features Raaji has to offer and the ways in which the users can interact with the chatbot. Building also on Winner's (1980) ideas about the politics of artifacts, we look at Raaji in the sociotechnical structure of Pakistan. We address how chatbots and other digital technologies can be used to empower women in the Global South and help in overcoming societal challenges.

Menstruation and, therefore, menstrual hygiene management (abbreviated hereafter as MHM) are the topics that do not get any attention in schools within Pakistan. The curriculum for grades 1 to 5 "does not refer to MHM," and the content covered in high schools is neither sufficient nor does it clearly address major health concerns (WaterAid, 2018, p. 2; Ali & Rizvi, 2010, p. 540). In the absence of any formal education, the only resource left for girls is the women of the family, mainly mothers and sisters (Ali & Rizvi, 2010, p. 537). However, in most cases, the information they get from family members "is not always timely nor is it adequate" (Chandra-Mouli & Patel, 2020, p. 616). Additionally, since the women in the household "shy away from discussing" menstruation and are not completely aware of the physiological processes, they end up passing on misinformation and "cultural taboos" instead of factual information (Garg & Anand, 2015, p. 185).

This lack of awareness also gives rise to bigger, systemic problems, thus neglecting the concerns of women when it comes to menstrual hygiene management. The recent 2022 floods in Pakistan, for example, highlighted "period poverty"[1] in the country (Mansoor, 2022). While there was a lot of talk about food shortage and loss of life, the needs and experiences of menstruating women during this time have been significantly underexplored. In the Internationally Displaced Persons (IDP) camps, women had to resort to unsafe and unhygienic practices, such as using cloth pieces during menstruation and washing those in potholes filled with rainwater, thus causing "serious health risks" (Amin, 2022). The lack of awareness and concern was so grave that when some organizations like Mahwari Justice and HER Pakistan started gathering funds and distributing menstrual products, people—mostly men—referred to these as a "luxury" (Yousaf, 2022; Panwar, 2022). Similarly, even in the western world, governments impose sales tax, referred to as "luxury tax," on tampons and other feminine hygiene products, thus categorizing menstrual products under luxury goods rather than necessary health products (Lafferty, 2019, p. 59). This "luxury tax," also known as the "pink tax" (Taylor, 2022), is an upcharge on products targeted at women, creating a gender divide. Most women have this lack of awareness of how they are being exploited by corporations that manufacture these products, thus contributing to a culture of gender inequity.

---

[1] The term "period poverty" refers to "a lack of access to menstrual products, education, hygiene facilities, waste management, or a combination of these" (Geng, 2021). The lack of awareness in the society and unavailability of menstrual hygiene products all contribute to the gravity of the situation.

The lack of awareness and stigma attached to the topic, along with gender inequality, exclusion of "women and girls from decision-making processes" (Mahon & Fernandes, 2010, p. 102), and social and cultural limitations (Ali & Rizvi, 2010, p. 540), never really allow a discussion, let alone a way to find possible solutions. According to a survey conducted by the Danish menstrual tracking application Clue, more than 90% of Pakistani women refrained from talking about periods with male members of the family (George, 2016). The impacts of little or no awareness, misconceptions, and a complete disregard for the problems faced by women are devastating. It is clear that there is an urgent need to raise consciousness about MHM, period poverty, and related concerns in Pakistani society. At the very least, it is critical to educate young girls and women in a way that they can adopt hygienic practices and feel free to discuss their concerns and worries in a safe environment where conversations about periods are welcomed.

It is important to note that Pakistan is not the only country where menstruation, menstrual hygiene, reproductive health, and related topics are stigmatized. Several countries in the Global South, mainly in the South Asian region, share similar—if not entirely the same—concerns. For example, Garg and Anand (2015) write about the myths and misconceptions in India; Mahon and Fernandes (2010) discuss the issues of sanitation and hygiene in Nepal, India, and Bangladesh; and Alam et al. (2017) report on the issues faced by schoolgirls in Bangladesh. In some of these areas, certain actions are being taken to educate young girls and women about menstrual hygiene management. Some notable examples include the production and distribution of affordable sanitary napkins by Aakar Innovations (n.d.) in India; the provision of menstrual hygiene supplies, along with dedicated MHM education by ZanaAfrica (n.d.) in Kenya; publication of two detailed guides by WASH United—Rosie's World and Ruby's World—for MHM education (WASH United, n.d.); organization of period workshops and publication of comic books for young girls and boys by Menstrupedia (n.d.).

In what follows, we survey some digital interventions introduced in Pakistan for women's health and explore the gaps in the existing knowledge networks. We then discuss the features and affordances of Raaji, the positioning of the chatbot, and its effects on Pakistani society. This chapter concludes with a brief discussion on the role of Raaji in providing agency to women and creating digital safe spaces, along with the future prospects of chatbots in FemTech.

Digital Interventions for Women's Empowerment and Health in Pakistan

Pakistani society is highly patriarchal, with a gender inequality index (GII) that is always above the global average. According to UNDP, the GII of Pakistan is one of the highest in South Asia—only lower than Afghanistan (United Nations Development Programme, n.d.). From households to social gatherings and educational institutions to workplaces, women do not get equal representation, putting them at a disadvantage (Hadi, 2017, p. 292). Since, in most cases, women do not have enough say in decision-making nor do they get access to education that could empower them, their voice remains unheard, even when their health is on the line. Religious factors, family "honor," and cultural norms make it hard for women to get even basic healthcare. Maternal health and family planning get even more challenging, as women, particularly in rural areas, have lesser mobility and little access to information (Khan, 1999, p. 40).

The nature of these problems is more pronounced when women do not have equal access to technology. For example, many women do not possess a mobile phone, and some who do, cannot use their phones at will. Instead, they need the permission of their husband, brother, or father to own, let alone use, a phone. Sultana et al. (2018) discuss financial issues, social challenges, and "insufficient support" in Bangladesh resulting from this restricted access (pp. 6, 7). The situation in Pakistan is no different. If anything, a greater GII brings more challenges for women. In such patriarchal societies, where dominating or subverting the system is not an option, safe spaces can be created to some extent by working within the system. Sultana et al. (2018) refer to this practice as designing "within the patriarchy" where the goal is to "empower women within the structures of their society, instead of trying to destroy those structures"

(p. 9). This attitude shifts the focus back to women, thus prioritizing their needs. There is a need for digital interventions to "define and empower" instead of "divide and conquer" (Lorde, 1984, p. 113). The affordances of existing sociotechnical systems can be leveraged to create safe digital spaces and provide women and young girls with helpful resources.

Several information and communication technologies (ICT) solutions have been implemented in Pakistan to give women some level of independence within the existing patriarchal structure. Even the government of Pakistan has created a few initiatives to educate and empower women. In one such program, 16 Community Technology Learning Centers (CTLC) were established throughout the country to provide technical knowledge and skills to women living in rural areas. According to Khalafzai and Nirupama (2011), this "project was not a national policy initiative, but a pilot [...] with a limited 0.5% budgetary allocation" (p. 91). Additionally, the definition of empowerment is only restricted to access to technology in this program, with the hope that this will help in overcoming the digital divide (National Commission for Human Development, 2021). As Eubanks (2012) notes, this limited view of ICT interventions, where the emphasis is only on access to technology, does not lead to justice; along with access to technology, improved political, social, healthcare, and financial conditions are needed for social justice (p. 8).

In a country where only "7% of women are included in the formal financial sector" and only 39% "own mobile phones," equality becomes a big challenge (Mustafa et al., 2019, p. 46). Projects such as CTLC can, therefore, only do so much, particularly when it comes to the health and hygiene of women. Research has shown that simple ICT interventions, such as the use of text messages to disseminate useful information to pregnant women, also run into several issues because of family dynamics and "gender boundaries" (Batool et al., 2017). Therefore, raising awareness about women's issues faces several roadblocks that cannot merely be addressed by introducing a new technological solution. It is critical to create digital safe spaces and sites where women can share their experiences and seek help from experts.

When it comes to menstrual hygiene management and reproductive health, women need awareness about menstruation and hygienic products so they can fight misconceptions regarding menstruation. Various discourses around menstruation deem women as "impure" and prevent them from taking part in various activities like playing games, cooking, going to religious sermons, and so on. Recently, some nonprofit organizations in Pakistan have started campaigns to highlight the problems faced by women and to provide them with the necessary resources. Baithak[2] and HER Pakistan[3] are two such initiatives that are creating awareness, particularly in the rural areas of the country. During the recent floods in Pakistan, another student-led platform, Mahwari Justice,[4] initiated a menstrual relief campaign.

Some attempts have also been made to create safe spaces on social media platforms, where women share their concerns anonymously, getting some advice and support. Women-only groups on Facebook are one such example. These groups allow women to discuss sensitive and taboo topics, such as abortions and sexual abuse (Younas et al., 2020). However, the use of social media for women is also monitored and restricted in most cases. Oftentimes, women have to convince their family members about the use of social media platforms or maintain an anonymous presence (Karusala et al., 2019). Additionally, the information received through these platforms is not always factual, since, more often than not, the comments are not coming from experts, but from other users. This can result in the dissemination of misinformation and myths, instead of useful knowledge.

It is important for young girls and women in Pakistan, especially those living in rural areas with restricted mobility and limited access to social media, to have an effective resource they can seek help from. ICT initiatives can help in creating safe spaces where women can not only talk

---

[2] "Baithak is a non-profit organization that advocates for gender justice, especially women's access to their reproductive rights in Pakistan through advocacy, education, and awareness." (Baithak—Challenging Taboos, n.d.)

[3] "HER Pakistan is a youth and women led organization that empowers individuals about menstruation through education, service and advocacy." (HER Pakistan, n.d.)

[4] Mahwari Justice is a "student led grassroot movement providing menstrual relief to flood affectees in Pakistan." (Mahwari Justice, n.d.)

about sensitive, private concerns but also find solutions that are otherwise nowhere to be found in a patriarchal society. In a society where there is no formal educational environment for MHM and reproductive health, digital media can play a critical role in overcoming misconceptions and creating awareness about this topic.

In certain areas, ICTs are being used to create awareness and educate young girls about menstrual hygiene management. One such technological intervention is the use of educational chatbots. These technologies can not only raise awareness about MHM but "also allow girls to discuss their menstrual issues and problems in private with their peers or experts" (Manzoor & Khurshid, 2021). Wang et al. (2022) discuss the usefulness of SnehAI—an artificial intelligence chatbot—in promoting "sexual and reproductive health (SRH)" and advocating "for the health and well-being of women and girls." The findings of their case study indicate that an educational chatbot can help in creating a "safe space for users to talk about otherwise sensitive topics," thus meeting the needs of vulnerable populations. Similarly, Rahman et al. (2021) developed and tested the prototype of AdolescentBot in Bangladesh. The prototype was also integrated with Facebook Messenger to reach out to the target audience. Their findings indicated that such a chatbot could raise awareness and "lessen mental stress," leading to better health for the users.

A similar solution is being implemented in Pakistan to educate girls and young women about sexual and reproductive health. Raaji is a chatbot that aims to create awareness regarding "reproductive health, especially menstrual hygiene" among the women of Pakistan (Aurat Raaj, n.d.). Raaji leverages the potential of digital infrastructures. The chatbot serves as an educational resource for women in rural areas of Pakistan, mainly in the Sindh region, where they can learn about MHM in a safe setting. Not only does this chatbot provide anonymity as women can access this chatbot without signing up or giving their personal information, but there are training sessions and lessons taking place within the house of women digital leaders called Raaji menstrual champions. Village women and girls gather in small groups in the houses of these leaders to discuss Raaji's content and follow it up with a discussion. These listening sessions are further explained under "connectivity" in this chapter (Aurat Raaj, n.d.).

Raaji: An Overview

Raaji is a rule-based chatbot[5] developed by Aurat Raaj. By raising awareness regarding menstrual hygiene and reproductive health, this conversational agent aims at bridging the menstrual education gap and breaking the stigma in Pakistan. Raaji is a free chatbot that can be accessed from any web browser. The users do not need to download an application and/ or any add-ons to interact with the chatbot. This makes it easier to access the chatbot from any device. The pilot tests for Raaji began in 2019, by recruiting students between the ages of 11 and 19 from four schools in Karachi, Pakistan. The initial tests found that young girls had numerous misconceptions about menstruation and menstrual hygiene and that the chatbot could be a good source of information for them (Aurat Raaj, 2019).

In Pakistan, as in most of the world, English is the language of the Internet and thus the global marketplace (Naviwala, 2017). Therefore, the initial design of the chatbot supported only the English language. However, the choice of this language was not ideal for the target audience, that is, women from rural areas, as people speak Urdu and other regional languages in these areas. Over time, support for more languages was added to Raaji. Now, in addition to English and Urdu, the users can communicate with the chatbot in four local languages of Pakistan (Pushtu, Punjabi, Balochi, and Sindhi), with slight variations in the interface. Raaji holds the promise of serving as an important pedagogical and gender equality tool in a society where women face numerous barriers to accessing the information on menstrual hygiene. Additionally, this chatbot is not just restricted to Pakistan but is "planning pilots in Ghana, Kenya, Uganda, and Rwanda" (Aurat Raaj, n.d.) to meet the specific educational needs of women in the Global South.

Raaji is a promising platform that can help in disseminating useful information to young girls and women in Pakistan—information that is otherwise inaccessible. The provision of factual content can help in

---

[5] A chatbot "based on a fixed predefined set of rules" with questions and answers already fed into the system is a rule-based chatbot. Such a chatbot typically does not accept text inputs from the users. Instead, the users can select from the options presented to them (Adamopoulou & Moussiades, 2020, p. 378).

overcoming myths and misconceptions. The affordances of Raaji discussed in this chapter highlight how such tools, developed in the Global South, can be used to empower marginalized communities and help them overcome societal challenges.

There has been a lot of criticism that these FemTech projects are shaped by neoliberal ideologies in which the state–corporate nexus shifts the burden of health management on the people, simultaneously deeming the users as being "empowered." Often these technologies are used for reproductive surveillance, coercing women not only to register and give their data but pay for many such female apps like Flo (Mishra & Suresh, 2021; Hendl & Jansky, 2022). However, Raaji is free of charge, and women do not have to register any of their data to use it. Hence, it is a beacon of hope and attempts to resist neoliberal ideologies as it is a tool for the Global South by the Global South.

A Walkthrough of Raaji

There are slight variations in the design of Raaji for different languages, primarily because of the scripts of languages and varying levels of support in the digital environment. We provide a brief walkthrough of a user journey, focusing on the English version of the chatbot in Fig. 9.1. The users are not required to create an account, log in, and/or provide any identifying information to interact with the bot. The flowchart in Fig. 9.1 shows the categorization of information into sections and subsections.

Raaji welcomes the users with a clear message about its identity and purpose (Fig. 9.2a). The initial disclaimer tells the users that they are talking to a chatbot, and not a human. When the users click on the "Let's talk!" button, the chatbot shares its name, providing them with more options to choose from (Fig. 9.2b). From here on, the chatbot also reads its responses out to the users, ensuring that the users who cannot read the text are not left behind. Throughout their journey, the users can select the options and learn about menstrual hygiene management. Some of the responses include images and animation to keep the users engaged and/ or to illustrate a concept (Fig. 9.2c). If at any point, the users have to go back, they can either scroll all the way up and click on the "Let's talk!"

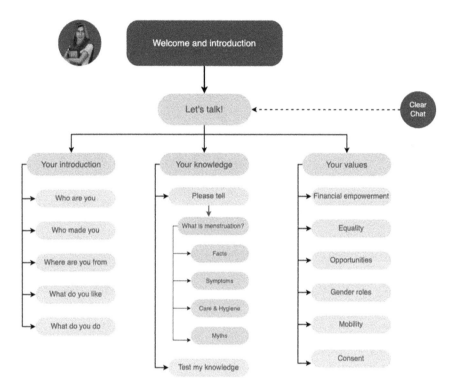

Fig. 9.1 An overview of the user journey when interacting with Raaji

button to restart the chat session or clear the chat by selecting the "Clear Chat" option (Fig. 9.2d).

Affordances and Limitations of Raaji

Raaji, like any other digital technology, has certain traits that allow users to interact with the chatbot. These distinguishing aspects—or affordances—aid or hinder the users as they try to accomplish their goals when interacting with the chatbot. Gibson (1979) points out that the affordance of any environment is "what it provides or furnishes" (p. 127). As the users interact with an artifact, these features help in building a relationship with the environment (Norman, 2013, p. 11). However, the

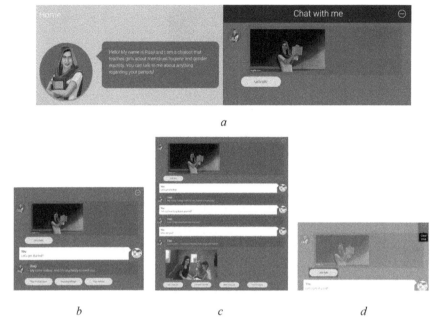

Fig. 9.2 The interaction of users with Raaji

affordances of any artifact might not always be visible. Instead, these become visible—or come alive—as a result of the interaction between the users and the technological artifact. Affordances, therefore, are not mere features or properties of a product, but "action possibilities" shaping the behavior of users by allowing them to act in certain ways as well as restricting their activities (Sun, 2012, p. 72). It must be noted that affordances do not necessarily consist of good aspects. The actions that an artifact allows—or does not allow—can impact the users in a good or bad manner, depending on the context and their needs.

Raaji, being a rule-based chatbot, has certain action possibilities for the target audience. These affordances, along with the chat prompts, guide the conversation, providing the users access to information, and restricting their actions at times. Wang et al. (2022) compiled a list of 15 functional affordances for a chatbot to analyze different ways in which the users can interact with such technology. Our discussion below is inspired by their work, borrowing 5 out of the 15 affordances that are most relevant to Raaji. These include glocalizability, connectivity, accessibility, multimodality, and interactivity. We discuss the possibilities for users, following into these categories, as they interact with Raaji. We also discuss the limitations of the chatbot that impact the users' experience.

Glocalizability

Glocalizability is a term derived from glocalization that is defined as a blend of the local and the global and was coined by sociologist Roland Robertson (1995). The creator of Raaji paid attention to the significance of glocalization in the rural settings of Pakistan. For instance, Raaji's avatar (from her clothes to her appearance) emphasizes the concept of glocalizability because a Pakistani woman wearing traditional Pakistani clothes would relate more to this avatar than one with a western appearance. The animated character or avatar of Raaji is designed so that it resembles a Pakistani woman.

Raaji was initially designed for the rural population of the Sindh province in Pakistan. In order to reach a wider audience, Raaji is also offered in multiple languages. These include four major regional languages of Pakistan (Pushtu, Balochi, Punjabi, and Sindhi), along with Urdu, English, Arabic, and French. However, the English version of the bot is the most developed with added features that are not available in other languages. For example, the category "Test my knowledge" is only accessible via the English version.

It is important to observe a few aspects of Raaji's Urdu version. The first thing to note is that the chatbot uses Latin characters to converse in Urdu. This is the type of text the youth is most familiar with, as they use Latin characters to type Urdu in text messaging. Additionally, Raaji uses a mix of Urdu and English to chat informally with the users. The use of English terms such as "topics," "female body," and "health systems" makes the bot relatable to a young audience (Fig. 9.3).

However, the use of Latin characters for Urdu conversation can lead to certain issues. Since the use of Latin characters for Urdu conversation is an approximation at best (Zaugg & Reeve, 2021), there is a lack of

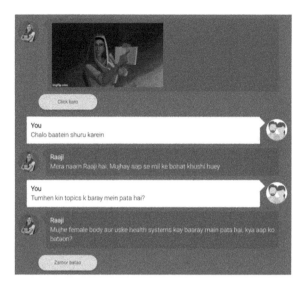

Fig. 9.3 Raaji conversing in Urdu

standard spelling, which can lead to wrong interpretations. Additionally, users who are not exposed to Latin characters cannot communicate with the chatbot in the Urdu language. Therefore, access to the Urdu version of the chatbot gets restricted only to those users who have some level of familiarity with the Latin characters and script. In order to converse with the chatbot in Urdu, the users need to know English phonetics which can be a hurdle for women, especially those in the rural regions of Pakistan.

Connectivity

The connection of women and young girls with Raaji is not restricted to their use of the chatbot. Instead, there is an effort to facilitate the creation of physical safe spaces where women can interact with the chatbot and get a better understanding of MHM. Rural women are invited to listening parties which are informal chat parties where the digital community leaders try to understand the needs, beliefs, attitudes, and practices of these women regarding menstruation. These listening sessions, called Raaji Rooms, are held in the homes of these community leaders and act as safe learning spaces for rural women (Fig. 9.4). The homes of these community leaders are more than just community centers but act as a sustainable digital solution for the rural community (Aurat Raaj, n.d.).

The hosts of these sessions—also referred to as digital champions—are much trusted in their community and act as opinion leaders. These digital champions are trained to use digital storytelling tools like PowerPoint presentations and a video introducing the chatbot (Khalid, 2021). Raaji Rooms are the resources that act as catalysts or enabling factors in the agentic process, thus fostering empowerment (Kabeer, 1999). These safe spaces facilitate women in setting their own personal health goals and enable them to act as agents of change.

Hendl and Jansky (2022) argue that the discourse of apps promises user empowerment because of gaining app-generated self-knowledge. Empowerment entails being in control of one's body and taking ownership of one's sexual, menstrual, and reproductive health. In the patriarchal society of Pakistan, where access to technology and resources is quite restricted for women, it is challenging to talk about topics related to menstrual hygiene and reproductive health. In such an environment, it becomes important to create tools that can dismantle this system and prioritize the needs of an underrepresented and marginalized

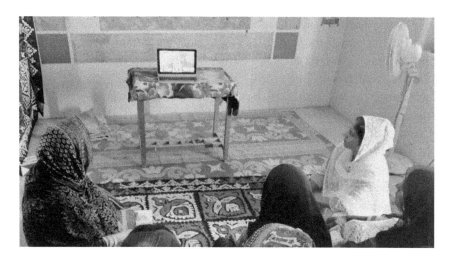

Fig. 9.4 Raaji rooms

community. Raaji rooms provide a conducive environment for such discussions. Initiatives such as Raaji are important to stand up against the existing sociotechnical systems where the designs are discriminatory. These tools based on "personal visions help lay the groundwork for political action" (Lorde, 1984, p. 113).

Accessibility

Raaji is available as a web application, accessible via any browser. The fact that the users do not have to sign up on the platform and/or create an account to interact with the chatbot adds to its accessibility. Given the lack of technological access, women in Pakistan might not have an e-mail address or a mobile number. The lack of such information, therefore, does not become a hurdle. Additionally, since Raaji is not hosted as a mobile application, users who do not own a smartphone can also interact with the chatbot, even when they are using a shared device.

Raaji provides young girls and women with a new medium that they can interact with, relate to, and learn from. The affordances of this chatbot can shape the behaviors of the target audience, providing them with factual information instead of myths and misconceptions. Raaji, being an informative and interactive tool, can reduce the stigma around MHM by employing methods of education and interaction (Madison, 2018, p. 2). By reaching out to young girls as well as elder women in the community, and conducting events such as Chatbot Parties, Raaji tackles myths at all levels in rural areas.

However, access to this chatbot is still restricted in various ways. Apart from smartphones, young girls and women in Pakistan do not have easy access to the Internet, particularly those living in rural areas. The state of digital literacy for women in Pakistan also poses a challenge as interacting with a new technology is in itself a learning process (Ali, 2021). Moreover, the chatbot discusses a taboo topic that the girls may not be exposed to before interacting with Raaji. Many mothers refrain from talking about menstruation with their daughters before they reach puberty, so teenage girls (who haven't had their period yet) may be excluded from such Chatbot Parties.

Multimodality

The information provided by the chatbot is mainly in the form of textual content. However, this is not the only mode of content delivery used by Raaji. In order to improve the user experience and illustrate some concepts, the chatbot shares images and animated content while responding to certain questions. For example, when introducing female reproductive health, the users see a diagram of the uterus that helps in illustrating the phenomenon of menstruation (Fig. 9.5).

All the questions answered by Raaji are accompanied by a voiceover. Every time the chatbot responds with a text, it is also read out loud by an automated voice. This also increases access by providing multiple ways to understand the content. The chatbot with its bright colors and relatable avatar is engaging and provides the user with exact answers rather than numerous options which would be the case had it been a random Google search. When the user asks Raaji about the myths around periods, Raaji responds by addressing the myths. For example, the chatbot busts common myths about showering, dietary concerns, and isolation while

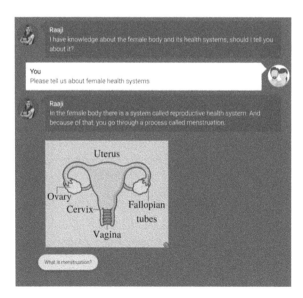

Fig. 9.5 Raaji uses a picture to explain the female reproductive system

menstruating. Hence, this information is specifically tailored to the myths around menstrual hygiene management in Pakistan.

Interactivity

The interaction with Raaji resembles text exchange on any instant messaging platform. When the users select a question, an animated typing bubble appears, indicating that Raaji is drafting the response (Fig. 9.6). Raaji's responses are quick, providing appropriate information without unnecessary delays.

Raaji is a rule-based chatbot with predefined questions and answers fed into the system. Therefore, the users cannot type in questions of their own and interact with this bot as freely as compared to an AI-based chatbot. The cost and resources could be one reason for creating a simple rule-based chatbot. Additionally, an AI-based chatbot "learns" from the users and can, therefore, be "taught" to "interact in racist and sexist ways" (Toupin & Couture, 2020, p. 738; Neff & Nagy, 2016). Therefore, with controlled interaction, a chatbot dealing with sensitive topics can be better monitored. A rule-based model works for Raaji as it was initially designed to remove any misconceptions surrounding menstruation. However, being a rule-based chatbot, Raaji offers little freedom to users during the interaction. The user journey is predetermined, where the users can only select the options and consume the information provided

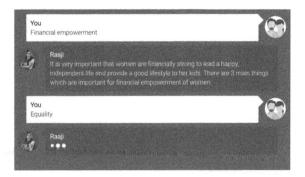

Fig. 9.6 Typing bubble to indicate that Raaji is responding to a question

to them. The users cannot jump to specific categories based on their needs and preferences. Instead, they have to stick to the flow presented by the chatbot.

One aspect of Raaji to improve the user experience and provide better interaction is the quiz offered under the "Test my knowledge" category. The chatbot asks a series of questions about menstruation (an example is shown in Fig. 9.7a). Toward the end of the quiz, the users are directed to Raaji's knowledge base (Fig. 9.7b). However, this quiz is only available in the English version of the chatbot. Users interacting with Raaji in other languages cannot access this interactive quiz. Moreover, the chatbot does not provide any feedback to the users on their responses. Even if all the answers are wrong, Raaji does not correct the users or provide factual information in response. The efficacy of the quiz can, therefore, be questioned, when it comes to clarifying misconceptions.

Another limitation or shortcoming of Raaji is that it does not lead the users to take any actions with the information provided by the chatbot. The information provided by the chatbot is limited to basic levels, and the users interacting only with the chatbot cannot do much with it. Once they have explored all the content provided by Raaji, the users are not directed to any resources where they can get further information, ask particular questions, and/or seek help regarding their specific needs.

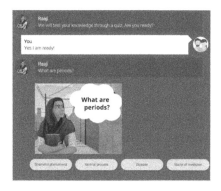
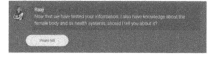

a   *b*

Fig. 9.7 Raaji asking questions to test a user's knowledge

Conclusion

Digital health technologies have been promoted as tools for women's empowerment claiming that by using these products, women will be able to "take ownership of reproductive health" (Hendl & Jansky, 2022). Raaji is the first AI chatbot in Pakistan to address Menstrual Hygiene Management. Despite being an exemplary solution for global problems like gender inequality and lack of education, this FemTech chatbot cannot solely be seen as the silver bullet for women's agency and empowerment.

Does the use of chatbots like Raaji increase women's agency? Will the master's tools ever dismantle the master's house? Or will these FemTech tools allow us to "beat him at his own game, but never enable us to bring about genuine change?" (Lorde, 1984, p. 110). There is no definitive answer. Several studies including that of Ali and Rizvi (2010), Chandra-Mouli and Patel (2020), George (2016), and Mahon and Fernandes (2010) as mentioned earlier in the chapter have shown that correct information on menstruation acts as an enabling factor in women's empowerment. However, one needs to be cautious about the power dynamics incorporated into these apps when looking at empowerment debates regarding FemTech and broader debates around equity and justice in healthcare.

It is also important to consider the aspect of control and discipline when interacting with such technologies. According to Hendl and Jansky (2022), the concept of empowerment is split into self-knowledge, self-management, and self-optimization. The significance of self-management in the discourse of apps is grounded in the notion that once the woman masters her menstruation, she can take control of her life. Such narratives of women having their cycles in control are based on a biologically deterministic notion whereby their body needs to be disciplined and follow a certain order (Hendl & Jansky, 2022). The notion of normative femininity is further reinforced by apps where women who do not menstruate or cannot conceive are excluded from the notion of a "normal" cycle (Corbin, 2019, p. 337). Mediated self-knowledge via these apps is framed as a tool for empowerment but simultaneously promotes biomedical bodily alienation (Hendl & Jansky, 2022).

Despite a lot of criticisms of FemTech projects, Raaji is the forerunner of such projects in Pakistan and the first of its kind. Raaji can be utilized as an important resource for the education of young girls and women in Pakistan. This tool can help in creating a digital space where women can learn about a crucial topic that is otherwise considered taboo. Raaji serves as an example of digital technologies serving as an agent of change. Looking at the "candidates for feminist technology" discussed by Johnson (2010), Raaji can be identified as a technology that is "good for women" and aims at constituting "gender equitable social relations" (p. 41). With its specific design and affordances, Raaji highlights the political nature of the existing structure, and the relationships of power and authority in society (Winner, 1980).

Johnson (2010) argues that technology may be deemed "feminist" when it increases women's sociopolitical status, improves gender power relations, and increases agency. However, the design of the technology sometimes reinforces dominant social inequalities and perpetuates sexist stereotypes as mainly men engineers are responsible for the design (Wajcman, 2006). Furthermore, the promises of empowerment made by the developers may not be that innocent as these apps are designed and marketed to serve vested interests and normalize certain desires, user identities, and health patterns as envisioned by the developers (Lupton, 2013). The tech industry is often considered the knowledge distributor from Global North to Global South whereby the latter is represented through a Western lens. The code of the AI system is permeated with western ideology and institutionalized into how technologies are shaped (Arora & Chowdhury, 2021).

Hence, future research should aim for a decolonial and intersectional feminist framework (Leurs, 2017; Costanza-Chock, 2020; D'Ignazio & Klein, 2020). Further studies should look at how the audience interacts with these messages and how the messages are read and interpreted to assess whether Raaji gives women agency. For a richer study, intended users of Raaji need to be surveyed or interviewed. The voices of the subaltern need to be incorporated, and it must be ensured that racial, colonial, and gender biases do not filter into the coding of the algorithm.

References

Aakar Innovations. (n.d.). *Aakar innovations*. Aakar Innovations | Transforming Lives through Innovations. https://www.aakarinnovations.com/

Adamopoulou, E., & Moussiades, L. (2020). An overview of chatbot technology. *IFIP International Conference on Artificial Intelligence Applications and Innovations*, 373–383.

Alam, M.-U., Luby, S. P., Halder, A. K., Islam, K., Opel, A., Shoab, A. K., Ghosh, P. K., Rahman, M., Mahon, T., & Unicomb, L. (2017). Menstrual hygiene management among Bangladeshi adolescent schoolgirls and risk factors affecting school absence: Results from a cross-sectional survey. *BMJ Open*, 1–10.

Ali, S. (2021, November 3). *Digital literacy in Pakistan: Where do we stand?* YourCommonwealth.   https://www.yourcommonwealth.org/editors-pick/digital-literacy-in-pakistan-where-do-we-stand/

Ali, T. S., & Rizvi, S. N. (2010). Menstrual knowledge and practices of female adolescents in urban Karachi, Pakistan. *Journal of Adolescence, 33*(4), 531–541.

Amin, A. (2022, October 6). *A small bit from a conversation from one of our visits to a flood IDP camp*. Facebook. https://www.facebook.com/story.php?story_fbid=pfbid0226hSQsyw4pNpvRGcCot3od4BCgqYFkopvRQjfqfW45hBg HvLxU1W9ZTGA18xFCWXl&id=100080503835493

Arora, P., & Chowdhury, R. (2021). Cross-cultural feminist technologies. *Global Perspectives, 2*(1), 25207.

Aurat Raaj. (2019, July 16). *Raaji goes into TESTINGs*. Aurat Raaj. https://auratraaj.co/blog/2019/7/28/raaji-goes-into-testings.

Aurat Raaj. (n.d.). *Aurat Raaj*. Aurat Raaj. https://auratraaj.co/

Baithak—Challenging Taboos. (n.d.). *Baithak—Challenging taboos—Home*. Facebook. https://www.facebook.com/baithak.pak/

Batool, A., Razaq, S., Javaid, M., Fatima, B., & Toyama, K. (2017). Maternal complications: Nuances in mobile interventions for maternal health in Urban Pakistan. In *ICTD '17: Proceedings of the ninth international conference on information and communication technologies and development*. https://dl.acm.org/doi/abs/10.1145/3136560.3136573

Chandra-Mouli, V., & Patel, S. V. (2020). Mapping the knowledge and understanding of menarche, menstrual hygiene and menstrual health among adolescent girls in low-and middle-income countries. In C. Bobel, I. T. Winkler, B. Fahs, K. A. Hasson, E. A. Kissling, & T.-A. Roberts (Eds.), *The Palgrave handbook of critical menstruation studies* (pp. 609–636). Palgrave Macmillan.

Corbin, B. A. (2019). Digital micro-aggressions and discrimination: Femtech and the 'Othering' of women. *Nova Law Review, 44*, 337.

Costanza-Chock, S. (2020). *Design justice: Community-led practices to build the worlds we need.* The MIT Press.

D'Ignazio, C., & Klein, L. F. (2020). *Data feminism.* The MIT Press.

Eubanks, V. (2012). *Digital dead end: Fighting for social justice in the information age.* The MIT Press.

Garg, S., & Anand, T. (2015). Menstruation related myths in India: Strategies for combating it. *Journal of Family Medicine and Primary Care, 4*(2), 184–186.

Geng, C. (2021, September 16). *What to know about period poverty.* Medical News Today. https://www.medicalnewstoday.com/articles/period-poverty

George, R. (2016, March 2). Bad blood: the taboo on talking about periods is damaging lives | Rose George. *The Guardian.* https://www.theguardian.com/commentisfree/2016/mar/02/taboo-period-menstruation-damaging-lives-euphemisms

Gibson, J. J. (1979). The theory of affordances. In *Ecological approach to visual perception* (pp. 127–137). Houghton Mifflin.

Hadi, A. (2017). Patriarchy and gender-based violence in Pakistan. *European Journal of Social Science Education and Research, 4*(4), 297–304.

Hafeez-Ur-Rehman, H. (2017, August 9). *U-report encourages menstrual health in Pakistan.* UNICEF. https://www.unicef.org/innovation/U-Report/menstrual-hygiene-innovation-challenge-pakistan

Hendl, T., & Jansky, B. (2022). Tales of self-empowerment through digital health technologies: A closer look at 'Femtech'. *Review of Social Economy, 80*(1), 29–57.

HER Pakistan. (n.d.). *HER Pakistan.* HER Pakistan. https://herpakistan.com/

Johnson, D. G. (2010). Sorting out the question of feminist technology. In L. Layne, S. Vostral, & K. Boyer (Eds.), *Feminist technology* (pp. 36–55). University of Illinois Press.

Kabeer, N. (1999). Resources, agency, achievements: Reflections on the measurement of women's empowerment. *Development and Change, 30*(3), 435–464.

Karusala, N., Bhalla, A., & Kumar, N. (2019). Privacy, patriarchy, and participation on social media. In *DIS '19: Proceedings of the 2019 on designing interactive systems conference* (pp. 511–526). https://dl.acm.org/doi/abs/10.1145/3322276.3322355

Khalafzai, A. K., & Nirupama, N. (2011). Building resilient communities through empowering women with information and communication technologies: A Pakistan case study. *Sustainability, 3*(1), 82–96. https://www.mdpi.com/2071-1050/3/1/82

Khalid, S. (2021, April 17). *Raaji & TRDP set off on menstrual education in Manjhand.* LinkedIn. https://www.linkedin.com/pulse/raaji-trdp-set-off-menstrual-education-manjhand-saba-khalid/

Khan, A. (1999). Mobility of women and access to health and family planning services in Pakistan. *Reproductive Health Matters, 7*(14), 39–48.

Lafferty, M. (2019). The pink tax: The persistence of gender price disparity. *Midwest Journal of Undergraduate Research, 11*, 56–72.

Leurs, K. (2017). Feminist data studies: Using digital methods for ethical, reflexive and situated socio-cultural research. *Feminist Review, 115*(1), 130–154.

Lorde, A. (1984). The master's tools will never dismantle the master's house. In *Sister outsider: Essays and speeches* (pp. 110–114). Crossing Press.

Lupton, D. (2013, June 13). *Digitized health promotion: Personal responsibility for health in the Web 2.0 era.* The Sydney Health & Society Group. https://ses.library.usyd.edu.au/handle/2123/9190

Madison, E. (2018). *How digital media is used to fight stigma.* https://www.ethanmad.com/post/digital_media_fight_stigma/digital_media_fight_stigma-madison.pdf

Mahon, T., & Fernandes, M. (2010). Menstrual hygiene in South Asia: A neglected issue for WASH (water, sanitation and hygiene) programmes. *Gender and Development, 18*(1), 99–113.

Mahwari Justice. (n.d.). *Mahwari justice (@MahwariJustice).* Twitter. https://twitter.com/mahwarijustice

Mansoor, S. (2022, September 14). Floods highlight period poverty in Pakistan. *Time.* https://time.com/6213181/period-poverty-pakistan-menstruation-floods/

Manzoor, S., & Khurshid, S. (2021). Role of ICT in promoting adolescent menstrual health. *Library Philosophy and Practice.* https://digitalcommons.unl.edu/cgi/viewcontent.cgi?article=11951&context=libphilprac

Menstrupedia. (n.d.). *Menstrupedia.* Menstrupedia Comic. https://www.menstrupedia.com/

Michael, J., Iqbal, Q., Haider, S., Khalid, A., Haque, N., Ishaq, R., Saleem, F., Hassali, M. A., & Bashaar, M. (2020). Knowledge and practice of adolescent females about menstruation and menstruation hygiene visiting a public healthcare institute of Quetta, Pakistan. *BMC Women's Health, 20*(4), 1–8.

Mishra, P., & Suresh, Y. (2021). Datafied body projects in India: Femtech and the rise of reproductive surveillance in the digital era. *Asian Journal of Women's Studies, 27*(4), 597–606.

Mustafa, M., Batool, A., & Raza, A. A. (2019). Designing ICT interventions for women in Pakistan. *Communications of the ACM, 62*(11), 46–47. https://dl.acm.org/doi/10.1145/3355696

National Commission for Human Development. (2021). *Annual Report 2021*. Ministry of Federal Education and Professional Training. http://www.nchd.org.pk/ws/downloads/annual_reports/NCHD_AR_2021.pdf

Naviwala, N. (2017, October 18). *Opinion | What's really keeping Pakistan's children out of school? (Published 2017)*. The New York Times. https://www.nytimes.com/2017/10/18/opinion/pakistan-education-schools.html

Neff, G., & Nagy, P. (2016). Talking to bots: Symbiotic agency and the case of Tay. *International Journal of Communication, 10*, 4915–4931.

Norman, D. (2013). *The design of everyday things: Revised and expanded edition*. Basic books.

Panwar, U. (2022, August 27). *Not necessity this is luxury*. Twitter. https://twitter.com/Uzairpanwar/status/1563538328712265733

Rahman, R., Rahman, M. R., Tripto, N. I., Ali, M. E., Apon, S. H., & Shahriyar, R. (2021). Combating adolescent sexual and reproductive health problems in Bangladesh. In *CHI '21: Proceedings of the 2021 CHI conference on human factors in computing systems* (pp. 1–15).

Rizvi, N., & Ali, T. S. (2016). Misconceptions and mismanagement of menstruation among adolescents girls who do not attend School in Pakistan. *Journal of Asian Midwives, 3*(1), 46–62.

Robertson, R. (1995). Glocalization: Time-space and homogeneity-heterogeneity. In M. Featherstone, R. Robertson, & S. Lash (Eds.), *Global Modernities* (pp. 25–44). SAGE Publications.

Singh, A., Kiran, D., Singh, H., Nel, B., Singh, P., & Tiwari, P. (2008). Prevalence and severity of dysmenorrhea: A problem related to menstruation, among first and second year female medical students. *Indian Journal of Physiology and Pharmacology, 52*(4), 389–397.

Sultana, S., Guimbretière, F., Sengers, P., & Dell, N. L. (2018). Design within a patriarchal society: Opportunities and challenges in designing for rural women in Bangladesh. In *CHI '18: Proceedings of the 2018 CHI conference on human factors in computing systems* (pp. 1–13). https://dl.acm.org/doi/10.1145/3173574.3174110

Sun, H. (2012). *Cross-cultural technology design: Creating culture-sensitive Technology for Local Users.* Oxford University Press.

Taylor, K. R. (2022, October 18). *CVS will pay "pink tax" and drop prices on period products.* Kiplinger. https://www.kiplinger.com/taxes/cvs-will-pay-pink-tax-and-drop%2D%2Dperiod-product-prices

Toupin, S., & Couture, S. (2020). Feminist chatbots as part of the feminist toolbox. *Feminist Media Studies, 20*(5), 737–740.

United Nations Development Programme. (n.d.). *Gender inequality index (GII).* Human Development Reports. https://hdr.undp.org/data-center/thematic-composite-indices/gender-inequality-index#/indicies/GII

Wajcman, J. (2006). Technocapitalism meets technofeminism: Women and technology in a wireless world. *Labour & Industry: a journal of the social and economic relations of work, 16*(3), 7–20.

Wang, H., Gupta, S., Singhal, A., Muttreja, P., Singh, S., Sharma, P., & Piterova, A. (2022). An artificial intelligence chatbot for young People's sexual and reproductive health in India (SnehAI): Instrumental case study. *Journal of Medical Internet Research, 24*(1).

WASH United. (n.d.). *mhm_guide.* WASH United. https://www.wash-united.org/mhm-guide/mhm-guide.html

WaterAid. (2018). *Menstrual hygiene management in schools in South Asia.* WASH Matters. https://washmatters.wateraid.org/sites/g/files/jkxoof256/files/menstrual-hygiene-management-snapshot%2D%2D-pakistan.pdf

Winner, L. (1980). Do artifacts have politics? *Daedalus, 109*(1), 121–136.

Younas, F., Naseem, M., & Mustafa, M. (2020). Patriarchy and social media: Women only Facebook groups as safe spaces for support seeking in Pakistan. In *ICTD2020: Proceedings of the 2020 international conference on information and communication technologies and development* (pp. 1–11). https://dl.acm.org/doi/abs/10.1145/3392561.3394639

Yousaf, S. (2022, August 29). Are period products a necessity or luxury for flood affected women? *Daily Times.* https://dailytimes.com.pk/989384/are-period-products-a-necessity-or-luxury-for-flood-affected-women/

ZanaAfrica. (n.d.). *ZanaAfrica.* ZanaAfrica Foundation. http://www.zanaafrica.org/

Zaugg, I. A., & Reeve, J. (2021). *The hegemony of keyboard defaults.* AoIR Selected Papers of Internet Research.

10

FemTech in (and for) Emerging Markets: Disruption in Kenya's "Silicon Savannah" Nairobi

Sarah Seddig

Introduction: FemTech, "a Really Good Market"?

"Last month, I counted three different IVF (In Vitro Fertilisation) clinics that had placements between my house and my office," says Evy, a Kenyan investor at a venture association based in Nairobi. As self-declared afro-optimist and champion for Africa's economic development, Evy's work revolves around building a network of investors across Kenya. Recently, she has become more attentive to gender-lens-investing by supporting female-led businesses and gender diverse agendas. Investing in women, as she puts it, allows to distribute capital more equally and to strengthen the creation of services and products for women's needs, that may be overlooked in a room full of male decision-making power. Evy carefully places both of her smartphones on the standing height table in front of us before

S. Seddig (✉)
Danish Institute for International Studies, University of Copenhagen, Copenhagen, Denmark
e-mail: ssed@diis.dk

© The Author(s), under exclusive license to Springer Nature Singapore Pte Ltd. 2023
L. Balfour (ed.), *FemTech*, https://doi.org/10.1007/978-981-99-5605-0_10

adjusting her tilted meet-and-greet tame tag on her white blouse. *"I live off Thika Road,"* she says, *"and recently, I saw a lot of billboards on fertilisation clinics and mHealth solutions catering [to] women—did you notice that?"* Evy's investment portfolio focuses on neither Female Technology (FemTech) nor HealthTech. Her trained eye as a young and successful investor, however, the new investment strategy, and perhaps her own experience as a young woman let her conclude:

> *It occurred to me, for someone to invest so much money putting up a billboard, several even, there must be a really good market. I use a period tracking app myself, but I was not aware of this scalability. Like, KFC[1] is competing with IVF?! That tells you that there's something. (Evy, Interview 2021)*

When leaving the start-up event later that evening, I take a detour via Thika Road up to Muthaiga and back to Kilimani neighborhood. Upon arriving at my apartment, I had counted three billboards advertising (in)fertility treatment clinics and five referring to digital and mobile health services (mHealth) for reproductive healthcare. Most of the billboards were advertising products from private companies. According to the companies' websites, all of them touted their product as specifically targeted toward women and girls in low-resource settings and as a *disruptive* force. The companies articulate their FemTech product has the potential to bring about a two-fold transformation. Firstly, they suggest that it has the capacity to *disrupt* the healthcare landscape in Kenya, simultaneously unlocking opportunities for emerging African markets. Secondly, they refer to it as *disrupting* a person's individual sexual and reproductive healthcare by challenging transitional forms of healthcare delivery, for example. This innovative approach promises to enable individuals to exercise greater control over their own health outcomes, thus facilitating a more proactive and empowering approach to healthcare.

With the rapid growth of "Information and Communications Technologies" (ICT) and mHealth services in Sub-Saharan Africa (Folaranmi, 2014), affordable and easily accessible FemTech solutions have been envisioned as an attractive resource in low-resource settings.

---

[1] Kentucky Fried Chicken.

This particularly applies to Africa's emerging markets. Considered under-served yet promising markets, they feature relevant technological and digital infrastructure, as well as the promise of considerable economic growth. While universal healthcare often remains limited in emerging markets, "girl-centered" and entrepreneurial approaches to development seem omnipresent phenomena (Caron & Margolin, 2015; Hayhurst, 2011, 2013, 2014). Over the past decade, national and international interest in tech-entrepreneurship within Kenya surged drastically. Particularly in Nairobi, technology enthusiasts seize market opportunities within the tech-sector. Often referred to as a tech-ecosystem, its network consists of diverse interconnected and interdependent business entities. Moreover, the high concentration of innovation hubs nurtures business incubation and acceleration. This has contributed to turning the country's capital into an attractive space for tech-entrepreneurs, data scientists, and private investors, such as venture capitalists and angle investors.[2] The reputation of Nairobi's tech-ecosystem has led the city to acquire the title "Silicon Savannah"—in reference to California's buzzing Silicon Valley.

When the private sector advertises FemTech as a novel and powerful driver of change for people living in contexts with limited resources, what are the underlying meanings and implications of the rhetoric of *disruption* associated with the development of the FemTech sector in Kenya's so-called "Silicon Savannah"?

Guided by the edited volume's overarching question "Who is FemTech for?", this chapter sheds light on the perspective of the people behind three FemTech companies situated in Nairobi's tech-ecosystem "Silicon Savannah." Rather than concentrating on a single FemTech solution, my

---

[2] Venture capitalists and angel investors are financial actors (individuals and firms) that provide investments to businesses in exchange for equity stakes or other financial returns. These investors differ in their investment approach and expectations. VCs manage institutional investors' funds and invest in early-stage companies with high growth potential by providing so-called "seed money," which is often used to cover the initial costs associated with starting a business, such as research and development, market analysis, and product development. They usually take an active role in company management and provide strategic advice and connections. Angel investors invest their own funds and typically take on more risk than VCs, investing in early-stage companies with less potential for high returns. While angel investors tend to have a greater inclination toward taking risks, VCs firms are typically more focused on evaluating the growth potential of a startup.

focus lies on enterprises that provide a variety of innovative products and services, such as portable ultrasound screening devices, mobile phone applications, and online platforms that are frequently linked to services offered at local private health clinics. Therefore, this contribution does not concentrate on one specific FemTech solution and its users; rather, it illuminates the viewpoints of entrepreneurs and investors, such as Evy, who perceive FemTech as a novel and favorable market for low-income settings. By critically examining the rhetorical dimensions in which "Silicon Savannah" operates in, I draw attention to the utilization of the rhetoric of *disruption* as a discursive strategy for capitalist expansion of FemTech in Kenya's burgeoning digitalized health sector.

Based on my PhD project "Bodies of Data," this contribution draws on eight months of qualitative multisited ethnographic fieldwork conducted in Kenya at the height of the COVID-19 pandemic between the beginning of 2021 and 2022. During this time, I followed entrepreneurs, data scientists, and investors working at or alongside HealthTech start-ups, innovation labs and accelerators in Nairobi. While I also interacted and accompanied health practitioners, such as clinicians, sonographers, community health workers, and patients in private health clinics situated in three informal settlements across Nairobi, for this contribution, I will mainly draw on the former. Communication with interlocutors continued even after the fieldwork was completed, using means such as phone calls, emails, and social media, until the time of writing this chapter. To maintain confidentiality, pseudonyms have been assigned to all interlocutors and organizations or companies referenced throughout this work. However, notable figures and widely recognized institutions, such as the World Bank Group, the Bill and Melinda Gates Foundations, or public figures such as names of politicians, whose actions are extensively documented, are exempted from this. The research's methodological approach and ethical considerations have been reviewed by the African Medical and Research Foundation (AMREF). AMREF granted the ethical approval for this research across the health sector and among vulnerable parts of the population during the height of the COVID-19 pandemic. Moreover, the project obtained a research permit provided by the Kenyan National Commission for Science, Technology and Innovation (NACOSTI).

Methodologically, I approached the field through participant observation, semistructured interviews, as well as informal conversations at (informal) events, companies' offices or coworking spaces. As a result of the introduction of COVID-19 restrictions, which promoted remote work, I complied with social distancing protocols and moved interviews to outdoor spaces such as cafés, restaurants, or Nairobi's Karura Forest. The majority of the entrepreneurs and investors mentioned in this chapter are more affluent than the people they intend to serve. Due to the availability of technologies such as Teams or Zoom, investors and entrepreneurs were able to transition to remote work arrangements and to continue their work with minimal disruption, also often from cafés. Not all the companies were clearly delineated as FemTech companies at the time of my fieldwork. While many entrepreneurs and investors were working on technologies that can be considered FemTech, only a few were using the term FemTech when I embarked on fieldwork. Yet, over the course of the following years, I witnessed a more frequent use of the term FemTech among the research's interlocutors as well as other actors in the Kenyan tech-ecosystem. While this may point to how my research has influenced the field, the adapted rhetoric more importantly points to the timely relevance of this chapter.

The chapter will open with an exploration of the context around the emergence of "Silicon Savannah" and its impact on the digital health sector. It will move on to examine the notion of disruption to provide insights on its contribution to shaping the discourse on FemTech in Kenya. Finally, it will conclude with an outlook on the FemTech market in and for emerging markets.

The Emergence of "Silicon Savannah"

When historians write Africa's digital story, Kenya will likely assume its place as the cradle of ICT revolution on the continent. Never before has an African nation gone through a disruption such as the digital transformation that is still underway in Kenya. With so much creativity and innovation going on, the nation is witnessing a gigantic paradigm shift. It is a revolution of a kind that is empowering ordinary citizens and reshaping their communities and lifestyles, heralding a new way of thinking about and understanding entrepreneurial opportunities and how to exploit them. (Ndemo, 2017, 4)

In his 2017 publication, *Digital Kenya. An Entrepreneurial Revolutions in the Making*, Bitange Ndemo, the former Permanent Secretary of the Kenyan Ministry of Information and Communication, accentuates the pivotal function that development of ICT has had in Kenya. Expounding on Kenya's position as a trailblazer in Africa, he portrays the digital transformation as a revolution and constructive *disruption* that facilitated innovation, empowerment, and opportunity. In his capacity as Permanent Secretary, Ndemo espoused the privatization and liberalization of the sector (Telkom Kenya, for instance). This agenda was well received, owing to the precedent set by former President Mwai Kibaki, who had advanced capitalist ideology during his tenure (Nyabola, 2018, 68).

With the onset of the second millennium and conversations about the continent's potential, the perception of Africa as the so-called *third world* underwent a significant transformation. No longer merely associated with debt, deprivation, and dystopia, Africa (among other continents, regions, and countries) was proclaimed a prosperous "emerging market". With great optimism and a bright future with unknown possibilities, emerging markets have come to be known as having the potential to flourish as the future for and of capitalism. As a more positive and invigorating alternative for a wide range of economies in Asia, Africa, Latin America, and Eastern Europe, Ravinder Kaur (2018a, 2018b) describes how the new concept, intended to connect the region to a more uplifting feeling, also creates a clean break from the negative connotations of the *third world*. The previously used rhetoric invoked a connection to the moment of decolonization, the global development aid regime, and the idea that less or underdeveloped nations failing to keep up with their developed northern or western counterparts. The defining characteristics of emerging markets include rapid population growth, increasing urbanization, a growing middle class, and a shift toward a market-based economy. In recent years, they have accounted for a significant proportion of global economic growth and have attracted substantial foreign investment.

The descriptions of Africa as an attractive investment location contributed to paving the way for the burgeoning tech-ecosystem "Silicon Savannah." As a nod to the technology hub Silicon Valley in California, the title grew in popularity between 2014 and 2017. Other African emerging technology ecosystems followed suit, gaining significant attention as evidenced by the growing number of innovation clusters in the region. Prominent examples include Lago's "Silicon Lagoon" (dubbed "Yaba Valley") in Nigeria or Cape Town's "Silicon Cape" in South Africa. These tech-ecosystems are seen to have the potential to tackle social and environmental challenges in Africa through scalable and profitable technological innovation. For instance, the World Bank Group and the Bill and Melinda Gates Foundation recognized these tech-ecosystems as aligned with their goals of reducing poverty and accelerating shared prosperity to transform an entire continent (Pollio, 2020, pp. 2716–2717). The recent Global Women's HealthTech Awards, presented jointly by the World Bank Group and the Consumer Technology Association (CTA) are another example of recognizing *"innovative startups that leverage tech to improve women's health and safety in emerging markets"* (International Finance Corporation, 2022). Kenya, however, stands out as one of the first countries in Sub-Saharan Africa with considerable progress in expanding internet access and digital infrastructure. This positioned Nairobi as an attractive location for tech companies seeking to establish a foothold on the continent.

As one of the largest economies in Central and East Africa (World Bank Group, 2019), this foothold has positioned Kenya among Africa's leading countries in technological innovation and progressive ICT growth (Ndemo & Weiss, 2017; Bramann, 2016; African Development Bank, 2019; African Development Bank Group, 2020; World Economic Forum, 2015). According to Waema and Ndung'u (2012), the augmentation of investments in the national fiber optic infrastructure, as well as the deployment of the fourth undersea cable, LION2, in 2012, resulted in a significant improvement in Kenya's bandwidth per user. With this ratio soaring to an impressive 24,000 mbps, Kenya's internet speed was unparalleled on the African continent at the time (Bramann, 2017, p. 233). This remarkable milestone can be attributed to a combination of amplified investment and expanded infrastructure. Compared to neighboring East African countries, the ubiquity of internet connectivity across the country, its high mobile phone penetration, and fast mobile internet speeds are still unmatched (Demombynes & Thegeya, 2012). This context allowed the Kenyan ICT-based mobile and virtual banking system M-Pesa to flourish in the everyday lives of millions of Kenyan citizens across the country. M-Pesa and other tech-innovations of the financial market, referred to as Finance Technology (FinTech), accelerated the mobile money penetration rate further. While M-Pesa emerged as a tech-success story that gained global recognition, it also contributed to drawing attention to Kenya's thriving tech industry and other tech-sectors respectively (Jack & Suri, 2011).

The success of M-Pesa motivated private sector investors to explore innovative ventures beyond the FinTech sector, for example the digital health market (Njoroge et al., 2017). With a surge in interest, the country was prompted to strengthen the integration of ICTs into the healthcare system (Mureithi, 2017). This leveraged telehealth and mHealth solutions, which are frequently reinforced by open data initiatives (Folaranmi, 2014; Ndemo, 2015). Health information for the public, the procurement and distribution of medicine, and increased attendance of mothers in pre- and postnatal care clinics improved notably. As part of the political agenda, Kenya implemented various policies and strategies on digital health. The policies ranged from the Kenya Government Vision 2030 (2007); the Kenya National e-Health Strategy (2011); the Sector Plan for Health (2013); the Kenya National ICT Master Plan 2014–2017 (2014); the Kenya Health Policy 2014–2030 (2014); to the Kenya e-Health Policy 2016–2030 (2016). While Kenya's political and infrastructural attention paved the way for advancing healthcare innovation, the surge of the COVID-19 pandemic drastically accelerated discussion in the ecosystem around the impact and value of HealthTech, including FemTech, for the overburdened public health sector.

Prior to the outbreak of the COVID-19 pandemic, there was a growing reliance on innovative technologies, particularly digital platforms, by individuals, businesses, and governments for a range of activities, such as financial transactions, logistics, commerce, education, and healthcare. Following the World Bank's report on *The Impact of COVID-19 on Disruptive Technology Adoption in Emerging Markets* (2020), many technology businesses adapted their business model further to rapidly respond to the crisis. The report presents the employment of disruptive technologies during the pandemic and discusses emerging market trends, and opportunities to maximize impact in emerging markets. Hospitals in high-income and upper-middle-income countries, for example, were able to promptly offer online healthcare services as part of their response efforts. This was facilitated by regulators who lifted restrictions on telemedicine (for example regarding contact-tracking-apps). Furthermore, users were inclined to adopt these technological solutions, many of whom were first-time users. Similarly, low-income countries also explored novel technologies, primarily digital financial services, as part of their response to the healthcare crisis. For instance, Kenya (as well as Rwanda) waived charges on M-Pesa payments, resulting in a considerable growth in peer-to-peer transfers, both in terms of volume and value (Strusani & Houngbonon, 2020, p. 5). All three companies that I was following were established before COVID-19 but implemented a tool to diagnose whether someone was suffering from COVID-19-related symptoms.

The COVID-19 pandemic has expanded existing disparities in healthcare, especially in the areas of sexual and reproductive health. While studies suggest that unwanted pregnancies, sexual and gender-based violence, and maternal and infant mortality increased during the pandemic in Kenya (Wangamati & Sundby, 2020; Ombere, 2021), the digital health industry and existing digital health practices such as telehealth or mobile health noticeably intensified due to the impacts of COVID-19 (Muli et al., 2021). FemTech solutions soon were discussed as having the potential to address existing and now intensified health disparities. While the accessibility of healthcare shifted to being gradually structured by the access to the digital, these new forms of digitization allow, and in the case of COVID-19 demanded, to deliver healthcare at a distance. The contrasting effects of the COVID-19 pandemic on the healthcare system in Kenya, as outlined in the previous two paragraphs, present a complex scenario. While the pandemic has negatively impacted sexual and reproductive health, the intensification of the digital health industry and the adoption of digital health practices such as telehealth and mobile health present an opportunity for innovation in healthcare. This underscores the focus on mitigating the negative impacts of the pandemic on the healthcare system while also capitalizing on the opportunities presented by the adoption of digital health practices. The ethnographic material discussed earlier, Evy's s statement, provides a glimpse into how actors in the tech-ecosystem are navigating this complex scenario. It offers insights into the challenges and opportunities that arise from the adoption of FemTech solutions in the health sector.

FemTech and the Rhetoric of Disruption in Kenya

One morning in March 2021, I drove to Evy's office, situated in a high-rise building overlooking South of Nairobi. According to HealthTech companies and investors I followed across Nairobi, COVID-19 was described to me as a *"catalyst for local innovations"* (Patrick, Interview 2022), a *"driver for Kenya's innovation"* (Timothy, Interview 2021), or an opportunity to generate funding to develop FemTech products further and to sustain the company and its employees. Amidst the pandemic, FemTech products, especially mobile phone applications, progressively incorporated supplementary COVID-19 features. The most common feature, a COVID-19 symptom tracker, was often incorporated into smartphone apps or through prompt messaging. Based on a digital questionnaire, the user would be able to assess whether they exhibited symptoms associated with the virus. The investor Evy (Interview 2022), for example, expressed her belief that in the future, people will reflect on how COVID-19 leapfrogged various innovations. The understanding of the pandemic as a trigger for healthcare innovation and opportunity for market expansion had been circulating in the tech-ecosystem with the onset of the pandemic. Indeed, interviews with Irene and Anna, who are both working within the HealthTech sector, confirm that the COVID-19 pandemic acted as an accelerant of their FemTech innovation in Kenya. One data scientist, employed at a Nairobi-based FemTech start-up, suggested that COVID-19 served as *"an accelerator because initially we weren't thinking about launching anytime soon"* (Anna, Interview 2021). One of the cofounders of this start-up, Irene, expanded on this. She recalled hearing the news of the first confirmed COVID-19 case in Kenya in 2020, and the feeling of urgency to act in response:

> I was like: 'Okay, guys, seriously, we need to do that—we can't afford. The government is mandating quarantine, people lock down and all, but we can't afford to do that. This is an opportunity for us to actually do something about it. So instead of people going home, we went to the office. We're in the office quarantining the whole time. The whole world, we had the whole world to ourselves. It was super quiet and nice. Everyone was just focused, they really wanted to do this. Within just two months, we were able to deliver a whole new product that can disrupt this upcoming market. (Irene, Interview 2021)

Disruption mostly carries a positive connotation among the people I interviewed. While it has become a distinct feature to the tech-ecosystem's rhetoric around companies' and their products' impact and value, the notion of *disruption* in innovation has also faced criticism. The concept of disruptive innovation, coined by Clayton Christensen, refers to a process where a product or service initially gains traction in the lower end or bottom of the market with simpler quality applications, and then aggressively moves up the market to eventually displace existing competition (Levina, 2017, p. 550). One major critique refers to the term itself. It is said to promote a view of disruptive innovation that is premised on the idea of "creative destruction," whereby new technologies and business models replace existing ones, and challenge established social and economic structures. Some critics contend that the term *disruption* valorizes certain forms of innovation, such as those that generate rapid growth and high returns for investors, while neglecting other forms of innovation that may be more incremental, sustainable, and socially beneficial. This narrow focus on *disruptive* innovation can lead to a short-term perspective that overlooks or disregards long-term societal benefits and sustainable development. Moreover, it can foster a culture of disregard for established norms, regulations, and ethics, particularly in the tech industry, where companies may seek to *disrupt* existing markets without considering the broader social and ethical implications of their actions. This view can be problematic, especially in the context of emerging markets in low-resource or underserved countries, where disruption can also exacerbate inequalities, particularly around sex and gender, or deepen poverty.

Considering the ongoing initiatives to digitalize and privatize healthcare delivery across Sub-Saharan Africa, data-driven technologies are increasingly filling the void of healthcare provision and offer promising avenues for exploration for investors. FemTech such as smartphone apps, wearables, and diagnostic devices are pertinent to discussions on how women's sexual and reproductive health "issues" can be addressed innovatively. Framed as *empowering* and *disruptive* solutions, FemTech tools are envisioned to provide insights into one's own biological processes. One of the most prevalent arguments is that based on the FemTech tool's information and analysis of personal data, users are provided with the ability to make informed and nuanced choices about their bodies and reproductive health (Nafus & Sherman, 2014; Ruckenstein & Pantzar, 2017; Tamminen & Holmgren, 2016). The prevalence of digital health practices and its reliance on digital technologies and data infrastructures, however, raises concerns about the implications of the tech-sector's use of private data. As Gina Neff (2019) notes, private companies are continuously developing novel methods of buying, selling, and sharing private data, making it essential to examine the ethical and regulatory frameworks for managing such data in digital health contexts (Neff, 2019, p. 283). This also applies to the FemTech industry, which relies on rapid and systematic data collection, monitoring, and analysis of personal information regarding the women's behavior as well as their bodily processes. Some scholars have raised their concern about modes of surveillance and the ownership of data in case data-driven technologies are being misused (Lupton, 2016a; Ruckenstein & Schüll, 2017; Zuboff, 2019).

Among tech-optimists and investors, however, discussions on the datafication of reproductive health have highlighted the nascent FemTech market as a valuable and "untapped opportunity." At this point in time, this "untapped market" has attracted millions of dollars of funding and revenue on a global scale. While it can no longer be considered a niche market across the northern hemisphere, companies and investors are increasingly shifting their focus to FemTech in and for other regions of the world, venturing into less explored terrains. Emerging markets seem especially interesting, where digital and entrepreneurial infrastructures support the development of those tools, while low resources and limited access to healthcare promise a great number of customers with unmet needs.

Like most of my interlocutors, Evy and Anna were critical of the term "Silicon Savannah." Anna, for example, working along start-ups and investors at an acceleration hub first felt indifferent toward the term: *"I guess if it puts us on the map and attracts capital, then great,"* she continues: *"I used to think without Africa in this perspective, but I think I am having a different perspective now. A lot of innovation is not new, like it's not original, not from scratch"* (Anna, Interview 2021). While she previously did not consider Africa in their viewpoint, she now recognizes that much of the innovation in Africa is not entirely new but instead builds upon existing innovation following a venture capital model that *"we've heavily borrowed from Silicon Valley. And I don't necessarily think there is a problem with that. The problem will be to copy and paste it, as opposed to building onto the innovation that is already there"* (Anna, Interview 2021). When making investment decisions, Evy, for example, not only has to consider whether an opportunity is investable, and has growth potential, but also whether it is attractive to other investors: *"Is that something the investors would have appetite in?"* (Evy, Interview 2021). Increasingly, she sees the focus on women's issues playing a more pertinent role among startups and investors that seek to venture into new markets. She notes that the increase interest in gender-lens-investing, along with the allocation of resources from the Global North, have a significant impact on investment decisions. She suggests that these factors may pose challenges in addressing issues related to resource allocation and reflect on the need to build upon existing innovation in Africa to consider local contexts in investment decisions, rather than simply adopting external models: *"because the money still comes from the Global North, it is still very much shaped by that kind of view. If resource allocation still happens from the Global North primarily, then I think disruption is a difficult thing to solve"* (Evy, Interview 2021).

To her, the idea of Kenya as the "Silicon Savannah" emerging market represents a western-centric view of the African technology industry. This echoes what other scholars and people in the tech-ecosystem critically voiced about the term "Silicon Savannah." It reduces the African technology landscape to a mere imitation of Silicon Valley, disregarding the unique context and dynamics of technology development in Africa, as well as the agency of African entrepreneurs and innovators. Moreover, the term may promote an oversimplified and one-dimensional view of African economies, emphasizing the technology industry's role in driving economic growth and development, while neglecting other critical sectors such as inequality, poverty, and sustainability. Additionally, some critics argue that the term reflects a neoliberal ideology that prioritizes entrepreneurship and innovation as the only solutions to development challenges. In several conversations with Evy, for example, she emphasizes that the term "Silicon Savannah" signals the need for more nuanced and context-specific approaches to the study of technology and development in Africa, and for greater attention to the complex social, cultural, and economic dynamics of technology development in the region:

> Just because there's a Silicon Valley? Why not be a Nairobi? Why do you have to be a Silicon Savannah? I have to put a disclaimer though, I'm very passionate about the continent of Africa. And when you see Silicon Savannah it almost seems like you're again, modelling to the West, instead of being innovative in doing your own thing. Have you heard of Ubuntu? Ubuntu is so African. Crowdfunding something else, but it's African! Like, why can't we have an Ubuntu for Silicon Savannah? I get it mostly from tech-based discussions, where we talk about Silicon Savannah; but why? We have Ubuntu and Ubuntu is successful in the world, embrace Ubuntu— and then Silicon Valley can adapt and become us. (Evy, Interview 2021)

In the African context, Ubuntu refers to a philosophy and way of life that emphasizes interconnectedness, community, and compassion for others. The term originates from various Bantu languages and is commonly used in southern Africa, particularly among the Zulu and Xhosa people. Ubuntu values emphasize the importance of treating others with respect and dignity, promoting harmony and cooperation within communities, and acknowledging the shared humanity that connects all individuals. It stresses the importance of relationships, family, and community, rather than individualistic pursuits. This can include acts of generosity, kindness, and compassion toward others, as well as a sense of responsibility toward the broader world. Ubuntu has become increasingly recognized as a valuable philosophy for promoting social justice, reconciliation, and sustainable development in Africa and beyond. It has been incorporated into various fields, including education, healthcare, and politics, with the aim of fostering greater social cohesion and collective well-being. Evy expressed this deep-seated commitment to local African solutions in the Kenyan context. Rather than simply modeling to the West and replicating (business) models and best practices, she argues that replicating a Silicon Valley in Africa is not innovative and does not embrace the uniqueness and potential of the African continent. Instead, she advocates for embracing existing African concepts like Ubuntu and creating innovative solutions that are tailored to the local context.

While most FemTech products cater primarily to people in the West, targeting white, middle-class affluent women, less investment and attention is drawn towards locally created solutions. Evy explains that most funding is allocated to entrepreneurs residing in the Global North aiming to disrupt their own market: *"This is where the money goes—unless you have a white co-founder or a good and sad story to tell"* (Evy, Interview 2021). This resonates with Ruth's critical observation of entrepreneurs' pitches to investors. Ruth works for a company that focuses on healthcare financing, data driven research, and that makes "inclusive health markets work in Sub-Saharan Africa" (Ruth, Interview 2022). "It is 'Poverty Porn' that sales," she says. In her point of view, some entrepreneurs perpetuate stereotypes by showing and telling exploitative imaginary or stories of people living in low-resource contexts to gain empathy and contributions from donors and investors.

> If you see that people are self-sufficient, they are taking care of or are figuring things out themselves, then there is no innovation that you can bring on board that can really change anything. You'd walk away if you're an investor. So you need to pitch that there is so much need that if you don't come now, the sky will fall on these people. At the end of the day, you have to show a gap that you want to be filled. (Ruth, Interview 2022)

Ruth notes that business development and fundraising professionals know how to communicate in the language that potential investors want to hear, but entrepreneurs themselves need to show evidence that their previous investments have yielded positive results. This will encourage investors to continue contributing to the business's mission. Moreover, Ruth accentuates that filling a gap with technology is not the only factor to consider when understanding underserved markets. She shares an example from her outreach to Mukuru, an informal settlement in Nairobi, where the lack of affordable and accessible health facilities is a major issue. While building a well-equipped facility in the area would be a good solution, she points to other more remote areas where the "brick and mortar system" might already be established, but professional medical staff are scarce. Ruth points out: *"what innovations are you bringing in to disrupt? Who are you serving, really?"* (Ruth, Interview 2022). Ruth invites to critically question whether emerging innovations like FemTech, have the potential to disrupt and serve people, or rather, help the entrepreneurs to sustain their own business ideas and developments.

Both, Evy and Ruth are concerned with this narration which seems detrimental and in opposition to the narrative of Silicon Savannah as emerging market. While Kenya is on the rise as a promising emerging market, women' sexual and reproductive health seems to be tied to discriminatory biases. During my fieldwork, many of the—mostly middle class—women explained that they were using period tracking apps to trace fertile days for conception, even though the FemTech solution was marketed to prevent unwanted and teenage pregnancy. When telling Evy about it, she laughed, *"that is what I mean, you sell the product as disrupting a novel market and helping the 'poor' African women to avoid pregnancy, when really many of us are using it not only for contraception but for fertility"* (Evy, Interview 2022).

Anna, who is also active within Nairobi's LGBTQ community, highlights the challenges of facing discrimination in accessing healthcare service more generally. She expressed her frustration with discrimination she, her community, but also pregnant teenagers face by individuals within the healthcare sector: *"Last month I experienced some problems. You know how many times I had to tell my gynecologist that there is no way I am pregnant? At first, he was convinced that my problems were related to a pregnancy"* (Anna, Interview 2021). She believes that it is crucial to build an environment without judgment in order to reduce misinformation and to promote the use of contraception. Anna highlights the fear of being judged by community health workers, doctors, and nurses when discussing intimate matters, which can deter individuals from seeking necessary medical advice or services. According to her, there is a huge potential for FemTech offering a less judgmental environment to discuss health matters.

During a conversation with Mary, I raised the aforementioned matter. Mary is a young Kenyan AI specialist who just graduated from Nairobi's Moringa School for technology education:

> Well, building a chat bot is not a problem as long as you have qualified professionals and verified information. But have you watched the Netflix documentary 'Coded Bias?' or 'The Social Dilemma'? There is a lot of racism and racists bias in our technology already, as the documentaries show. Especially in the health sector, it is not only about how the data is being coded or by whom with which purpose—but also the very data itself. (Mary, Interview 2022)

Mary refers to the fact that while women account for half of the world's population, yet most medical and health research is conducted with men. While the female body is a more complex organisms to study and test medication on due to physiological changes associated with the menstrual cycle, contraceptive use, and menopause, research tends to be more time-consuming and expensive. This also applies to other demographic factors represented in applied data and clinical trials, including the underrepresentation of people of colour. A presumed due to While medical mistrust has been cited as a reason for low participation in clinical trails, for example, evidence suggest systemic racism and structural factors as contributing factors. Hence, it could be argued that the data embedded to design FemTech tools does not universally apply to all individuals.

Disrupting healthcare delivery, access to health information and services therefore needs to include emerging markets and low-resources settings from the onset. This also applies to linguistic bias, since the dominance of English datasets for language processing often prohibits the "digital inclusion" of people who do not speak English. After confirming that the FemTech company she works for operate their digital tools in English only, Mary questions *"whether those FemTech solutions really address low-resource settings or primarily people from the middle-class, I do not know… When these technologies want to disrupt the space, then this is only possible by including the context. Modeling it to the West or the Global North, its bodies, and language will not be truly innovating the space"* (Mary, Interview 2021).

The context of Silicon Savannah as an emerging market has created an enabling environment for the development and potential impact of FemTech in the region. The conversations around Silicon Savannah's potential facilitated a surge in attention and influx of funding, support, and access to resources such as talent and infrastructures contributing to the growth of the digital health industry, including FemTech for sexual and reproductive health in Kenya and beyond. The context of Silicon Savannah has provided a fertile ground for this disruption, enabling the emergence of a community of innovators and entrepreneurs who are challenging established healthcare practices and developing new solutions to address the sexual and reproductive health issues. This disruption has created opportunities for new actors, such as FemTech startups, to enter the healthcare market and offer innovative solutions to long-standing sexual health challenges. At the same time, it has also challenged existing actors in the healthcare system to adapt to new technologies and models of healthcare delivery. In the case of FemTech in Kenya, the emergence of digital health solutions has disrupted traditional models of healthcare delivery, creating new opportunities for innovation and entrepreneurship.

The uncritical acceptance of digital health technologies as an empowerment tool for women, as well as the assumption that access to technology equals empowerment, however, warrants critical examination. Drawing on Deborah Lupton's (2013, 2015, 2016b) critique of digitized health promotion, she reminds us that digital health technologies, such as mHealth, privilege a rational consumer who prioritizes health over other aspects of their lives. Most of the time, this user needs to be competent in using digital technologies and is willing to take responsibility for their own self-care and preventive health efforts. This suggests, however, that those who lack access to digital technologies, and are not proficient in using them, are automatically excluded from the benefits of digital healthcare delivery. Moreover, access to digital health technologies is often contingent on one's ability to afford often expensive data plans to run FemTech applications and to have the time to do so, which privileges those who have not only financial resources *"but also, and more important, access to leisure time in which to track your glucose, analyze data logs for patterns, contact and develop a relationship with a health coach, or even to have a glass of orange juice or go for a walk"* (Levina, 2017, p. 559).

Conclusion: FemTech in (and for) Emerging Markets

The rapid growth of information and communications technologies and mHealth services in Sub-Saharan Africa has made affordable and easily accessible FemTech solutions an attractive resource in low-resource settings. Emerging markets in Africa have been considered underserved yet promising, and they have relevant technological and digital infrastructure that promises considerable economic growth. While universal healthcare remains limited in most of these emerging markets, girl-centered and entrepreneurial approaches to development are omnipresent phenomena. As such, private companies are advertising FemTech as a novel and powerful driver of change for people living in contexts with limited resources.

Emerging markets like Kenya, with rapid population growth, increasing urbanization, a growing middle class, and a shift toward a market-based economy, have accounted for a significant proportion of global economic growth and have attracted substantial foreign investment. This has led to the emergence of tech-ecosystems like "Silicon Savannah," with significant potential to tackle social and environmental challenges in Africa through scalable and profitable technological innovation. Kenya stands out as one of the first countries in Sub-Saharan Africa with considerable progress in expanding internet access and digital infrastructure, positioning it as an attractive location for tech companies seeking to establish a foothold on the continent. With its unmatched ubiquity of internet connectivity, high mobile phone penetration, and fast mobile internet speeds, Kenya has emerged as a leading country in technological innovation and progressive ICT growth in Africa.

While the COVID-19 pandemic acted as an accelerant for FemTech innovation in Kenya, with HealthTech companies and investors viewing it as an opportunity for local innovations and market expansion. Digital COVID-19 tools, such as smartphone apps and online platforms, became a common feature in FemTech products, with users being able to assess their symptoms of the virus through a digital questionnaire. Disruption was seen as a positive notion in the tech-ecosystem's rhetoric, but it also faced criticism for promoting a view of disruptive innovation that neglects other forms of innovation and disregards long-term societal benefits and sustainable development. While FemTech tools are envisioned to empower women and to address their sexual and reproductive health issues innovatively, the reliance on digital technologies and data infrastructures raises concerns about the implications of the tech-sector's use of private data. The term "Silicon Savannah" has been critically analyzed by various scholars and people in the tech-ecosystem. Mary, Anna and Evy, for example, all agree that the term represents a Western-centric view of the African technology industry and overlooks the unique context and dynamics of technology development in Africa.

Additionally, the term may promote an oversimplified and one-dimensional view of African economies, emphasizing the technology industry's role in driving economic growth and development, while neglecting other critical sectors such as inequality, poverty, and sustainability. Rather than copying and pasting external models, they advocate for embracing existing African concepts and creating innovative solutions that are tailored to the local context.

References

African Development Bank. (2019). African economic outlook 2019. Macroeconomic performance and prospects; jobs, growth and firm dynamism; integration for Africa's economic prosperity. https://doi.org/10.1007/978-1-349-74024-6_59.

African Development Bank Group. (2020). African economic outlook 2020. Developing Africa's workforce for the future. *Annual Yearly Review Study*. https://www.afdb.org/fileadmin/uploads/afdb/Documents/Publications/African_Economic_Outlook_2018_-_EN.pdf

Bramann, J. U. (2017). Building ICT entrepreneurship ecosystems in resource-scarce contexts. Learnings from Kenya's 'silicon savannah.' In *Digital Kenya. An Entrepreneurial Revolution in the Making* (pp. 227–264). https://doi.org/10.1057/978-1-137-57878-5.

Bramann, J. U. (2016). *The emergence of Kenya's „silicon Savannah". Building ICT entrepreneurship ecosystems in resource-scarce contexts and Mobile technology's potential to tackle unemployment.* Leipzig Graduate School of Management.

Caron, C. M., & Margolin, S. A. (2015). Rescuing girls, investing in girls: A critique of development fantasies. *Journal of International Development, 27*(7), 881–897. https://doi.org/10.1002/jid.3146

Demombynes, G., & Thegeya, A. (2012). *Kenya's mobile revolution and the promise of mobile savings.* World Bank Policy Research Working Paper. Vol. 5988. http://econ.worldbank.org/external/default/main?pagePK=64165259&piPK=64165421&theSitePK=469372&menuPK=64166093&entityID=000158349_20120306084347.

Folaranmi, T. (2014). MHealth in Africa: Challenges and opportunities. *Perspectives in Public Health, 134*(1), 14–15. https://doi.org/10.1177/1757913913514703

Hayhurst, L. M. C. (2011). Corporatising sport, gender and development: Postcolonial IR feminisms, transnational private governance and global corporate social engagement. *Third World Quarterly, 32*(3), 531–549. https://doi.org/10.1080/01436597.2011.573944

Hayhurst, L. M. C. (2013). Girls as the 'new' agents of social change? Exploring the 'girl effect' through sport, gender and development programs in Uganda. *Sociological Research Online, 18*(2), 1–12.

Hayhurst, L. M. C. (2014). The 'girl effect' and martial arts: Social entrepreneurship and sport, gender and development in Uganda. *Gender, Place and Culture, 21*(3), 297–315. https://doi.org/10.1080/0966369X.2013.802674

International Finance Corporation, World Bank Group. (2022, January 5). *World Bank Group and CTA announce winners of Global Women's HealthTech Awards.* https://pressroom.ifc.org/all/pages/pressdetail.aspx?id=26778

Jack, W., & Suri, T. (2011). *Mobile money. The economics of M-Pesa* (pp. 1–30). NBER Working Paper Series.

Kaur, R. (2018a). Southern futures. Thinking through emerging markets. *Comparative Studies of South Asia, Africa and the Middle East, 38*(2), 365–376. https://doi.org/10.1215/1089201x-6982134

Kaur, R. (2018b). World as commodity. Or, how the 'third world' became an 'emerging market'. *Comparative Studies of South Asia, Africa and the Middle East, 38*(2), 377–395. https://doi.org/10.1215/1089201x-6982145

Levina, M. (2017). Disrupt or die: Mobile health and disruptive innovation as body politics. *Television & New Media, 18*(6), 548–564. https://doi.org/10.1177/1527476416680451

Lupton, D. (2013). Quantifying the body: Monitoring and measuring health in the age of MHealth technologies. *Critical Public Health, 23*(4), 393–403. https://doi.org/10.1080/09581596.2013.794931

Lupton, D. (2015). Quantified sex: A critical analysis of sexual and reproductive self-tracking using apps. *Culture, Health and Sexuality, 17*(4), 440–453. https://doi.org/10.1080/13691058.2014.920528

Lupton, D. (2016a). The diverse domains of quantified selves. Self-tracking modes and dataveillance. *Economy and Society, 45*(1), 101–122. https://doi.org/10.1080/03085147.2016.1143726

Lupton, D. (2016b). *The quantified self. A sociology of self-tracking.* Polity Press.

Muli, E., Waithanji, R., Kamita, M., Gitau, T., Obonyo, I., Mweni, S., Mutisya, F., Kirira, P., Nzioka, A., Figueroa, J. D., & Makokha, F. (2021). Leveraging Technology for Health Services Continuity in times of COVID-19 pandemic. Patient follow-up, and mitigation of worse patient outcomes. *Journal of Global Health, 11.* https://doi.org/10.7189/JOGH.11.05024

Mureithi, M. (2017). The internet journey for Kenya. The interplay of disruptive innovation and entrepreneurship in fueling rapid growth. In *Digital Kenya. An entrepreneurial revolution in the making* (pp. 27–53). https://doi.org/10.1057/978-1-137-57878-5.

Nafus, D., & Sherman, J. (2014). This one does not go up to 11: The quantified self movement as an alternative big data practice. *International Journal of Communication, 8*(1), 1784–1794.

Ndemo, B., & Weiss, T. (2017). *Digital Kenya. An entrepreneurial revolution in the making.* Palgrave Macmillian. OriginURL. https://link.springer.com/book/10.1057/978-1-137-57878-5

Ndemo, B. (2017). The paradigm shift: Disruption, creativity, and innovation in Kenya. *In Digital Kenya. An Entrepreneurial Revolution in the Making,* 1–12.

Ndemo, E. B. (2015). Political entrepreneurialism. Reflections of a civil servant on the role of political institutions in technology innovation and diffusion in Kenya. *Stability, 4*(1), 1–14. https://doi.org/10.5334/sta.fd

Neff, G. (2019). The political economy of digital health. *Society and the Internet, 281–92*. https://doi.org/10.1093/oso/9780198843498.003.0017

Njoroge, M., Zurovac, D., Ogara, E. A. A., Chuma, J., & Kirigia, D. (2017). Assessing the feasibility of EHealth and MHealth. A systematic review and analysis of initiatives implemented in Kenya. *BMC Research Notes, 10*(1), 1–11. https://doi.org/10.1186/s13104-017-2416-0

Nyabola, N. (2018). *Digital democracy, analogue politics*. Bloomsbury Publishing.

Ombere, S. O. (2021). Access to maternal health services during the COVID-19 pandemic: Experiences of indigent mothers and health care providers in Kilifi County, Kenya. *Frontiers in Sociology, 6*(April), 1–8. https://doi.org/10.3389/fsoc.2021.613042

Pollio, A. (2020). Making the silicon cape of Africa: Tales, theories and the narration of startup urbanism. *Urban Studies Journal Limited, 57*(13), 2715–2732. https://doi.org/10.1177/0042098019884275

Ruckenstein, M., & Pantzar, M. (2017). Beyond the quantified self: Thematic exploration of a Dataistic paradigm. *New Media and Society, 19*(3), 401–418. https://doi.org/10.1177/1461444815609081

Ruckenstein, M., & Schüll, N. D. (2017). The datafication of health. *Annual Review of Anthropology, 46*, 261–278. https://doi.org/10.1146/annurev-anthro-102116-041244

Strusani, D., & Houngbonon, G. V. (2020). *What COVID-19 means for digital infrastructure in emerging markets*. World Bank Publications.

Tamminen, S., & Holmgren, E. (2016). The anthropology of wearables: The self, the social, and the autobiographical. *Ethnographic Praxis in Industry Conference Proceedings, 2016*(1), 154–174. https://doi.org/10.1111/1559-8918.2016.01083

Waema, T. W., & Ndung'u, M. N. (2012). Understanding what is happening in ICT in Kenya. *Policy Paper, 52*(9), 1–56.

Wangamati, C. K., & Sundby, J. (2020). The ramifications of COVID-19 on maternal health in Kenya. *Sexual and Reproductive Health Matters, 28*(1), 69–71. https://doi.org/10.1080/26410397.2020.1804716

World Bank Group. (2019). *Kenya economic update. Securing Future Growth. Policies to Support Kenya's Digital Transformation*.

World Economic Forum. (2015). *The global information technology report 2015. ICTs for inclusive growth*.

Zuboff, S. (2019). *The age of surveillance capitalism. The fight for a human future at the new frontier of power* (1st ed.). PublicAffairs.

Part III

FemTech to (Over)come: "New Methods, Technoselves and Data Sovereignty"

11

Wearing Danger: Surveillance, Control, and Quantified Healthism in American Medicine

Rebecca Monteleone and Ally Day

Introduction: A Story of Electronic Medical Records and Inequality

The third-floor offices of the 1920s' building in the midwest United States where the community health center rented us doula space were overly air-conditioned—outside it was over 100 degrees but inside I was shivering. I (Ally) was here making phone calls to potential clients, searching all people in the electronic medical record (EMR)[1] database who have had recent positive pregnancy tests and OB/GYN exams. According to the new grant received to counter the disproportionately high rates of infant and maternal mortality in our community among

---

[1] In this article, we refer to Electronic Medical Records at EMRs as opposed to the more general Electronic Health Record (EHR) for two reasons: It is the term used by the researchers we cite, and it highlights EMRs relationship to the larger Medical Industrial Complex. However, later in the article, we will cite an instance where a researcher chooses to reimagine the use of these kinds of records and names them Electronic Health Records (EHR).

R. Monteleone (✉) • A. Day
University of Toledo, Toledo, OH, USA
e-mail: Rebecca.Monteleone@UToledo.Edu

© The Author(s), under exclusive license to Springer Nature Singapore Pte Ltd. 2023   **237**
L. Balfour (ed.), *FemTech*, https://doi.org/10.1007/978-981-99-5605-0_11

African American people, all clients receiving care through the agency were entitled to free doula support, which includes prenatal education, physical labor and delivery support, and postnatal lactation support. I was working as one of these two free doulas. It was my fourth call of the day; according to the EMRs, this client was in their second trimester. I was taken aback when a deep assertive voice answered the phone—not because it was presumedly-male so much as because the phone was answered at all. I was used to leaving messages. I asked to speak to the client and, when asked who is calling, explained I am from the community health organization offering doula services. I heard a throat clearing and several voices muffled in the background. "My son was a still-birth," the voice explains. "And my wife still had to go through labor. Now is not a good time. We are going to the funeral." I quickly offered condolences and hang up, checking the chart again. Did I make a mistake? Did I miss a note? An "event" of labor and delivery?

No. Nothing. The last notation was a regular 15-min office exam, no complications noted. A few days later, I mentioned this interaction to my boss, the midwife running the new program. "This is the problem," she said. "The hospital EMRs can't talk to the clinic's EMRs so we never know if there were deliveries or emergencies with clients unless they come for a follow-up. And they never do."

"Why don't the EMRs talk to each other?" I asked.

"Because the hospitals have expensive EMRs that are used only within their closed system. And the clinic can't afford that infrastructure—it's too expensive for a nonprofit serving a low-income community." How can two EMR systems be so incompatible that we cannot have a clinic coordinate with an area hospital to capture all care received? It seems like a low bar to have a hospital delivery recorded in the database of the serving primary care physician.

The above example illustrates several key problems with the implementation of medical technology: the growing divide between those who can afford it (for profit hospitals) and those who cannot (nonprofit clinics); the limited opportunity to record a full client experience; and the increased probability of user mistakes or occlusions. In addition, those who are marginalized bear the disproportionate weight of these issues, in part because they may lack access to the most innovative and up to date technologies, and in part because of existing racist and ableist biases that shape the technology and the environment in which it is deployed. In the following article, we explore the technological innovations and fault-lines around medical and wellness technologies that standardize and quantify technologies that form the cornerstone of FemTech. Analyzing Electronic Medical Records and wearable data trackers, we place their development in a larger historical context, questioning their efficacy in our current sociopolitical context of deep structural inequality in relation to medical care, and interrogating the futures their use anticipate. We analyze this technology from our expertise in critical disability studies, a field that centers not just the experience of disability, but the ways in which social, political, and medical systems construct disabled subjects in the first place. Critical disability studies ask us to reject simple categorization of able-bodied and disabled and to instead unpack the power dynamics that create those categories in the first place. Interrogating who creates technology, and who benefits from technology's use, is a project of critical disability studies.

Recent technological innovations have allowed EMRs to integrate data from wearable health devices such as activity trackers, leading to new technological and ethical concerns, which include, but are not limited to, data overload and interpretation, data management and storage (and environmental considerations of cloud storage) and user confidentiality and consent. While visions of utopian technologically driven futures among healthcare providers and engineers undergird these innovation projects, we question the efficacy and ethics of this most recent material transformation. How will it affect what we deem knowledge about bodies and Medicine[2]?

Recent conversations in Feminist Science and Technology Studies and feminist health highlight how our current neoliberal medical system no longer serves patients in need of care but consumers in search of a product (Dubriwny, 2012). In this chapter, however, we argue that with the advent and utilization of commercialized healthcare technologies such as EMRs, medical consumers are no longer in search of products;

---

[2] We capitalize Medicine to connote the systemic and institutionalized practice of Medicine and not individualized treatments and care per se.

they become the product through their data; the new consumers in this system are the hospitals, clinics, and commercial entities that collect data to be bought and sold in a medical marketplace. When it comes to community health clinics that serve a population reliant on Medicaid in the United States, such as the one referred to above, the valuable data accrued by the clinic come from people who have little agency within the larger medical system (an assumption we will return to in this article's conclusion); pregnant people must procure prenatal care or they risk further intervention of state systems once their child is delivered. Seeking care at a community health clinic is often the only viable option for poor pregnant people, and so their engagement with these technical systems is not optional. In the process of this transformation from patient to consumer to product, a knowledge transformation also occurs. Embodied knowledge (what a person knows, feels, conveys about themselves) is supplanted by clinical knowledge (what the practitioner assumes, deduces, records), which is then supplanted by algorithmic calculations (what a technological system measures, records, reduces, and analyzes). At the same time, new regimes of power emerge, creating expectations of optimization and self-management through datafication. As such, the bodies of those most marginalized (femme bodies, bodies of color, disabled bodies, poor bodies) become *dis*embodied and fragmented data sets, where an agonizing stillbirth becomes just another occlusion.

From Bedside to Lab to Everywhere All at Once: Medical Transformations in the Twentieth Century

Women, femmes, and female-bodied people are increasingly turning to technologies to monitor and manage their health needs. In this section, we address two historical decades that offer us ruptures, opportunities and lenses through which to view the most recent technological developments; doing so, we argue that historical precedents of techno-optimism—or the belief that technological innovation is central to creating better futures—coupled with the promise to provide individualized care while extracting data, can provide an entry point to understanding this current technological moment.

Roughly 100 years ago, the United States marked a significant historical shift in both how its citizens practiced medicine and how medicine itself was understood. As historian Nancy Tomes (2016) writes, the "old-style family doctor" was being replaced by a "better kind of medical man" in the 1920s (p.48). This new medical doctor expected patients to pay more for his services; in exchange, he offered "increasingly sophisticated, technologically advanced services, the need for which they [the patients] could not easily judge for themselves" (p. 48). This generation of doctors faced "higher educational standards" than the previous generation's family doctors, and tougher licensing laws (p. 49). In addition, by eliminating house calls, doctors could also provide more "technological marvels" from their office or their local hospital (49). The American Medical Association, still in its adolescence, continued to market these new doctors with a techno-optimism despite a much more varied reality. "Not only was the upgrading of new standards more slow and uneven than they admitted," writes Tomes, "but the profession was also unsettled by the rapid advance of specialization. [...] The public had been promised a more 'standardized profession' than could actually be delivered" in the interwar years (p. 50). During this time period, it was economically much more advantageous to be a specialist than a general practitioner and these doctors benefited from new technologies such as electrocardiograms, blood tests for chemical analysis (complete with advanced microscopes and slide-making equipment), autoclaves for equipment sterilization, x-ray units, physiotherapy equipment, clinical thermometers, steel needles, surgical knives, and syringes. By the 1930s, doctors appeared to have a much more objective and measurable means to assess patient health, all through the creation and aggressive advertisement of medical technology. Tomes argues that it is within this time period that patients were truly transformed into consumers, encouraged by popular magazines to doctor shop, which in turn led to "buyer's remorse" when patient-consumers reviewed bills and were unable to assess the necessity of a particular technological intervention. In sum, during the interwar years, Americans became more expectant of advanced medical technologies in their doctor visits while remaining skeptical of its cost and value.

The late-twentieth century marked another transformation in American medicine, characterized by an expansion of medical authority out of the clinic and into everyday life. Rapid innovation in biomedical technologies paired with an increasing social pressure to self-govern in pursuit of optimal health produced a context in which all embodiment came under the jurisdiction of the medical establishment. In the preceding years, the role of the doctor had moved from one of cognitive authority at the bedside to what Jewson (1976) dubs "Laboratory Medicine" through the medical technologies mentioned above, which jettisoned observational and clinical judgment in favor of scientific and statistical analysis. Pathology became contingent on identification through testing and quantification of bodily processes, and a physician's role shifted to one of data interpretation.

In essence and as argued throughout this volume, the body became datafied. Information and data management—including management through standardized medical records and diagnostic codes—became central to healthcare (Bowker & Star, 1999; Clarke et al., 2003). Simultaneously, greater ability to screen, record, and compare health data, couched in the emerging rhetoric of preventative medicine, established new categories of risk. Prevention justified expanded authority to monitor not just the unwell, but the always-potentially-unwell, ushering in an era of surveillance (Armstrong, 1995). New identities and social positions emerged as the boundaries between healthy and unhealthy blurred. One became at-risk through the identification of genetic markers or new classifications such as "pre-diabetic" (Aronowitz, 2009). And, as Clarke and colleagues write (2003), citing the work of Deborah Lupton (1995, 1999) and Alexandra Howson (1998), "risks are calculated and assessed in order to rationalize surveillance, and through surveillance risks are conceptualized and standardized into ever more precise calculations and algorithms" (p. 172). Under this new biomedical political economy, risk is not *discovered*, but *induced* through new means of testing, measuring, and quantifying life. This process pathologized (and therefore authorized the surveillance of) the entire population.

Surveillance medicine, a term coined by sociologist David Armstrong in 1995, did not limit itself to what could be measured via blood tests, body measurements, or karyotypes, but expanded into all aspects of one's lifestyle. As Armstrong writes of health promotion strategies after the Second World War, "concerns with diet, exercise, stress, sex, etc. became vehicles for encouraging the community to survey itself. The ultimate triumph of surveillance medicine would be its internalization by all the population" (1995, p. 400). Coupled with the powerful discourse of neo-liberal self-responsibility, this focus on self-monitoring and management moralized health. As Robert Crawford (1980) writes, "healthy behavior has become the paradigm for good living," a concept he dubs "healthism" (p. 380).

The transformation of medicine to one that a) relies on the accumulation of data via technoscience, b) produces new identities and categories of risk, expanding the authoritative reach of medicine, and c) moralizes health and optimization as individual responsibilities, lays the groundwork for increasingly invasive, oppressive, and standardized means of surveillance (Clarke et al., 2003). By couching this transformation in a discourse of self-empowerment and techno-optimism, medical and tech industries deceive and coerce users, extracting and profiting from their data on the unfulfilled promise of meaningful, personalized care. This process enables the emergence of biomedical technologies such as EMRs and wearable data trackers that reduce and make commensurate diverse bodily experiences.

Reduction and Responsibility: Calculating Embodiment

In this section, we look at how the development and implementation of EMRs and wearable data trackers fit into a larger historical pattern of techno-optimism and ethical duplicity, tracing some of the particular narratives embedded in both technologies that produce and reproduce conditions that confer agency and authority only to professionals, reduce and undermine embodiment, and moralize the quantification of health.

Put simply, EMRs work to standardize records across healthcare professionals, allowing data input in one computer to be accessible across a building or medical campus by another professional. Rarely do nonclinicians have the opportunity to access this data, let alone self-report (Day, 2021). Additionally, what medical professionals' input are often medical codes for billing information or short-hand responses to demographic or symptom data; there is rarely a way these symptoms can capture longer narratives or medical observation, which elides the complex embodied knowledge of the person seeking care (Day, 2021). As a result, treatment plans are prescriptive and standardized, leaving little room for individual assessment and leading to a moralizing of patient noncompliance (Day, 2021).

The first three years of the COVID-19 epidemic have exposed large-scale technological and procedural shortcomings in the US health systems, ushering in another important moment in medical technology and its material transformations. For example, news reports have called for a significant upgrade to EMRs, noting that while 96% of hospitals and 84% of medical offices use EMRs, they lack ability to transfer data outside of the on-site server, leading to a fragmentation of user data as seen in the opening vignette. Additionally, because EMRs require manual input and interpretation, they are insufficient for providing real-time treatment needed in times of COVID-19 diagnosis and care (Pryor et al., 2020; Shulte, 2020). While EMRs have been in operation since the mid-1960s, it was not until the passage of the Affordable Care Act in 2011, which included a "Meaningful Use" provision for technological development in care coordination and quality as well as security of data, that EMR usage significantly increased.

In calling for an overhaul of EMRs (instead referring to these as Electronic Health Records), John Glaser writes that we are "beyond fixing user interface or interoperability [...] The overhaul must also support the ability of providers to adopt the new value-based-care business model of healthcare—one that rewards providers for outcomes rather than the volume of services and that shifts their focus from reactive sick care to the proactive management of health" (Glaser, 2020, p. 3). While Glaser highlights a key ideological problem with the commercialization of American Medicine, his call to action relies on an understanding of preventative medicine that authorizes surveillance in the pursuit of bodily optimization.

One approach to this "proactive management of health" that has gained traction in the past decade is the integration of wearable data into EMRs. Broadly defined as electronic tools that can be worn via clothing, accessories (watches) or skin adhesive, wearable data trackers these devices collect data and analyze data from the user in real time while they are doing their daily tasks (Al-Azwani and Aziz, 2016, p. 151). These devices are portable, accessible, and multifunctional; some, such as insulin monitors or vital sign monitors, are approved in the United States by the Food and Drug Administration, but most are not (ibid). The most popular wearable devices, such as fitness trackers, have no responsibility or way to ensure accurate data collection, and no responsibility to data security (ibid).

In 2019, there were more than 400 commercial wearable tracking devices that are compatible with EMRs, and that number continues to grow (Dinh-Le et al., 2019). Apple and Google have both developed products, interfaces, and storage solutions specifically aimed at integrating and collating health data (Apple Healthkit and Google Cloud Healthcare API). Enabled through a collaboration with several major EMR companies, users of Apple's Health app, for example, can share biodata such as heart rate, menstrual cycle, steps, and sleep patterns directly with their clinicians (Apple, 2021). We contend that the integration of wearable technologies into this overhaul does not meet the standards of "value-based care" that Glaser calls for, in part due to the historical precedent of techno-optimism and ethical duplicity in healthcare, but also due to the increasing unreliability of user data and fragmentation of patient identity. Like EMRs, wearable data trackers serve to reduce embodiment to a discrete set of standardized measurements. Not only does this process create roadblocks to holistic care, but it also deepens the disconnect between a person and their body by interpreting the ostensibly objective data from trackers as more "real" than embodied experience (Del Busso et al., 2021; Lupton, 2016). An extension of what Susan Wendell (1996) describes as an "alienation from our bodies and our bodily experiences" through the privileging of scientific medical authority and subsequent invalidation of embodied knowledge, data trackers displace self-narratives of bodily experiences in favor of data accumulation (p. 119). Ultimately, quantification and standardization through data trackers produce an illusion of control. This control, however, is applied inequitably. Women's bodies, for example, are targeted due to the historic perception that they are "difficult to make sense of and in need of discipline and augmentation, particularly in relation to women's biology, size/surface and comportment" (Del Busso et al., 2021, p. 18). Marginalized, unpredictable, and unruly bodies—fat bodies, disabled bodies, queer, and trans bodies—are those most subject to the processes of surveillance, reduction, and commensuration enabled by the tracking technologies.

As mentioned above, bodily quantification is not just a tool applied by the medical establishment as seen with EMRs, but one that has become internalized as necessary for managing and perfecting oneself. Self-monitoring and quantification in pursuit of individual perfection is deeply entangled in the fabric of the American imagination. In the eighteenth century, Benjamin Franklin diligently tracked his pursuit of "moral perfection" through a physical chart (Neff & Nafus, 2016). In the early twentieth century, calorie tracking for weight loss exemplified the positivist ideals embraced in the Progressive Era (Jou, 2018). Now, your Apple Watch encourages you to "close your rings" by reaching (often arbitrary) goals around calorie consumption, standing, and exercising. The quest for health optimization by means of self-monitoring and data tracking have come to be understood in American culture as righteous and virtuous: To pursue health is to assert oneself as a responsible, manageable citizen (Cardell, 2018; Goodley, 2016; Wernimont, 2018). The consequences of this moralization are manifold. If one's body cannot be "made perfect" through these self-governing processes, it is understood as a moral failing, particularly if that body is a gendered or racialized one. This is true regardless of whether the expectations of health optimization are even possible within the constraints of the technology. In a literature review of women's experiences of self-tracking devices, Del Busso et al. (2021) found that women commonly reported that when wearables gave them feedback for improvement, they felt as if they were "failing at being healthy," even when the data interpreted by the wearables failed to account for exigencies such as pregnancy or recent surgery (p. 15). The rhetoric of self-optimization through data tracking, which promotes self-control and restriction as virtues, can also be observed in pro-eating disorder online communities (Greene & Brownstown, 2021). In a 2021 study conducted with young women with eating disorders in college or university settings, Elizabeth Eikey found that the emphasis on quantification in diet and fitness apps exacerbated disordered eating, led to obsessive thoughts, and provided a rigid and rewarding structure for caloric restriction. Ultimately, these technologies create a standard of personal accountability that attributes blame when someone does not meet health optimization standards while at the same time ceding authority to interpret embodiment to a clinical or (often obscured, often decontextualized) algorithmic authority.

Becoming Profitable Data: New Identities Through Quantified Healthism

In this section, we will explore the emergence of new regimes of authority and identity through what we dub "quantified healthism," exemplified through the integration of wearable tracking data into EMRs. Throughout this analysis, we interrogate how the consequences of the surveillance, consumption, and commensuration of bodies come to bear especially on women, femmes, and disabled people, those who interact with medical authority most often on behalf of themselves or as caretakers.

Anticipating futures of reductionist and datafied health technologies means recognizing the ways in which these futures are already upon us. In September 2022, Google Cloud partnered with Fitbit to produce Device Connect, which streamlines the process of providing tracking data to health organizations. With the aim of "support[ing] care teams and empower[ing] patients to live healthier lives," Device Connect creates a frictionless system for consenting users to share data with healthcare organizations, as well as for those organizations to collate, visualize, and analyze it (Lynch & Mcdonough, 2022). While couched in the rhetoric of patient-centered care, citing examples like the management of chronic disease and postoperative recovery, the true value of Device Connect lies in the ability to leverage large data sets for research and population-level study. The immediate extraction and abstraction of data away from individual user and toward aggregation reveals a new major technoscientific identity transformation: users as *data*.

Clarke et al. (2003) argue that the contemporary healthcare landscape is ripe for producing new technoscientific identities. The rise in surveillance medicine marks us all as in a constant state of uncertainty, on the cusp of disablement: We become "pre-symptomatic," "high risk," "patients-in-waiting" (Timmermans & Buchbinder, 2010), or the "worried well" (Garfield, 1970). As our biological data is extracted and interpreted, our bodies are not just standardized, but replaced entirely by what Stephen Horrocks (2019) dubs "datafied body doubles." Writing about technological interventions for Type 1 diabetes, Horrocks states that these "numerical stand-ins for the body…construct them as both usable and controllable," by users and clinicians (p. 2). As our experiences of embodiment become replaced by numerical models, our alienation from our bodies grows, as does the subsequent invalidation of our self-knowledge. We no longer simply rely on professionalized clinicians and their scientific authority to explain our bodies to ourselves, but on black-boxed and proprietary software that both determines what metrics are meaningful and how to make sense of them. What cannot be quantified is dismissed. Quantified healthism is rooted in these dual forces of neoliberal self-responsibility, which confuses health with virtue, and the abdication of authority to biomedical technologies, which reduces health to the discrete and measurable.

Furthermore, these data are valuable. Health data, particularly data collected by commercial entities through consumer products like data tracking devices, contributes to the multibillion-dollar data brokerage industry (Federal Trade Commission, 2014). Datafication makes disabled and nonnormative bodies legible—and therefore both manageable and profitable—to hegemonic power structures. The reduction of embodiment to a discrete set of measurements, erasing complex lived narratives, is essential for this process. As an analytic, quantified healthism contextualizes disembodiment through datafication in the ableist and capitalist structures that drive us to produce and use new biomedical technologies. Once bodies become calculable, they become profitable.

Biomedical Luddites? Resisting Technological Transformations Through Noncompliance

In 2018, disabled scholar Gabi Schaffzin co-opted data from his Fitbit and 23andMe profile to highlight the contradictions and neoliberal control inherent in the quantification of bodies. Taking the data produced by his Fitbit, he creates visual, auditory, and 3D artwork, exposing how abstract and arbitrary these metrics are. By reclaiming and reimagining these data, however, Schaffzin doesn't just critique quantification of bodies, he also reclaims ownership over his body. As he writes of his art, it is "useless as a means of training and diagnosis, but also completely valueless to those who may want to appropriate my condition for their gain" (p. 10).

Technological progress in the United States has become synonymous with social progress, creating a moral imperative to innovate and adopt ever-evolving tech (Marx, 1987). Paired with the neoliberal demand to optimize one's health through individual interventions and the integration of biomedical technologies into routine care, it is difficult to imagine futures where these technologies are not ubiquitous. If, as we propose, quantified healthism carries with it a dangerous practice of surveillance and control that converts consumers into simplified and sellable data points sans narrative, then the question becomes how does one resist what seems like the inevitable adoption of these technologies. Drawing on Schaffzin's example above, the antihegemonic concept of crip technoscience and two historical examples of resistance, we propose a communitarian response of noncompliance to quantified healthism that co-opts and crips datafication while resisting a libertarian, individualized opting out.

How can we imagine a technological future that does not seek to control, make docile, or eliminate marginalized, disabled and nonnormative bodies? Aimi Hamraie and Kelly Fritsch (2019), for example, suggest doing so involves centering disabled knowledge in order to "harness technoscience for political action, refusing to comply with demands to cure, fix, or eliminate disability" (p. 2). They coined the term "crip technoscience" to describe this framework, distinguishing it from the science and technology that has oppressed nonnormative and marginalized bodies. Rather than rejecting technology out of hand, they argue that technology produced and deployed by and for disabled people, resisting neoliberal ideals such as independence and productivity, can work toward justice. Such an approach also requires shifting from thinking about the individual to thinking about (and with) the collective. M. Remi Yergeau (2013) provides an example of this kind of transformation in their critique of the disability-focused "hackathon." Moving away from technological innovations aimed at assimilating or fixing disabled and nonnormative bodies, they instead call for a "criptastic hacking" that "rails against forced normalization, one that moves from body-tweaking to something collective, activist, and systemic" (para 23). In other words, pushing past the intense individualization of medical technologies— which aim to make sense of and manage discrete bodies—we can make our way toward a technological future in which the target for intervention is eliminating systemic oppression.

In the 1960s and 1970s, feminist self-help movements became a popular way for women and female people to claim their rights to reproductive freedom, from forming and utilizing an underground phone tree in Chicago to access abortion providers (Jane Collective) (Kaplan, 1995) to forming self-help groups in California that, among other things, taught about and performed menstrual extraction (usually to avoid unwanted pregnancy) (Ruzek, 1978). Most sustaining of this movement was the creation of the Boston Women's Health Collective and their infamous collation of health advice and first-person accounts that became known as *Our Bodies, Ourselves* (OBOS), a volume that has endured 8 general editions and been translated into 34 languages as of 2022 (Boston Women's Health Collective, 2022; Kline, 2010). There are few important legacies here that are central to our argument: the first, this movement did not neglect technology but instead advocated for better technology, more user-friendly technology, technology for the use of individuals to be shared with medical providers at the consumer's discretion. This legacy can be understood through the many ways that women and femme body people have been encouraged to gain knowledge and advocate for themselves in OBOS writings and consciousness-raising groups. We propose that by providing technology to users to be utilized at their leadership with medical professionals, we invert the power dynamic of medical exceptionalism and data ownership. Second, the feminist health movement emphasized the importance of simple technology (see menstrual extraction devices, for instance) to be used in communitarian settings for individual health and community empowerment. This ideology shifts a focus in technological development from creating the most complex and expensive devices to that which is accessible, inexpensive, and long-lasting.

One might argue that if we improve wearables (to make them less expensive, e.g.) and create EMRs that are shared with patients, we could fulfill the ideology of the women's health movement. The problem is that this in and of itself does not solve the problem of datafication. Here, we may turn to the Luddite movement of the early nineteenth century. While the term Luddite is often thrown around to refer to someone who is opposed to or unfamiliar with the latest technology, the original Luddites, textile workers in Britain known for destroying newly introduced machines in factories, were most concerned with the kinds of technology that stripped workers of their rights. They were not against technology wholesale, but against that which would make human lives and communities more precarious (Conniff, 2011). What we can understand from this movement is not a solution that requires opting out of technology all together but rather, a lifestyle within which we opt-in but in haphazard and disruptive ways. We could, like Schaffzin's subversion of algorithmic certainty through the appropriation of his biodata into artwork, reclaim ownership of our body minds through individual disruption. To claim ownership over one's own body, however, one subverts the capitalist systems of diagnosis for the means of Medicine while still buying into (pun intended) the idea that a body is something to be owned, useless data and all.

Following the examples of criptastic hacking, Luddites and health activists before us, we call for a collective refusal of quantified healthism. For example, we may choose to wear an Apple Watch for its GPS capacity for a daily bike ride or run but refuse to wear it for most of the rest of the day. Thus, the data acquired (i.e., steps taken, heart rate, etc.) is incomplete—the data becomes part of Apple's data set, so to speak, but meaningless. Another way to think of this is by utilizing community health services for necessary prenatal care but refusing follow-up visits, creating open-ended patient records. In order to resist becoming another data point through which Medicine can profit, we propose that the best way to move forward in relation to medical technology is by embracing non-compliance. This embrace of noncompliance can come at the individual level but, perhaps more importantly, at a community level. We can see this kind of subversion of institutional structures that track and monetize data through movements such as mutual aid, which is an informal network that emerges where individuals provide for the immediate needs of one another while also demanding change at the structural level (Mendez, 2022). This kind of network has already been embraced by disabled people in larger urban areas (Piepzna-Samarasinha, 2018; Nishida, 2021) and can provide a template for noncompliance as a community project.

Through noncompliance, we resist becoming data.

References

Al-Azwani, I., & Aziz, H. (2016). Integration of wearable technologies into patients' medical records. *Quality in Primary Care, 24*(4), 151–155.

Apple. (2021, June 7). Apple advances personal health by introducing secure sharing and new insights. [Press Release]. https://www.apple.com/news-room/2021/06/apple-advances-personal-health-by-introducing-secure-sharing-and-new-insights/

Armstrong, D. (1995). The rise of surveillance medicine. *Sociology of Health and Illness, 17*(3), 393–404.

Aronowitz, R. (2009). The converged experience of risk and disease. *Milbank Quarterly, 87*(2), 417–442.

Boston Women's Health Collective. (2022). History and legacy. *Our Bodies Ourselves Today*. Retrieved November 15, 2022, from https://www.our-bodiesourselves.org/about-us/our-history/

Bowker, G., & Star, S. L. (1999). *Sorting things out: Classification and its consequences.* MIT Press.

Cardell, K. (2018). Is a fitbit a diary? Self-tracking and autobiography. *M/C Journal, 21*(1). https://doi.org/10.5204/mcj.1348

Clarke, A., Shim, J., Mamo, L., Fosket, J. R., & Fishman, J. (2003). Biomedicalization: Technoscientific transformations of health, illness, and US biomedicine. *American Sociological Review, 68*(2), 161–194.

Conniff, R. (2011). What the luddites really fought against. *Smithsonian Magazine.* https://www.smithsonianmag.com/history/what-the-luddites-really-fought-against-264412/

Crawford, R. (1980). Healthism and the medicalization of everyday life. *International Journal of Health Services, 10*(3), 365–388.

Day, A. (2021). *The political economy of stigma: HIV, memoir, medicine, and crip positionalities.* Ohio State University Press.

Del Busso, L., Brottveit, G., Løkkeberg, S. T., & Gluppe, G. (2021). 'Women's embodied experiences of using wearable digital self-tracking health technology: A review of qualitative research literature. *Health Care for Women International, 26*, 1–25.

Dinh-Le, C., Chuang, R., Chokshi, S., & Mann, D. (2019). Wearable health technology and electronic health record integration: Scoping review and future directions. *Journal of Medical Internet Research mHealth and uHealth, 7*(9). https://doi.org/10.2196/12861

Dubriwny, T. N. (2012). *The vulnerable empowered woman: Feminism, postfeminism, and women's health.* Rutgers University Press.

Federal Trade Commission. (2014). *Data brokers: A call for transparency and accountability.* https://www.ftc.gov/system/files/documents/reports/data-brokers-call-transparency-accountability-report-federal-trade-commission-may-2014/140527databrokerreport.pdf

Garfield, S. (1970). The delivery of medical care. *Scientific American*, April 1.

Glaser, J. (2020). It's time for a new kind of electronic health record. *Harvard Business Review: Analytics.* Retrieved November 2, 2022, from https://hbr.org/2020/06/its-time-for-a-new-kind-of-electronic-health-record

Goodley, D. (2016). *Disability studies: An interdisciplinary introduction* (2nd ed.). Sage.

Greene, A., & Brownstown, L. M. (2021). "Just a place to keep track of myself": Eating disorders, social media, and the quantified health. *Feminist Media Studies*, 1–18.

Hamraie, A., & Fritsch, K. (2019). Crip technoscience manifesto. *Catalyst: Feminism, Theory, Technoscience, 5*(1), 1–33.

Horrocks, S. (2019). Materializing datafied body doubles: Insulin pumps, blood glucose testing, and the production of usable bodies. *Catalyst: Feminism, Theory, Technoscience, 5*(1), 1–26.

Howson, A. (1998). Surveillance, knowledge and risk: The embodied experience of cervical cancer. *Health, 2*, 195–215.

Jewson, N. D. (1976). The disappearance of the sick-man from medical cosmology, 1770–1870. *Sociology, 10*(2).

Jou, C. (2018). The progressive era body project: Calorie-counting and "disciplining the stomach" in 1920s America. *The Journal of the Gilded Age and Progressive Era, 18*(4).

Kaplan, L. (1995). *The story of Jane: The legendary underground feminist abortion service*. University of Chicago Press.

Kline, W. (2010). *Bodies of knowledge: Sexuality, reproduction, and women's health in the second wave*. University of Chicago Press.

Lupton, D. (1995). *The imperative of health: Public health and the regulated body*. Sage.

Lupton, D. (1999). *Risk*. Routledge.

Lupton, D. (2016). *The quantified self*. Wiley.

Lynch, A. H., & Mcdonough, A. (2022, September 27). Introducing device connect for fitbit: How google cloud and fitbit are working together to help people live healthier lives. Retrieved November 18, 2022, from https://cloud.google.com/blog/topics/healthcare-life-sciences/device-connect-for-fitbit-powered-by-google-cloud

Marx, L. (1987). Does improved technology mean progress? *Technology Review*, 33–41.

Mendez, V. (2022). What does mutual aid mean, and how can it transform our world? globalgiving.org. Retrieved February 20, 2023, from https://www.globalgiving.org/learn/what-is-mutual-aid

Neff, G., & Nafus, D. (2016). *Self-tracking*. MIT Press.

Nishida, A. (2021). *Just care: Messy entanglements of disability, dependency and desire*. Temple University Press.

Piepzna-Samarasinha, L. (2018). *Care work: Dreaming disability justice. Arsenal Pulp Press.*, 2018.

Pryor, R., Atkinson, C., Cooper, K., Doll, M., Godbout, E., Stevens, M., & Bearman, G. (2020). The electronic medical record and Covid-19: Is it up to the challenge? *American Journal of Infection Control, 48*(8), 966–967.

Ruzek, S. (1978). *The women's health movement: Feminist alternatives to medical control*. Praegar Publishers.

Schaffzin, G. (2018). Reclaiming the margins in the face of the quantified self. *Review of Disability Studies: An International Journal, 14*(2).

Shulte, F. (2020, April 30). As coronavirus strikes, crucial data in electronic health records hard to harvest. *Kaiser Health News.* Retrieved November 18, 2022, from https://khn.org/news/as-coronavirus-strikes-crucial-data-in-electronic-health-records-hard-to-harvest/

Timmermans, S., & Buchbinder, M. (2010). Patients-in-waiting: Living between sickness and health in the genomics era. *Journal of Health and Social Behavior, 51*(4).

Tomes, N. (2016). *Remaking the American patient: How Madison Avenue and modern medicine turned patients into consumers.* University of North Carolina Press.

Wendell, S. (1996). *The rejected body: Feminist philosophical reflections on disability.* Routledge.

Wernimont, J. (2018). *Numbered lives: Life and death in quantum media.* MIT Press.

Yergeau, R. M. (2013). Disability hactivism. In M. Hocks & J. Sayers (Eds.), *Hacking the classroom: Eight perspectives.* Retrieved November 18, 2022, from http://cconlinejournal.org/hacking/

12

Between Liberation and Control: Mixing Methods to Investigate How Users Experience Menstrual Cycle Tracking Applications

Lisa Stuifzand and Rik Smit

Introduction

Around one-third of American women use a Menstrual Cycle Tracking Application (MCTA), and the most popular applications, Flo and Clue, have more than 55 million users combined (Garamvolgyi, 2022). In May and June 2022, that number started to go down, as many women discontinued and deleted these applications from their phones. The main reason for this was a leaked document that said the US Supreme Court would overturn *Roe vs. Wade* and thereby the federal right to abortion. Many users were afraid that their menstrual cycle data would be used against them in court if they chose to access abortion care. When the Supreme Court did, indeed, overturn the famous 1973 decision, this led to even more public scrutiny of period and health tracking apps for women (Torchinsky, 2022). Even if this concern might be hypothetical for now,

L. Stuifzand (✉) • R. Smit
University of Groningen, Groningen, Netherlands
e-mail: p.h.smit@rug.nl

commentators and experts pointed toward many of the unexplored risks of trusting one's intimate data to commercial tracking applications.

This chapter engages with users' experiences of, thoughts about, and attitudes toward MCTAs before (rumors of) the overturning of *Roe vs. Wade*. As a specific, but popular, form of FemTech, MCTAs allow for the tracking, monitoring, and quantification of the menstrual cycle and its associated symptoms. This input is then used by the app to provide predictions about the menstrual cycle (Bhimani, 2020; Karlsson, 2019; Kressbach, 2021; Levy & Romo-Avilés, 2019). This process can be referred to as the datafication (Van Dijck, 2014) of menstruation. Linked to ideas stemming from the quantified-self movement (Wolf, 2010), MCTAs are marketed as providing objective insights into the menstrual cycle, similar to other self-tracking technologies (Kressbach, 2021; Lupton, 2016). The numerical presentation of information in the form of analytics and data visualization makes it seemingly trustworthy (Lupton, 2015, 2016; Kressbach, 2021; Van Dijck, 2014). Through such representations, menstruators may view and even experience their own bodies and natural cycles in new ways.

The large-scale datafication of menstruation, as the introductory example shows, leads to new, critical questions and reinvigorates older debates concerning the relationship between the female body and (intimate) technology, biomedicalization, (self) surveillance, and control. In the first part of this chapter, we will (re)visit these questions and concerns. This is followed by a discussion of the methodology employed to answer our research question:

How is the female body datafied and commercialized through MCTAs, and to what extent are users experiencing these applications in terms of liberation and control?

In addition, this research question will be divided into three subquestions: (1) In what ways do MCTA users quantify themselves, and what are the reasons they quantify their menstruation? (2) How does the interface of MCTAs reflect different perspectives on the menstrual cycle, gender, fertility, and sexuality? (3) How do users of MCTAs experience both liberation and control through these applications, and what can cause those experiences?

After recapping the main issues surrounding MCTAs discussed in the previous chapter, this chapter in particular will showcase how a unique combination of quantitative and qualitative research methods can help shed a different light on FemTech research. Through a combination of quantitative Reddit content analysis and qualitative focus group research, the research questions will be answered. Hereby, we aim to provide empirically grounded analysis of user experiences and showcase work on the intersections of humanities and social science research.

The Datafication of Menstruation

MCTAs are often advertised as "empowering" tools that enable users to understand their cycle and body better and take control over their menstrual health (see Figs. 12.1 and 12.2). Beyond PR, some research has also demonstrated the positive effects of MCTAs. Levy and Romo-Avilés (2019), for instance, have pointed out that these applications help menstruators to improve their menstrual cycle and health literacy, making MCTAs, possibly, a promising tool for female empowerment. As

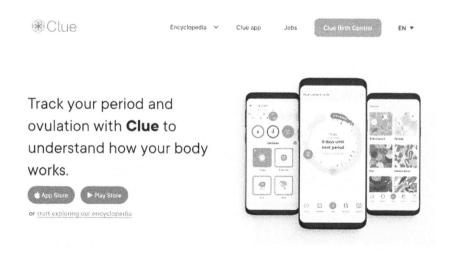

Fig. 12.1 Screenshot of the Clue website homepage

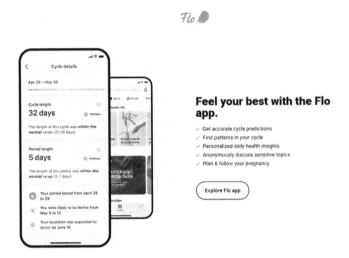

Fig. 12.2 Screenshot of the Flo website homepage

menstruators learn more about their cycle and become more confident in them and their bodies, chances are that they will want to share it with others, both online through these applications, on other platforms, and offline, decreasing the shame and taboo around menstruation (Kressbach, 2021; Verstappen, 2018). This has been confirmed by various studies on MCTAs (Hohmann-Marriott, 2021; Karlsson, 2019), which point out that users experience MCTAs as a means to push back on cultural norms surrounding the menstrual cycle and use algorithmic predictions to gain back control over their bodies. In addition, as women get more comfortable within their menstrual cycle, they tend to have a more positive body image, show more sexual assertiveness, have more sexual experiences, and simultaneously take fewer sexual risks (Schooler et al., 2005).

In addition to MCTAs, older menstrual technologies, such as tampons, pads, or planners, take such a prominent role in the bodily experience of menstruation that the menstruating body becomes socially constructed by culture rather than biologically determined (Haraway, 1991). Consequently, through the usage of technology, menstruators have the power to have more liberty and agency to construct themselves and their bodies. When data is entered into MCTAs, the body and the self become intertwined in human-data assemblages, making the body and self both the subject of scientific management and the product that results from it (Lupton, 2016). These assemblages are constantly modified as users enter new data into the MCTA, either manually or automatically, or when different data sets interact together (Lupton, 2015, 2018, 2019). MCTA users can try to take control of this assemblage by continuously working on their "data sense," as they combine personal information, generated by self-tracking practices, with their bodily sensations, affective responses, and the various cultural, personal, and spatial contexts in which they take place (Hohmann-Marriott, 2021; Lupton, 2018, 2019, 2020). As this menstrual self-tracking data becomes integrated into the user's life, the data in these applications is imbued with meaning and comes to matter (Lupton, 2018, 2019).

Through the "objective" representation of menstrual information, the menstrual experience is not only part of the body itself, but also of the MCTA. As the data materializes, feelings and bodily experiences become part of the MCTA, detached from personal and bodily experience. Therefore, the distance between the body and one's actual feelings increases; the body is rendered into a data object that may lead to a kind of self-estrangement (Bhimani, 2020; Lupton, 2015). The conversation is not about one's subjective experiences anymore, but about data on menstruation, a distanced object. Therefore, MCTAs have the power to transform menstruation, that was previously considered "unclean," into something "clean": data. As menstruation is datafied, and therefore not part of one's subjective experiences anymore, on which the taboo rests, it can help women to talk more easily about their menstruation (Bhimani, 2020). Seen in this light, and taking the idea of the cyborg as a potentially liberating assemblage, MCTAs can have positive consequences for menstruators' self-perceptions. However, the studies mentioned above do not account for the larger structures of power in which women using MCTAs are embedded. We will turn to this topic now.

Biomedicalization and Technologies of the Self

Medical discourses surrounding menstruation are not solely produced by medical experts, but by a "public health establishment" existing of the pharmaceutical industry, media companies, the feminine hygiene industry, online "health" experts, and the companies developing MCTAs (Ayo, 2012; Wood, 2020). This discourse supports forms of self-discipline related to lifestyle changes. Instead of performing strict control on its citizens like previous power systems, "biomedicalization" instead "governs at a distance" (Sanders, 2017), meaning that it shapes its subjects' behavior by sanctioning expert knowledge that articulates "objective" norms of a healthy lifestyle. It frames its subjects as self-managing, self-surveilling individuals who freely regulate and monitor themselves in accordance with these norms (Ayo, 2012; Foucault, 2000; Lupton, 2016; Wood, 2020). Within this power system, individuals themselves are held responsible for their own health and well-being, and inequalities in physical and mental health are seen as a consequence of badly made individual choices (Ayo, 2012; Levy & Romo-Avilés, 2019). If one is not able to conform to being a "healthy" citizen or does not engage in self-monitoring of health-related behaviors, it can lead to the stigmatization and discrimination of these individuals (Ayo, 2012; Lupton, 2016).

However, a menstruator cannot be in complete control of their menstruation, and therefore, the perception that one should be in control of it distances the woman from her own body (Buckley & Gottlieb, 1988; Ussher, 2006). The biomedicalization of menstruation creates new menstrual stigmas and taboos surrounding menstrunormativity, further controlling women's bodies and lives (Wood, 2020). Premenstrual syndrome (PMS), for example, which depicts the female body as an unruly entity controlled by hormones, is a case in point. Symptoms associated with PMS that were previously an experience now turn into an illness or condition, something that can be objectively defined and evaluated (Buckley & Gottlieb, 1988; Kressbach, 2021; Ussher, 2006).

If menstruators want to pursue a healthy menstruating and reproductive body, they can use various "technologies of the self," like MCTAs. These technologies "[…] permit individuals to reflect and act on their own bodies and souls, thoughts, conducts, and way of being, so as to transform themselves in order to attain a state of happiness, purity, wisdom, perfection, or immorality" (Foucault, 1997, p. 225). Through MCTAs menstruators perform self-surveillance and discipline themselves according to the patriarchal and medical notions of femininity and menstruation. While app usage may lead to insight or empowerment at first glance, disciplinary forces lead to their use in the first place. Because everyone's menstrual cycle is different, chances are that a user is not conforming to the normalized expectations of menstruation presented in the app through medical knowledge and data visualizations, leaving the user feeling as if there is something wrong with their bodies (Wood, 2020). This reinforces bodily alienation, where the woman's subjective experiences of her own body are trusted less than the data presented in the app, even though the medical concepts that they are built upon can be inaccurate (Buckley & Gottlieb, 1988; Wood, 2020).

Self-Surveillance and the Male Gaze

Not only do biopower and biomedicalization exercise power over women's self-surveillance practices, they also intertwine with patriarchal conceptions of femininity and menstruation (Bartky, 2014; Sanders, 2017). With power being everywhere yet nowhere in particular, feminist critiques of Foucault note that women, in addition to conforming to health norms, are also internalizing a panoptical male gaze within themselves, a gaze that becomes part of how a woman thinks, structures and judges herself (Bartky, 2014; Foucault, 1979; Ussher, 2006; Wood, 2020). Women continuously apply various disciplinary techniques in order to produce a "feminine body" that conforms to the female beauty standards of a given time (Bartky, 2014; Wood, 2020).

This objectification of their own bodies can contribute to women's bodily alienation from their own subjective experiences (Wood, 2020), something that is intensified once the body is datafied (Webster, 2017). Self-objectifying behaviors can be particularly harmful to a woman's mental health. Women have to conform to certain behavioral norms, like using euphemisms to hide the word "menstruation" and, most importantly, to hide the fact that they are on their period (Kissling, 2006; Ussher, 2006; Wood, 2020). Apart from contributing to more negative attitudes toward menstruation, these behaviors can also lead to women shaming their own bodies, decreased sexual experience, and loss of confidence (Fredrickson & Roberts, 1997; Wood, 2020). This leads to what Houppert (1999) called a "culture of concealment."

In this culture of concealment, menstruators govern themselves through various commercial control technologies, like soaps, make-up, razors, menstrual products, birth control, and MCTAs in addition to mastering various skills and gaining specialized knowledge to operate these devices (Bartky, 2014; Sanders, 2017). Digital self-tracking technologies, like MCTAs, provide women with a new way of monitoring and analyzing themselves. MCTAs encourage rigorous self-policing mentalities by suggesting the sense of constant visibility to an all-knowing surveillance apparatus, coercing women to internalize a disciplining and normalizing gaze (Lupton, 2015; Sanders, 2017). Therefore, instead of dealing with the problem of breaking the taboo around menstruation, MCTAs can simply relocate the problem of self-policing to a new apparatus (Karlsson, 2019).

Dataveillance and Privacy

Not only do women surveil themselves through MCTAs, so do companies who can exploit the data for commercial purposes. This "dataveillance" monitors citizens for specific purposes, does not state these beforehand, and is "built into" the flows of ordinary life rather than being organized into disciplinary institutions. Users frequently have no idea who conducts dataveillance or how their personal information is used (Lupton & Michael, 2017). The concept of dataveillance, therefore, fits well into the system of biopower, as control is exercised in every aspect of everyday life. Because of the individualized nature of these technologies, as well as the fact that they are wearable, they feel physically close and confidential to the individual, making dataveillance a normative experience that makes life more convenient and efficient, leading many people voluntarily subject themselves to surveillance (Best, 2010; Sanders, 2017).

Trading metadata in exchange for different online services has become the norm; only a few users appear to be ready to pay for privacy (Best, 2010; Van Dijck, 2014). Individuals are typically hesitant to share their data, but neither are they really concerned about sharing it (Hohmann-Marriott, 2021). While most people say that they are concerned about their privacy, their actual behavior appears to contradict this, a contradiction known as the "privacy paradox" (Best, 2010; Nissenbaum, 2010). Users of internet services, on the other hand, frequently do not have a choice because participation in monitoring is frequently a prerequisite for using that technology. Users may not even realize what they are agreeing to, or they may be forced to use technology in order to function properly as members of an increasingly digitized society (Best, 2010; Nissenbaum, 2010; Ostherr et al., 2017). Because these transactions operate within a "black box," and consumers sometimes have no understanding of how they function, it may hide the true nature of the transaction, leading users to feel that they cannot opt-out of surveillance activities (Ostherr et al., 2017; Pasquale, 2015).

When considering privacy in the context of feminism, it is the tagline "the personal is the political" that questions the divide between private and public life (Friedan, 1963; Hanisch, 1970; Karlsson, 2019). While for men, privacy was connected to the home, for women, the "privacy of the home" served as a possible cover-up for domestic violence and repression happening in the household (Hanisch, 1970). As a result, finding "a room of one's own" has always been difficult for women, especially for lower-class women (Woolf, 1929). Total interference of the state in the private sphere, however, is not a better alternative, as shown by the governmental control of the female reproductive body. On the one hand, MCTAs offer this "room" for women, where they can escape the menstrual stigma they face in daily life. On the other hand, they subject themselves to their own control and that of digital health companies (Healy, 2021; Karlsson, 2019; Lupton, 2015; Sanders, 2017).

When it comes to menstrual data, users do not seem to be that concerned about their data. Users believe that they have more privacy online. Karlsson (2019) notes that users feel that they have more privacy online as their menstruation turns into datafied traces of blood that are separated from their bodies, clinging to the notion that their data is anonymized and disappears into the abundance of data. Therefore, users show much more concern about the stigma around menstruation and people in their private lives seeing when they menstruate than the potential loss of their data in cyberspace (Karlsson, 2019; Kressbach, 2021). It may be argued that MCTAs, unlike many other female products, are capitalizing on the societal and cultural taboos connected with the female body, providing women with an opportunity to escape these taboos (Karlsson, 2019).

Methodology

Research Design

Through a combination of quantitative and qualitative analysis we aim to empirically investigate and ground the theoretical topics covered in this chapter so far. Moreover, the goal here is to showcase what shape research into FemTech might take. For the quantitative research part, subreddits that discuss MCTAs are used as data. Because of its anonymous nature, Reddit offers a platform for menstruators where they can freely express their feelings and experiences about their menstrual cycles and the apps that they are using. Therefore, when researching user experiences, Reddit offers a critical platform in providing insights into the discourse on these experiences. By using R, data was extracted from various subreddits after which frequency analysis, sentiment analysis, and automated topic modeling were conducted. Following this, the outcomes were incorporated into the second part of the analysis, which consisted of a qualitative thematic analysis of data from two focus groups with people using MCTAs. This combination of quantitative and qualitative research methods gives us a deeper understanding of and insight into the experiences of and discourses surrounding MCTAs.

Sample

Using the RedditExtractoR package, data was extracted from three different subreddits, r/Periods (45.5K members), r/TwoXChromosomes (13.2M members), and r/birthcontrol (84.2K members). These subreddits were chosen based on a search for "period tracking" in the Reddit search engine. After sorting on relevancy, the subreddits that were on the first page and mentioned period tracking were noted. Afterward, the subreddits that were specifically geared toward medical conditions or specific issues—like miscarriages, infertility, or PCOS—were filtered out, only including those that were as "general" as possible in order to avoid any specific bias in the data toward a specific situation or condition and its discourse. After the list was generated, an initial search in R using the RedditExtractoR package was performed in order to look for the three subreddits that include the most posts on MCTAs, resulting in the three subreddits mentioned above.

Data was extracted from subreddits by using the keywords period, menstruation, cycle, track, tracking, and tracker to search for relevant Reddit posts. After that data was collected and combined, it was again filtered with a list of keywords and names of popular MCTAs and to only include posts from the years 2018 until 2021. For the final step, the data was manually filtered by looking at the titles of the Reddit posts and filtering out those that did not fall in line with our research. This manual filtering process led to the removal of nine posts in r/Periods, 14 in r/TwoxChromosomes, and nine in r/birthcontrol, leaving a total of 139 posts and 1988 comments ready to be analyzed.

Automated Analyses

The research took an inductive approach (Schwartz & Ungar, 2015) and explored the discourse around MCTAs through various forms of automated content analysis. In order to perform this automated content analysis, the *quanteda* package was used. This package is specifically developed for the quantitative analysis of textual data, ranging from data preprocessing to data visualization (Benoit et al., 2018). After the data was cleaned and tokenized, the tokens were counted for their frequency and visualized in frequency plots and word clouds. Because Clue and Flo were the two MCTAs most mentioned in the posts and have quite different designs, sentiment analysis was performed to research the general consensus in the discourse on these two apps. The sentiment analysis gauged the sentiment of the discourse based on the standard Lexicoder Sentiment Dictionary 2015 which includes negative, positive, negative-positive, and negative-negative words and is used to calculate a sentiment score. Lastly, an exploratory automated topic model analysis was conducted on the Reddit data. Through performing topic modeling, a list with keywords grouped together into topics was generated. These themes were then given their own names based on the keywords. After exploring the discourse around MCTAs on Reddit, the results, together with insights from the theoretical framework, were used in order to prepare and conduct the focus groups.

Focus Groups[1]

For this study, two reconvening focus groups were held, the first one consisted of seven women and the second one consisted of six of those same seven participants. There were not many requirements when selecting the participants, except for the fact that they had to use MCTAs on a relatively frequent basis. Participants have been sampled through "snowball sampling," a nonprobable sampling technique that is particularly helpful when dealing with a specific sample group, like the one necessary

---

[1] Before the start of the focus groups, participants were asked to fill in a consent form, in which they consented to the voluntary nature of the research, the recording and transcription of the focus groups, and the usage of anonymized quotes. The audio files and transcripts were encrypted and stored on a separate USB drive in order to limit the risk of a data breach as much as possible. During transcription, the names of participants were changed to keep the data anonymous. As the focus groups dealt with a sensitive topic, there was a chance that participants might overshare, referring to a situation where respondents present more information, express views or mention experiences in the group setting that they eventually feel uncomfortable about sharing with the group. While it provides reassurance to individuals that others may express the same feelings, behaviors, and uncertainties, it can also make them feel very uncomfortable (Bloor et al., 2001). Therefore, in the same form of consent, the purpose of the research was clearly stated and its voluntary nature was emphasized. Next to that, it was noted that if participants wanted a specific part of the interview to be deleted from the transcript, they had the power to do so.

for this research (Goodman, 1961). For the sampling process, one of the authors employed her social network and posted a message on her Instagram story, asking contacts if they knew people that used MCTAs and wanted to participate in the research. Throughout the research, we will refer to the participants by their given alias.

The focus group is rather homogenous; all participants identified as female, were between the ages of 22 and 26, and lived in the Netherlands. Because of the similarity in age, the participants shared similar experiences around menstruation and its social discourse, allowing for a fruitful conversation about the different topics discussed. What is particularly noticeable is that those who are single are not using hormonal birth control at the moment, while those in relationships do. While the homogeneous nature has been very beneficial for the course of focus groups and openness among the participants, it can also provide a one-sided view of MCTAs (Morgan, 1997).

The two focus groups each lasted about sixty minutes. The first focus group was held on December 2nd, and the second one on December 15th, 2021, leaving a period of approximately two weeks in between. Because of Covid-19 lockdown regulations, the focus groups were held online. Before the first focus group, participants were asked to fill in a small survey that asked for their basic demographic information, their history of taking birth control, and a few short questions about their experience with MCTAs (see Appendix 2). The first focus group focuses primarily on the menstrual taboo and user experiences, moderated through five different statements:

1. There is still a taboo on menstruation, and this reflects itself in small adjustments I make in my daily life.
2. I trust the predictions and additional information that are provided to me through these apps.
3. Information generated by menstrual cycle tracking apps has an influence on how I arrange my life.
4. I have the feeling that I am more in control of my own body now that I use a menstruation cycle tracking app.
5. I worry about my privacy when using menstruation apps.

In addition to these statements, questions were asked based on previous answers given by the participants in the focus group itself or in their survey, while leaving room for discussion. At the end of the first focus group, they were given the exercise of sending screenshots of things that stood out to them concerning the design or language use in their preferred MCTA. While they did this, they were asked to take into consideration different perspectives on fertility, sexuality, and gender. In the second focus group, a PowerPoint presentation containing the screenshots was made, and the design of the app, usage of symbols, and features were discussed.

Results

Automated Content Analysis on Reddit

The following section will present the results of three different automated content analysis methods that were performed on the Reddit data: frequency analysis, sentiment analysis, and automated topic modeling.

The frequency analysis showed that the apps Clue (239 times) and Flo (183 times) are most often mentioned in Reddit discourse (see Figs. 12.3 and 12.4). It seems that they are appreciated, as words like "good" (190 times), "love" (90 times), and "great" (79 times) appear with significant frequency in Reddit posts. The high occurrence of the word "symptoms" (157 times) suggests that the Redditors were either discussing symptoms in relation to menstruation or potentially asking for suggestions about which apps allowed for the tracking of certain symptoms or appreciating an app for the variety of symptoms that could be registered. With "ovulation" (139 times), "pregnancy" (100 times), and "fertility" (97 times) showing its significant presence, it can be suggested that MCTAs are discussed in the light of fertility and pregnancy, potentially suggesting the usage of the app as a tool in fertility awareness-based methods. On the other hand, the words "pill" (101 times) and "birth control" (75 times) suggest conversations around birth control, either discussing various types of birth control, or the possibility to register birth control in the

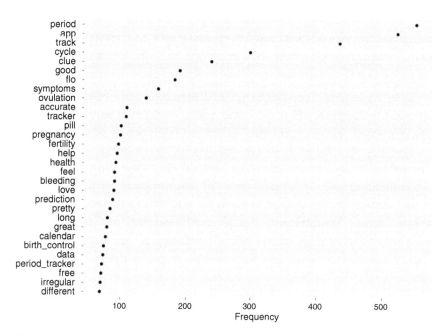

Fig. 12.3 Frequency plot of tokens used

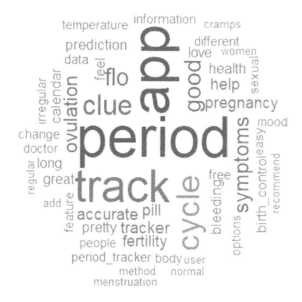

Fig. 12.4 Word Cloud of tokens used

app. The sentiment analysis shows that the sentiment score of Flo (0.82) was higher than that of Clue (0.68), suggesting that the discourse around Flo was more positive than the discourse around Clue (see Figs. 12.5 and 12.6).

When comparing the frequency of the tokens used in the discourse around both apps (see Figs. 12.7 and 12.8), we see that words like "accurate," "pretty," "great," and "love" occur more frequently in the discourse around Flo. For Clue, however, the word "recommend" occurs more often than it does in the discourse around Flo, suggesting that Clue is recommended more on Reddit than Flo. The design of both applications is also somewhat represented in the discourse. While the presence of the words "data," "information," "easy," and "calendar" in Clue discourse suggests the minimalistic and scientific design of the app, "easy" and "pink" suggest the easy, but very female-oriented design of the app.

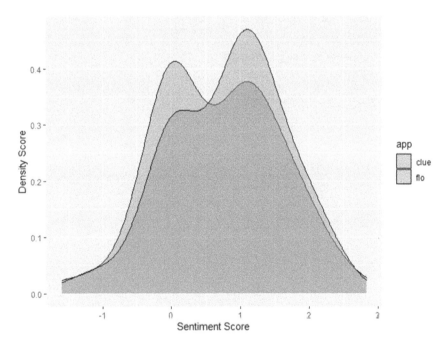

Fig. 12.5 Density plot of sentiment score

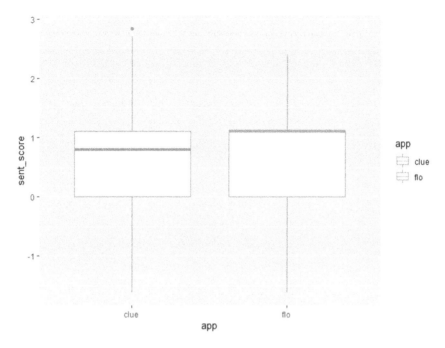

Fig. 12.6 Boxplot of sentiment score

Finally, the data suggests that the two apps are being compared a lot, as both MCTAs occur often in each other's frequency plot.

The results of the automated topic model analysis show that many different topics concerning MCTAs are being discussed within the various subreddits. While some themes were a bit vague and hard to define with a name, others were very clear from looking at the keywords. Three prominent conversations around MCTAs on these three subreddits stand out. The first, and probably the main one, is about asking and providing recommendations on MCTAs. This theme reflects Reddit's nature as a forum and social media platform, one that one uses to ask questions and receive answers from strangers. Flo, Apple Health, and Clue seem to be the main recommended apps, and overall, it is suggested that the Redditors share an overall positive outlook on MCTAs. The second main theme discusses the menstrual cycle and menstrunormativity. It is suggested that Redditors ask each other for information about what is

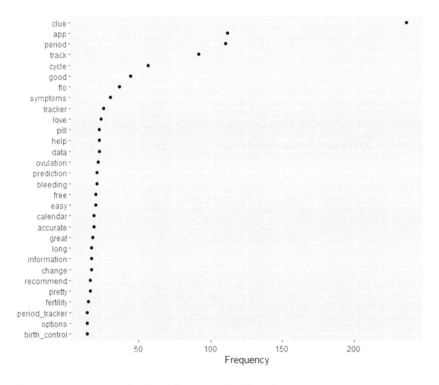

Fig. 12.7 Frequency plot for tokens used in Clue discourse

normal and what is not concerning the menstrual cycle and discuss the course of the cycle by discussing hormones, fertility, ovulation, and medical conditions like PCOS. In relation to that, Redditors discuss the reliability and accuracy of the fertility awareness-based method. Lastly, Redditors discuss the various different features of the app. They discuss the possibility of tracking menstruation, symptoms, moods, and pain, and talk about the wanted feature to turn on/off notifications and reminders that the app gives them. It also suggests that information provided by MCTAs is useful to Redditors. Finally, the freemium model is being discussed, suggesting a discussion about whether it is worth getting the paid version or sticking to the free one.

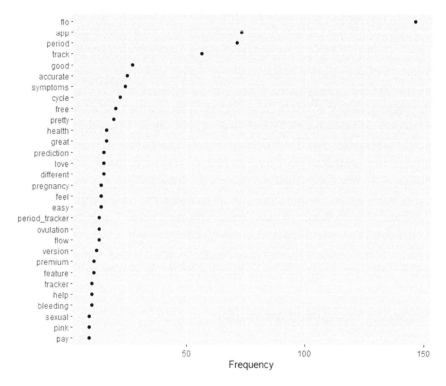

Fig. 12.8 Frequency plot for tokens used in Flo discourse

Thematic Analysis in Focus Groups

In this section, we report on the attitudes and practices related to four themes that emerged during the focus group sessions. These themes will be discussed in relation to the theory in the next section. The themes are:

Quantification and Cycle Tracking

As no participants tried to get pregnant during the time the focus groups were held, participants used MCTAs for two reasons. The main reason was to keep track and prepare for the next menstrual cycle. The other one was to find patterns in their cycle. In the prefocus group survey, all participants noted that they use MCTAs to not only track their blood loss, but also to track various symptoms associated with the menstrual cycle, moods and activities. Within the process of quantification, it was the app's customizability that was mentioned and widely appreciated by six out of seven participants. They also mentioned that they appreciated the information that MCTAs provided them through its data visualizations and additional articles and deemed it to be trustworthy. However, participants also expressed concerns with inaccurate or inappropriate information presented in the app. One of the participants filed a complaint with Flo for providing inaccurate information on washing the vulva with soap. In addition, the placement of "face slimming" and "weight loss" workouts in the Period Tracker–Period Calendar app was found inappropriate. Finally, participants did not appreciate the cluttered and childish design of the Simple Design–Period Tracker application and rather preferred a cleaner design like that of Apple Health or Clue.

Normative Design and Annoyance

When discussing the design of the different applications, various worries were expressed when it came to the representation of the menstrual cycle in these applications. It seems that if the participant had a regular cycle, either natural or through birth control, the app would be most accurate. If the cycle was irregular, the predictions seemed less accurate, or the app used did not allow for the registration of various birth control methods.

Worries were expressed when it came to the representation of gender, sexuality, and fertility within the design of MCTAs. Participants noted that most apps stereotyped its user as the heterosexual woman through the pink design, gendered language, and the focus on pregnancy. When it comes to registering sexual activity, it was concluded that most apps contained similar options, and that the symbols used for registration were gender-inclusive. However, one of the participants noted that there was no option to mention with which gender you had sex with. This conversation also started some confusion as to what is defined as "protected" and "unprotected" sex, as it can have two different meanings concerning preventing pregnancy and preventing Sexual Transmitted Diseases

(STDs). Several participants were annoyed with the focus on pregnancy, expressing their concerns concerning language use and the nonexisting option to edit whether you can actually get pregnant or not. Apps that took a more gender neutral approach, like Clue and Apple Health were appreciated by the users.

When discussing privacy, the overall consensus was that there was little concern for privacy. Many participants had never thought about it before or had never looked into it. Some had more knowledge about privacy but still did not care enough to take rigorous measures and adjust their behavior, as "their data was already out there anyway." Instead, users mainly expressed their annoyance with in-app advertisements, which affected their user experience. However, when hypothesizing about the potential use of this data by health insurers, participants seemed more worried, especially about it potentially having consequences for the way in which risk is assessed.

Feelings of Liberation

All participants expressed feeling somewhat more "free" in their menstrual cycle because of the application. We will explicitly pick up on this important theme in the conclusion of this chapter. For now, it is important to mention that many expressed learning more about their menstrual cycle and its associated symptoms through the insights provided by the apps, increasing their menstrual literacy.

Participants mentioned that MCTAs gave them more insight into what symptoms and moods can actually be associated with different phases of the menstrual cycle, information that was previously unknown to them. The app is often used by the participants as a guideline for when their period is supposed to start, in order to better prepare themselves and be kinder to themselves once their period arrives. Three participants also expressed that MCTAs gave them some form of peace regarding symptoms that they felt as they combined data from self-tracking practices with their own subjective experiences in order to better understand the self. For those three participants that quit hormonal birth control, the MCTA functioned as a tool to better understand their natural cycle.

Many of the participants expressed that they felt like the MCTA made it easier for them to understand their period and talk with their friends about it. One of the participants, Eva, even adopted a very period-positive approach to her menstruation, even posting about her experience using an MCTA on her Instagram story.

Feelings of Bodily Alienation

While participants were overall very positive about the relationship between themselves and the app, it does seem that MCTAs can induce feelings of health or pregnancy anxiety among the participants. The app here often confirms notions of menstrunormativity and therefore confirms that anxieties and insecurities women already have when it comes to their menstruation. In addition, the app can contribute to bodily alienation as the app can help women invalidate their own subjective experiences of the body. Five out of seven participants noted that they used their apps to reaffirm their symptoms or moods, risking the formation of a placebo effect, where the app might confirm certain thoughts that might not even be true.

Discussion

As the Reddit analysis suggests and the focus group research confirms, MCTA users use the application not only to track their menstruation but also other symptoms and factors that they deem significant in the process of gaining more knowledge about their menstrual cycle. This includes the tracking of certain symptoms, moods, vaginal discharge, contraceptive use, sexual activity, and hours of sleep. Users appreciate the ways in which information about their menstruation is datafied and presented to them in the form of statistics, data visualizations, and additional articles, appreciating minimal design over overly cluttered and girly designs. Generally, participants believe in the accuracy and objectivity of data, reflecting the ideology of dataism. They incorporate this data further into their lives by using it to help them prepare for different phases of their menstrual cycle or by using the data to gain more knowledge about the menstrual cycle and its associated symptoms. However, while quantifying menstruation may feel empowering because it gives the woman more control over her own body, it also demonstrates her commitment to using these MCTAs for self-surveillance and management of her menstrual cycle, feeding into neoliberal and patriarchal society's expectations of femininity (Hohmann-Marriott, 2021; Lupton, 2015; Sanders, 2017).

As participants were all of a younger age group, none of them were using MCTAs for the purpose of achieving pregnancy or keeping track of fertility in relation to that. Instead, participants noted two main reasons for using MCTAs: (1) in order to keep track and prepare for their next menstrual cycle and (2) to find patterns within their own menstrual cycle. The Reddit analysis, though, does suggest that MCTAs are used for fertility purposes. It can potentially even be used as a tool for fertility-awareness-based methods, as the topic model suggested. It is suggested here that women feel the need to be in charge of their own fertility and should intensely surveil themselves to fulfill their role as "digital reproductive citizens," reflecting the prescribed role of a woman as a mother (Healy, 2021; Lupton, 2016). Both the extent of datafying the menstruating body and the self-policing of one's fertility show how using these applications can coerce women to internalize a disciplining gaze upon themselves and fulfill their role as "digital reproductive citizens" (Lupton, 2015; Sanders, 2017).

While MCTAs have the potential to transform users into "cyborgs" (Haraway, 1991), which enables users to eliminate the traditional binary notion of gender in the digital realm, research shows that MCTAs do not fulfill this potential. Rather, they are "technologies of the gendered body" that are embedded in and reinforce normalized conceptions of femininity (Balsamo, 1996). The designers of these applications seem to have a stereotypical woman in mind as their target subject. There was a general consensus among the focus group participants that the MCTAs were particularly made for heterosexual women who love pink and use the app in order to manage fertility and, sooner or later, want to get pregnant.

Clearly, a set of "truths" based on patriarchal taboos and the medicalization of the female body, sexuality, and menstrual cycles are embedded in these MCTAs (Buckley & Gottlieb, 1988; Foucault, 1978; Ussher,

2006). These "truths" are also reflected in the binary gender identity that is further reinforced through the use of gendered language, such as the Flo app, that always refers to its users as women rather than using a gender-neutral term (Balsamo, 1996; Healy, 2021). In addition, sometimes the information and advertisements, like the promotion of weight loss in the Simple Design Period Tracker and the Period Tracker–Period Calendar app, capitalize on women's insecurities during the different phases of the cycle. These features show no care for the user's mental health, but instead seem to be designed to commodify the menstruating body. Another possibility is that the designers of the app actually think that this is what users want to see during their menstrual cycle, having no idea what women are looking for in these applications (Fox & Epstein, 2020; Epstein et al., 2017). In this case, social media research, like presented in this chapter, could help designers with designing the application to make it appeal more to their target audience.

While all of the applications' symbols were gender-neutral, there was no option to specify what the gender of your sex partner was. While this already verifies notions about heteronormativity that are embedded in these apps, it also leaves the definition of "protected" and "unprotected" sex open to question. The MCTAs relate this back to the protection of pregnancy, which means that it does not take into consideration the transmission of STDs, leading to confusion among the participants about what to fill in when registering sexual activity. Therefore, the lack of options for registration of sexual activity does not only show a bias toward heteronormativity but also toward fertility, identifying the female body as a maternal one (Balsamo, 1996; Ussher, 2006; Healy, 2021). Lastly, it shows that the designers are unconcerned with the sexual health of their users.

When it comes to the representation of menstruation in the app, it was found that the app's predictions worked better for those with regular cycles than for those with irregular cycles. This is not surprising, as irregularity makes it more difficult for the algorithms to predict those periods. However, in the case of one participant, the app Clue had trouble adapting its algorithm to a consistent but longer and less normal cycle. It is unclear if this demonstrates the algorithm's dysfunctionality, given the participant's previous "normal" cycle length, or whether it demonstrates the app's inherent conceptions of menstrunormativity. However, the fact that certain applications do not appear to operate with less common birth control, such as the injectable pill, demonstrates the app's incorporation of menstrunormative norms. The app of another participant did not allow her to disable period tracking or record the fact that she takes the injection pill. This indicates that the app is largely aimed at people who do not use birth control or who use the more well-known methods, such as the contraceptive pill or IUD. Similarly to Fox and Epstein's (2020) study, it was also found that the design of the application could have a significant role in "dumbing down" the menstrual cycle, as participants expressed their annoyance toward the usage of childish characters in a serious health tracking app.

When one does not conform to these menstrunormative conceptions, one may be notified or alarmed when the period is irregular. This is sometimes accompanied by a recommendation to see a doctor, despite the fact that it could simply be a part of one's menstrual cycle. This shows that the apps are embedded in the biomedical power system, influencing the way participants think about menstruation and the associated symptoms. While both users' cycles are similar in duration and variance, Flo considers one user's irregular cycle to be significantly more problematic than Clue considers the other user's irregular cycle to be. Flo uses words like "normal" and "irregular," implying a negative connection with an irregular cycle, while Clue makes no such association. The use of language shows how menstrunormativity is embedded in the language used in these applications.

The biomedical power system can also be found within the discourse around MCTAs. First, the automated topic model suggests that menstrual normativity is a hot topic on the three subreddits, indicating concerns about how users perceive their cycle in comparison to others. Also in the focus group, Sophie noted that when she knew she was experiencing PMS, she considered her body to be somewhat of an unruly entity, one that could not be controlled as much as in other phases of her cycle. She believes that she is not fully in control of her body at those times, signaling the increased distance between her body and mind (Buckley & Gottlieb, 1988; Ussher, 2006).

While users tend to trust the information that is developed through these applications, they do not *blindly* trust it. They often combine the knowledge gained from MCTAs with their own knowledge about the menstrual cycle and their bodily sensations, developing a data sense (Hohmann-Marriott, 2021; Lupton, 2018; Lupton, 2019). The development of this data sense seems to be greater for those that have irregular cycles and cannot rely on the app's predictions. Therefore, they have to rely more on their own bodily cues. Yet, when this balance is disturbed by either inaccurate self-tracking data or not listening to bodily sensations well enough, the app can help reinforce bodily alienation, where the woman subconsciously sees the subjective experiences of her own body as something that cannot be trusted and instead trusts the app more (Buckley & Gottlieb, 1988). This can sometimes be the case, as these apps confirm users' feelings or increase health and pregnancy anxieties when the body does not align with the information provided in the application.

Even though some rely more on the app's information and recommendations than others, all participants showed that they in some way critically thought about the data that was presented to them. Participants mainly use MCTAs as a tool to better understand their menstrual cycle and body, increasing their menstrual and body literacy (Bobel, 2010; Hohmann-Marriott, 2021). These perceptions reflect the marketing of MCTAs as empowering tools (Kressbach, 2021). Participants in the focus groups acknowledged the wide range of symptoms that can be tracked, some of which they had no idea that they could be related to the menstrual cycle (Levy & Romo-Avilés, 2019; Verstappen, 2018). In relation to that, participants said that these applications gave them new insights into their cycle and symptoms, allowing them to better prepare for upcoming cycle phases and be more kind and less critical of themselves. In addition, MCTAs provide a tool for those who recently quit hormonal birth control to get to know their natural cycles. As MCTAs allow the participants to "distance" themselves from their subjective feelings, understand themselves better and be more in control and at peace with their cycle, one's increased menstrual literacy can also provide a tool in menstrual activism and resist self-surveillance, control, and concealment (Bhimani, 2020; Bobel, 2010; Hohmann-Marriott, 2021).

Even though participants might be quite active in fighting patriarchal taboos concerning menstruation, they show less concern when it comes to systems of power such as dataveillance. Reflecting the findings by Karlsson (2019) and Kressbach (2021), participants express far greater concern about the stigma of menstruation in their private lives than the potential loss of their menstrual data in cyberspace. In addition, participants seem to value personalization a lot more than privacy. All six participants of the focus group showed their appreciation for customization and personalization features, and two expressed annoyance over in-app advertisements in their MCTAs. While there was somewhat of a concern when it came to targeted advertisements, none of the participants cared about privacy enough to take rigorous measures, like limiting the amount of data they entered into the app or using an app that does not require an account. Most of them never really thought about it, or thought that their data was not interesting to anyone beyond themselves (Best, 2010; Hohmann-Marriott, 2021). Only one participant did a Google search before downloading an app to see which one had the best privacy policies, but never thought about it since.

The lack of care for privacy seems to simply come from a lack of knowledge. They do not really know who is conducting this dataveillance and what it is supposed to be used for (Lupton & Michael, 2017). The "privacy paradox," as mentioned by Nissenbaum (2010), however, is not present in this study. Participants simply expressed that they do not necessarily care about privacy, because their data was out on the streets anyways. Perhaps this generation has grown up with social media platforms and has been giving away their data since childhood. In some ways, participants voluntarily subject themselves to surveillance (Best, 2010; Sanders, 2017). However, simultaneously, giving away your data is deemed necessary in order to have access to online services. They express that they feel it is already too late to start caring about privacy, as many big tech companies have all their data already (Ostherr et al., 2017). Participants voluntarily subject themselves to surveillance (Best, 2010; Sanders, 2017). However, they do express concern when it comes to health insurance companies having access to their data, fearing the potential discrimination they might face in the future.

Conclusion

How is the female body datafied and commercialized through MCTAs, and to what extent are users experiencing these applications in terms of liberation and control? We know that the menstruating body is datafied and commodified in a variety of ways, but that it is often done through datafying both menstruation and associated symptoms. However, the way in which menstruation and associated symptoms are datafied mostly reflects normative notions of femininity, menstruation, sexuality, and fertility—notions that are rooted in neoliberal and patriarchal ideologies. Participants primarily view MCTAs in the light of liberation, as they believe it helps them increase their menstrual literacy, be more considerate of themselves during different phases of the menstrual cycle, and is used as a tool in regaining control over the natural cycle and in menstrual activism. While there were some concerns about bodily alienation and a loss of data sense, participants were not particularly worried about these forms of control. Participants felt controlled in two ways: through the menstrual taboo that is still present in their everyday lives; and through patriarchal notions of femininity and sexuality that are embedded into the design of the app. While these control systems are rather prevalent in the users' daily lives, other power systems like those of neoliberalism, biomedicalization, and dataveillance remain hidden in the background and are subconsciously influencing their usage of MCTAs.

Through this mixed-methods approach using social media and focus group data, we have novel insights into how users experience MCTAs and how these experiences fit into biomedical, patriarchal and capitalist power systems. Especially when it comes to the liberation vs. control debate, we see that Reddit users and participants of the focus groups are inherently liberating themselves through discussing their experiences with MCTAs both on- and offline. It shows how an app can help menstruators to understand their cycle better and use this information on their cycle to discuss their experiences of the app.

While the study highlights various aspects of MCTAs, it also leaves us with a general overview of various different topics that could be explored more in-depth. Therefore, for further research, it is suggested to explore any of the abovementioned topics and the relationship of MCTAs to the three power systems more in-depth. Secondly, the research was focused on a specific age group, which resulted in the fact that the research lacked certain perspectives from menstruators from different age groups, ethnicities, and gender identities. Therefore, focusing on a different target group could provide interesting insights into using the MCTA as a tool in fertility measurement or discuss different representations of menstruation, gender identity, and sexuality more in-depth.

Future app developers are encouraged to use more inclusive language in their applications, like by changing "high chance of getting pregnant" to "fertility is high" and offering more customizable options for the design and features of the app, so it can fall in line with anyone's gender identity or sexuality. Additionally, there is a need for a clearer disclosure of privacy policies, explicitly stating in what ways data will be shared with third parties, making it easy to understand for everyone. Lastly, future apps should be developed using a period-positive approach so that, instead of relying on neoliberal and patriarchal notions of femininity, they should take on discourses from menstrual activism in their design.

Future research on FemTech, and specifically MCTAs, can benefit from approaches that mix distant reading of large social media data sets to reveal trends and sentiments of specific populations of users with in-depth qualitative methods to engage with experiences, practices, and attitudes of individual users. This will yield results that show how individual users are shaped by socially shared norms and attitudes, but also how individual experiences and practices deviate from these. Applying such an approach, future research could focus on the political–economic dimensions of FemTech and how, for example, app stores and digital marketplaces set standards for such technologies. Also a research focus could be on practices of resistance or nonuse and the motivations that drive this. As menstruation will become increasingly datafied and part of a broader platform economy, such directions in future research are pertinent.

References

Ayo, N. (2012). Understanding health promotion in a neoliberal climate and the making of health conscious citizens. *Critical Public Health, 22*(1), 99–105.

Balsamo, A. (1996). Introduction. In *Technologies of the Gendered Body* (pp. 1–16). Duke University Press.

Bartky, S. L. (2014). Foucault, femininity, and the modernization of patriarchal power. In R. Weitz & S. Kwan (Eds.), *The politics of women's bodies: Sexuality, appearance, and behavior* (4th ed., pp. 64–85). Oxford University Press.

Benoit et al. (2018). Quanteda: An R package for the quantitative analysis of textual data. *Journal of Open Source Software, 3*(30), 774, https://doi.org/10.21105/joss.00774

Best, K. (2010). Living in the control society; Surveillance, users, and digital screen technologies. *International Journal of Cultural Studies, 13*(1), 5–24.

Bhimani, A. (2020, May 4). Period-tracking apps: How femtech creates value for users and platforms. *LSE Business Review.* http://eprints.lse.ac.uk/104770/1/businessreview_2020_05_04_period_tracking_apps_how_femtech_creates.pdf

Bloor M., Frankland J., Thomas M., & Robson K. (2001). *Focus groups in social research.* Thousand Oaks, CA: Sage.

Bobel, C. (2010). *New blood: Third-wave feminism and the politics of menstruation.* Rutgers University Press.

Buckley, T., & Gottlieb, A. (1988). *Blood magic: The anthropology of menstruation.* University of California Press.

Epstein, D. A., Lee, N. B., Kang, J. H., Agapie, E., Schroeder, J., Pina, L. R., Fogarty, J., Kientz, J. A., & Munson, S. A. (2017). Examining Menstrual Tracking to Inform the Design of Personal Informatics Tools. Proceedings of the SIGCHI conference on human factors in computing systems. CHI Conference, 2017, 6876–6888. https://doi.org/10.1145/3025453.3025635

Foucault, M. (1978). *The history of sexuality volume 1: The will to knowledge* (R. Hurley, Trans.). Penguin Random House.

Foucault, M. (1979). *Discipline and punish: The birth of the prison.* Vintage.

Foucault, M. (1997). Technologies of the self. In M. Foucault & P. Rabinow (Eds.), *Ethics: Subjectivity and truth. The essential works of Michel Foucault, 1954–1984* (pp. 223–252). The New Press.

Foucault, M. (2000). Governmentality. In J. D. Faubion (Ed.), *Power: The essential works of Foucault, 1954–1984* (pp. 201–222). The New Press.

Fox, S., & Epstein, D. A. (2020). Monitoring menses: Design-based investigations of menstrual tracking applications. In C. Bobel, I. T. Winkler, B. Fahs, et al. (Eds.), *Handbook of critical menstruation studies* (pp. 733–750). Palgrave Macmillan.

Fredrickson, B., & Roberts, T. (1997). Objectification theory: Toward understanding women's lived experience and mental health risks. *Psychology of Women Quarterly, 21,* 173–206.

Friedan, B. (1963). *The feminine mystique.* Norton.

Garamvolgyi, F. (2022, June 28). *The Guardian.* https://www.theguardian.com/world/2022/jun/28/why-us-woman-are-deleting-their-period-tracking-apps

Goodman, L. A. (1961). Snowball sampling. *Annual Mathematical Statistics, 32*(1), 148–170.

Hanisch, C. (1970). The personal is political. In S. Firestone & A. Koedt (Eds.), *Notes from the second year: Women's literation: Major writings of the radical feminists* (pp. 76–78). Radical Feminism.

Haraway, D. (1991). A cyborg manifesto: Science, technology and socialist-feminism in the late twentieth century. In *Simians, cyborgs and women: The reinvention of nature* (pp. 149–181). Routledge.

Healy, R. L. (2021). Zuckerberg, get out of my uterus! An examination of fertility apps, data-sharing, and remaking the female body as a digitized reproductive citizen. *Journal of Gender Studies, 30,* 400–416.

Hohmann-Marriott, B. (2021). Periods as powerful data: User understandings of menstrual app data and information. *New Media & Society,* 1–19.

Houppert, K. (1999). *The curse: Confronting the last unmentionable taboo: Menstruation.* Faraar, Strauss, and Giroux.

Karlsson, A. (2019). A room of one's own? Using period trackers to escape menstrual stigma. *Nordicom Review, 40,* 111–123.

Kissling, E. A. (2006). *Capitalizing on the curse: The business of menstruation.* Lynne Rienner.

Kressbach, M. (2021). Period hacks: Menstruating in the big data paradigm. *Television and New Media, 22*(3), 241–261.

Levy, J., & Romo-Avilés, N. (2019). "A good little tool to get to know yourself a bit better": A qualitative study on users' experiences of app-supported menstrual tracking in Europe. *BMC Public Health, 19*(12–13), 1–11.

Lupton, D. (2015). Quantified sex: A critical analysis of sexual and reproductive self-tracking using apps. *Culture, Health and Sexuality, 17,* 440–453.

Lupton, D. (2016). *The quantified self.* Polity Press.

Lupton, D. (2018). How do data come to matter? Living and becoming with personal data. *Big Data & Society*, July–December, 1–11.

Lupton, D. (2019). *Data selves: More-than-human perspectives.* Polity Press.

Lupton, D. (2020). Data mattering and self-tracking: What can personal data do? *Continuum, 34*, 1–13.

Lupton, D., & Michael, M. (2017). 'Depends on who's got the data': Public understandings of personal digital dataveillance. *Surveillance and Society, 15*(2), 254–268.

Morgan, D. L. (1997). *Focus groups as qualitative research.* Sage Publications.

Nissenbaum, H. (2010). *Privacy in context: Technology, policy and integrity of social life.* Stanford University Press.

Ostherr, K., Borodina, S., & Bracken, R. C. (2017). Trust and privacy in the context of user-generated health data. *Big Data & Society, 4*(1), 1–11.

Pasquale, F. (2015). *The black box society.* Harvard University Press.

Sanders, R. (2017). Self-tracking in the digital era: Biopower, patriarchy, and the new biometric body projects. *Body & Society, 23*(1), 36–63.

Schooler, D., Ward, M. L., Merriwether, A., & Caruthers, A. S. (2005). Cycles of shame: Menstrual shame, body shame, and sexual decision-making. *The Journal of Sex Research, 42*(4), 324–334.

Schwartz, H. A., & Ungar, L. H. (2015). Data-driven content analysis of social media: A systematic overview of automated methods. *The Annals of the American Academy of Political and Social Science, 659*, 78–94.

Torchinsky, R. (2022, June 24). *NPR.* https://www.npr.org/2022/05/10/1097482967/roe-v-wade-supreme-court-abortion-period-apps

Ussher, J. M. (2006). *Managing the monstrous feminine: Regulating the reproductive body.* Routledge.

Van Dijck, J. (2014). Datafication, dataism and dataveillance: Big Data between scientific paradigm and ideology. *Surveillance and Society, 12*(2), 197–208.

Verstappen, I. J. (2018). *Qualitative health and quantified cycles: The use of menstrual self-tracking apps in a neoliberal context.* University of Utrecht. https://dspace.library.uu.nl/handle/1874/369202

Webster, S. B. (2017). *The history of the curse: A comparative look at the religious and social taboos of menstruation and the influence they have on American society today.* The University of North Carolina.

Wolf, G. (2010, April 28). The data-driven life. *The New York Times*. http://www.nytimcs.com/2010/05/02/magazine/02self-measurement-t.html

Wood, J. M. (2020). (In)visible bleeding: The menstrual concealment imperative. In C. Bobel, I. T. Winkler, B. Fahs, et al. (Eds.), *Handbook of critical menstruation studies* (pp. 319–336). Palgrave Macmillan.

Woolf, V. (1929). *A room of one's own*. Harcourt Brace & Co.

13

Using and Interpreting FemTech Data: (Self-)Knowledge, Empowerment, and Sovereignty

Stefano Canali and Chris Hesselbein

Introduction

As this volume has shown, 'FemTech' seeks to take seriously the long-neglected issue of women's health not only by developing medical technologies that address female-specific conditions as well as general health conditions that differently or disproportionally affect women, but also by having women—as designers, investors, and recipients—lead the way in producing and using such technologies. FemTech, in other words, is supposed to be both *by* women as well as *for* women. An underlying assumption is that women's health needs are fundamentally different to those of men, and that medical technologies need to be reshaped to facilitate the inclusion of women and their specific needs in order to achieve a greater degree of gender equality in healthcare as well as beyond. According to a recent report by consulting firm McKinsey, FemTech attends to 'women's unmet health needs' and provides 'better outcomes for women patients and consumers', it is claimed, by 'disrupting healthcare' and improving

S. Canali • C. Hesselbein (✉)
Politecnico di Milano, Milan, Italy
e-mail: stefano.canali@polimi.it

care delivery and diagnosis as well as by addressing stigmatized areas and enabling self-care (McKinsey, 2022, 2–5). FemTech, in short, is a crucial means of empowering women to gain knowledge about and take control over their own bodies and health.

At its very core, FemTech—particularly in the guise of self-tracking devices and apps—focuses on as well as relies upon the female body and its experiences, practices, and processes. These phenomena, indeed the very body itself, provide the data that are being collected, counted, and analysed, and these outputs are subsequently used as the basis upon which FemTech products can be manufactured and marketed. The female body is therefore both the source of data that enables FemTech products as well as the target that FemTech products seek to monitor, aid, care for, and improve. However, women's bodies have long been a site of techno-scientific contestation, control, and exploitation (Martin, 1987; Wajcman, 1991), not just through direct medical interventions and healthcare policies, but also more subtly and indirectly through marketing narratives of self-care and empowerment. It is important to note that the majority of FemTech products that are currently offered to consumers focus on reproductive health, and generally in the form of apps for menstrual- and fertility tracking (FemTech Analytics, 2021). For this reason, it is of key importance to analyse the emergence of FemTech through a critical lens that remains focused on the relationships between data, knowledge, embodiment, and power (D'Ignazio & Klein, 2020). What kinds of (self) knowledge do FemTech self-tracking devices provide and to whom? What degrees of control over one's body and health do these forms of knowledge facilitate? How do these processes play out on the level of technology design and usage as well as data collection and interpretation? How are knowledges and practices being (re)configured and how do they inform individual as well as collective agency or empowerment? Finding answers to these questions is critical not just for interrogating the current promises and pitfalls of FemTech but will remain a pertinent issue as developments in digital health continue to unfold in the future.

This chapter focuses on two issues that are pertinent to these questions as well as other issues discussed in this volume. The first revolves around the usage of FemTech products and how these may provide or (re) configure self-knowledge. The second centres upon a keyword that is defining our current technoscientific era, namely 'data', and how this is being collected, interpreted, mobilized, and put to new uses. Taken together, both issues confront the relationship between knowledge and empowerment.

The first set of issues involves questions surrounding the design and usage of FemTech and how these inform (self-)knowledge as well as individual or collective empowerment. As noted just above, FemTech products are generally marketed as providing women with better insight into the working of their bodily functions, and therefore also giving them—individually as well as more broadly—a greater degree of control over their own body and health. It is less often noted, however, that FemTech products can downplay the experiential and embodied knowledge of women. In a nutshell, FemTech frames the body itself not as a sensing entity through which one gains self-knowledge, but as a source for the generation of data that requires analysis by a device in order to be known. Self-knowledge, in other words, shifts from being produced by the self to being produced by the device or application of the FemTech developer, from which it can, retranslated into numbers and graphs, be represented back to the consumer (Schüll, 2016). Although ethnographic research on users of self-tracking devices indicates that this is not necessarily an issue for self-trackers, and indeed often seen as offering exactly the types of insights that are sought after (e.g. Lupton, 2019; Pantzar & Ruckenstein, 2017), it also shows that self-tracking can lead to doubt and ambivalence about one's own body and experiences (Lomborg et al., 2020) as well as 'alienate' users from their own practical and experiential understanding of body and self (Kressbach, 2021; Smith & Vonthethoff, 2017). This suggests that the usage of FemTech can have implications that might diverge from or even run counter to the feminist goal of 'elevating' knowledge that emerges from embodied experience (D'Ignazio & Klein, 2020), which problematizes FemTech's potential for empowerment. Furthermore, given the co-constructive relationship between bodies and technologies, this shift from sensing body to sensory device is likely to have implications for the (self-)perceptive abilities of the body as well as its agency.

Second, as has been noted in multiple critiques of datafication in healthcare (Lupton, 2016; Neff & Nafus, 2016; Ruckenstein & Schüll,

2017), personal data, which form the basis for the development of FemTech products as well as the health solutions for which consumers turn to such devices, are highly contested as well as lucrative goods. The datafication and digitalisation of health are often presented as movements towards more precise, personalized as well as higher-quality evidence for biomedical research and clinical care, and this is echoed in discussions on FemTech. However, the variability of FemTech products and lack of access to the ways in which data are collected, classified, and interpreted create obstacles to determining and assessing the quality of FemTech data. In most cases, it remains unclear to users how and which data are collected, and this lack of clarity extends to the ways in which inferences and predictions are made, under which conditions they are established as accurate, and therefore to what extent they are valid.

Furthermore, the sharing of personal data with third parties, whether for scientific research, targeted advertising, or the marketing of healthcare products and services, has given rise to concerns about security, privacy, surveillance, commodification, and exploitation (Mehrnezhad et al., 2022; Mishra & Suresh, 2021). For FemTech, datafication emerges at the intersection of conflicting tendencies: The creation of FemTech data can be seen as a way of empowering women and producing quantitative and concrete evidence about their health concerns, which have traditionally been underrepresented in biomedical research and healthcare; yet, this data is also extremely valuable to the biomedical industry as well as big tech companies.

In the critical literature on the datafication of health, one solution has been proposed to address both sets of concerns: data sovereignty. Data sovereignty seeks to extend the legal concepts of 'self-determination' and 'property' and principles of individual or collective agency and autonomy to digital practices (Gurumurthy & Chami, 2021; Hummel et al., 2021). In the context of FemTech, one could also see this as an extension of the concept of 'bodily sovereignty' to the data that bodies produce. Greater control over one's data, it is thought, can thus lead to greater control over one's body and self. However, access to and sovereignty over one's data are not unmitigated goods, as will be discussed below.

This chapter thus confronts the question 'Who is FemTech for?' by focusing both on how such devices or applications may (not) produce (self-)knowledge as well as on the data practices that surround FemTech products. By combining approaches from the philosophy of medicine, critical data studies, and feminist science and technology studies, we seek to address issues of usage and data interpretation in wearable FemTech and how these problematize FemTech's capacity to 'empower' women and their health.

FemTech and Its Critics

It is a common assertion that FemTech self-tracking devices facilitate the production of knowledge, and therefore provide users with a greater degree of control over their body and health (e.g. FemTech Analytics, 2021; McKinsey, 2022). In particular, wearables, such as menstruation- and fertility-tracking devices connected to smartphone apps, are accompanied by claims that are reminiscent of a central tenet of the Quantified Self, namely the idea that self-knowledge can be obtained through numbers (Lupton, 2016). More precisely, aspects of daily life that are usually known from an experiential and qualitative perspective—or that are not consciously known because they are part and parcel of our invisible bodily functions—are self-reported or measured via biosensors and converted into quantitative variables that are scrutinized for correlations and patterns that would otherwise remain obscured. This datafication of our bodily functions is claimed to produce more objective insights into our body and health, provide users with a greater degree of control and self-determination, and ultimately also benefit women's healthcare more broadly through the collection of data for scientific research.

As introduced by proponents working in the field, FemTech is a system of tools that provides more empowerment and autonomy to individual users, in this way contributing to research on issues that are particularly pressing to women. For example, wearable and tracker devices sold by Bloomlife monitor maternal and foetal health parameters, thus expanding the availability and limits of monitoring that can be done remotely and at home. According to the company, this is a way of 'increasing access' to health parameters, 'empowering women' thanks to real-time feedback, as well as improving risk stratification, personalizing prenatal care, and improving research outcomes (https://bloomlife.com, accessed December 23, 2022). Similarly, according to a recent report by management consulting company McKinsey, FemTech directly addresses issues and aspects of health that affect women disproportionately or predominantly, including menstrual health, sexual health, pelvic care, and menopause (McKinsey, 2022). In turn, the empowerment and improved autonomy enabled by FemTech is considered a way of catalysing additional social changes, such as the increasing presence of women in leading and senior positions in various industries. For example, according to McKinsey, menopause 'frequently occurs when women are most likely to step into senior roles. Its effects can have an impact on the number of women in top positions and the quality of women's experiences throughout organizations'. The idea here seems to be that more data on issues that are particularly pressing for female health can lead to more knowledge on these issues and thus empower women in terms of their health and beyond. On the face of it, this linear model that connects data, knowledge, and empowerment seems to go in a direction that is generally favoured by feminist discourses on health and empowerment. Products such as those designed by Bloomlife thus have effects that extend beyond immediate health outcomes and into social and cultural practices including work and family life.

However, FemTech products, and particularly the burgeoning subset of self-tracking devices and apps that focus on sexual and reproductive health, have attracted the attention of critical scholars from various backgrounds. As we have seen throughout the volume, an emerging critical literature on FemTech has discussed various issues that have emerged against the backdrop of narratives promoted by the FemTech industry on inclusion, diversity, and feminism. While the collection of data performed by FemTech products can be seen as a way of empowering users and supporting female well-being, it can also have ambivalent consequences and lead to misuse. Perhaps unsurprisingly, many of these studies have observed that FemTech tracking devices may repeat many of the issues that have been encountered in the Quantified Self community—such as the exertion of disciplinary power and control through surveillance techniques as well as the enforcement of individualizing rationalities (Ruckenstein & Schüll, 2017), and the exploitation of asymmetric power relations and biocapital (Neff & Nafus, 2016). Yet, there seem also to be a number of important additions.

First, FemTech products are targeted mainly at healthy, young, cis heteronormative women with a relatively high level of income and education, thus excluding older, less health literate as well as less wealthy women as well as populations with relatively more marginalized illnesses (Krishnamurti et al., 2022). Next, FemTech products often focus on fertility or contraception, and tend to rely on language and imagery that reproduces and reinforces traditional, heterosexual, or stereotypical conceptualisations of womanhood and femininity as well as neoliberal ideals of self-regulation and optimization (Epstein et al., 2017; Roetman, 2020; Sanders, 2017; Vallor, 2016; Wilkinson et al., 2015). In other words, some FemTech products not only run the risk of maintaining or reproducing traditional conceptualizations of women's roles and femininity, but also of reaffirming or exacerbating unequal social relations among different groups of women. Furthermore, some FemTech products have been accused of extracting invisible labour from their users, and of disciplining them into the maintenance of bodies and social relations that are amenable to post-feminist and capitalist structures, for example, by linking menstrual health to work productivity (Lupton, 2016; McEwen, 2018).

Others have moreover asserted that FemTech can be understood as a form of reproductive self-surveillance that commodifies and 'datafies' the lived experiences of female users under the guise of empowerment while harnessing such data for profit (Healy, 2021; Mishra & Suresh, 2021). In this direction, Teresa Almeida and colleagues have also argued that FemTech applications and devices can lead to significant violations of individual and group privacy (Almeida et al., 2022). Several FemTech companies still do not abide by data collection regulations such as the GDPR (the General Data Protection Regulation), which has been in force in Europe since the 2018 and places significant restrictions on the collection and use of personal data, particularly health data (Mehrnezhad et al., 2022). Instead of complying with these requirements, FemTech products and services frequently share vulnerable data with other commercial entities in ways that are often not transparent to individual users (see, e.g. the case of Flo Health, as discussed in the Introduction to this volume, and Shipp & Blasco, 2020).

Similarly to other digital health technologies, the FemTech industry tends to operate in grey areas of regulation, where traditional regulatory approaches and bioethical principles are often not considered (Faubion, 2021; Predel & Steger, 2021). As a result, FemTech can lead to more marginalization and discrimination of users, as the data collected by FemTech products and services—especially when shared with third parties and commercial entities—can expose vulnerable aspects of the menstrual cycle, infertility, or pregnancy. Inferences based on access and use of these data, in turn, can marginalize FemTech users, as data on menstrual cycles can deprive them of their reproductive rights, expose abortion in areas where this is illegal, and signal pregnancies in the workplace (see Introduction to this volume; Fox & Spektor, 2021; Brown, 2021). It has also been noted that the development and usage of FemTech can lead to more algorithmic bias, as the databases assembled through FemTech products and services fail to include the needs of individual users, such as privacy and data sharing. These biased and insecure datasets can thus perpetuate discrimination while simultaneously leading to more forms of social profiling and exploitation that harm discriminated social groups and users for the benefit of big tech companies.

Bodily Self-Knowledge and Control Through Datafication

Despite the trenchant criticisms we have discussed in the previous section, the FemTech sector is predicted to continue growing at a fast pace in the upcoming years (McKinsey, 2022). It is therefore of key importance to ask what might be underpinning the continuing success of FemTech in light of these scholarly criticisms and why people continue to welcome such technologies into their lives. A crucial part of this question is to examine the core assertion that FemTech can lead to more and better self-knowledge as well as control over one's body and health. An entry point into evaluating this assertion is to examine the growing body of qualitative research on self-tracking and FemTech devices that has emerged over the past decade, which provides a nuanced discussion of how datafied bodily processes come to matter in the lives of self-trackers, how they interpret, value, or reject such insights, and how self-tracking data might enliven or impoverish one's sense of self and one's embodiment. Such studies therefore manage to avoid overly celebratory accounts of the liberatory potential of self-tracking devices as well as more negative accounts that grant insufficient agency to self-trackers and frame them as 'dupes' of systems of surveillance and marketing narratives. Examining the findings of ethnographic studies will allow us to better understand the 'as yet undetermined individual and collective possibilities' (Schüll, 2018, 28) of FemTech, and particularly on the level of embodied self-knowledge as well as of the implications this has for women's empowerment in health issues.

In contrast to biomedical perspectives—which place negative emphasis on the asymmetrical power relations between producers and users of self-tracking devices, the extraction, commodification, and exploitation of intimate data, and the threat of 'dataveillance' and 'neoliberal subjectification' (Ajana, 2017; Neff & Nafus, 2016; Ruckenstein & Schüll, 2017; Van Dijck, 2014)—ethnographic studies show that self-tracking devices and the personal data they produce can 'render aspects of a private, subjective, and somewhat inaccessible world of feelings and problems more tangible and comparable' (Sharon & Zandbergen, 2017, 1705). In short, self-tracking allows users to see processes, patterns, and rhythms that would otherwise remain 'below the threshold of perception' (Schüll, 2019, 919). Importantly, it is often argued that self-tracking data does not simply displace or negate previous conceptualisations of the self and its experiences, but is translated by people to fit their cultural understandings and expectations as well as their everyday experiences in an eclectic and 'situated' manner (Pantzar & Ruckenstein, 2017). Moreover, the datafied bodily processes that are visually re-represented to self-trackers are often valued because they can initiate a process of critical reflection and provide the basis for the changing of habits or tendencies that are perceived to be infelicitous, and even free people from the sense of being caught in a fixed or essential identity (Ruckenstein, 2014; Schüll, 2016). Self-tracking practices can therefore be understood as providing a 'laboratory of the self' in which the 'qualified' body and self can be explored and reflexively brought into conversation with the metrics and experiences of others (Kristensen & Ruckenstein, 2018). The transformation of ambiguous and messy bodily processes and experiences into visualized and controllable 'life slices' (Pantzar & Ruckenstein, 2017) promotes a 'move away from embodied and emotional dimensions of the self' and allows for the 'mutual constitution of self and technology' (Kristensen & Ruckenstein, 2018, 3629–3635, see also Lupton, 2019; Mopas & Huybregts, 2020). As these ethnographic studies show, self-trackers are frequently motivated to engage in datafication practices because they appreciate the complementary insights that tracking devices and apps can provide in addition to that of their lived experiences.

Even critical studies of self-tracking therefore appear to back up the assertion, although with a number of important qualifications, that self-tracking can lead to improved self-knowledge about the body, its functioning, and its health status, and thus also provide a greater sense of self-control. Several studies on the use of FemTech products and apps for self-tracking bear out similarly positive accounts. For example, research on devices and apps used for monitoring reproductive and sexual health have examined the multiple and varied reasons why users engage in such practices. Various studies of menstruation- and fertility-tracking apps (Epstein et al., 2017; Gambier-Ross et al., 2018) find that menstruators use these not only to gain a general understanding of their bodily and emotional states but also to practically plan their daily lives, achieve the goal of achieving or avoiding pregnancy, and to inform conversations with healthcare providers. It is important to note that in contrast to self-tracking practices that focus on lifestyle or health behaviours that can be controlled and altered, such as certain eating habits for example, menstrual cycles are a lot less amenable to such interventions beyond that of hormonal birth control. That is to say, menstrual tracking cannot show one how to change this process, but menstruators can 'learn how to adjust their thoughts and behaviours around [menstruation]' (Epstein et al., 2017, 6885). Knowing one's menstrual cycle and being able to prepare and plan around this process is considered valuable not just to those who wish to conceive (and who might be undergoing infertility treatment, which is a complex and emotional intervention), but also for those who wish to gain greater control in the planning of their professional and social activities.

Other studies have similarly found that period-tracking devices and apps can be used in ways that neglect the 'reproductive imperative' altogether and instead provide the basis for negotiating one's 'mood, energy, or mental health' as well as broader health infrastructures (Ford et al., 2021, 54). Self-tracking can help users manage the disruptive potential of 'hormones' to one's daily life, but also create a deeper understanding and indeed even appreciation of these deeply intimate interactions between body, mind, and self, as well as suggest techniques for managing and anticipating their effects. In short, menstrual tracking reveals patterns of relations between one's cycle and one's mood, and can thus better 'attune' users to their body than before. The self-knowledge that emerges from the information provided by self-tracking technologies and the interpretation by users can provide a greater feeling of control and therefore empowerment, but this is achieved at the cost of participating in systems that surveil and exploit personal health data as well as neoliberal and post-feminist discourses that emphasize stereotypical femininity, self-optimization, and individual resilience rather than communal healthcare (Roetman, 2020; Sanders, 2017).

From this brief overview of existing studies on self-tracking and FemTech products and their usage, it appears that they can provide significant insights into understanding one's body and self. Users of such technologies can gain self-knowledge about their body and therefore attain a greater sense of control of their lives, even if this is provided with significant and sometimes negative trade-offs. Moreover, self-tracking technologies frame the production of self-knowledge not as something that is done by the self but as something that emerges from the datafication of bodily processes and their mediation of this information by FemTech products back to the user. This translation of bodily processes and behavioural patterns into numbers and visual representations is not only valued by self-trackers for its potential to uncover hidden and potentially problematic health issues, but sometimes also for the sheer pleasure of gaining a greater understanding about one's own body through data and the comfort that a greater sense of predictability and control can provide (see also Lupton, 2015, 2019 on this point). Analysts have therefore evaluated this technologically mediated process of self-discovery rather positively as a form of 'everyday sensemaking' and as allowing for 'the mutual constitution of self and technology' (Kristensen & Ruckenstein, 2018, 3635), or even as an 'everyday cyborg' (Ruckenstein, 2022) or 'post-human cyborgs' who are merely seeking a 'more holistic sense of what they are experiencing' (Mopas & Huybregts, 2020). Such references to the 'cyborg'—one of the central metaphors of feminist science and technology studies—recall both the optimistic accounts by (cyber)feminist scholars celebrating the hybridity that digital technology purported to offer (e.g. Plant, 1998) as well as more pessimistic critiques (e.g. Wajcman, 2004). The latter have underscored that digital technologies do not necessarily represent a radical rupture with older technologies, and that liberatory promises of empowerment as well as celebrations of the collapse of boundaries between body and technology are perhaps overblown, particularly considering the ways in which digital technologies continue to be imbricated in the essentialization of gender identities as well as the policing of bodily differences. These considerations make it especially relevant to examine how self-tracking and FemTech technologies might subvert or displace self-knowledge that arises from bodily experiences, which is a form of knowledge central to feminist theory.

A starting point, therefore, for discussing how self-tracking devices might problematize rather than foster the creation of self-knowledge is that self-tracking data does not always make sense to users, particularly in relation to the senses and lived experience of users, and can therefore lead to anxiety and doubt rather than actionable insights (Lomborg et al., 2018; Pink et al., 2018). For example, when the data that is produced about a particular activity differs from the perception and experience of that activity, users may either start to question the accuracy and validity of the performed measurements or that of their own evaluative capabilities. Moreover, because information about the body and one's health carries a strong affective dimension, such personal data can be experienced as insightful and motivating, but equally also as troubling or demotivating (cf. Hamper, 2020). Particularly the latter instantiation of them can lead to 'data anxiety' (Pink et al., 2018) or to 'data ambivalence' (Lomborg et al., 2020) in which users are called to choose between placing hope and trust in the data produced by a device or in the perception and experience by and of their own body. Making sense of data and applying its insights as a form of self-knowledge that can be mobilized towards achieving self-care is, in other words, not always straightforward. The actions and behaviours of users are certainly not necessarily determined by the potential inaccuracy or ambiguity of self-tracking data; they can critically engage with such data and use the information and suggestions that emerge from the quantification process in a selective and purposive manner, thus retaining a sense of control and agency. But the mismatch between one's knowledge, sensations, or experiences and the data provided by self-tracking devices can leave users 'stuck with meaningless data' and thus significantly increase their sense of anxiety and uncertainty about their body and health as well as the device (Lomborg et al., 2020, 8–9).

In addition to potentially creating doubt and anxiety among users, self-tracking devices and data can also have 'addictive' qualities and start to become 'fetishized' by users as providing seemingly objective insights that speak on behalf of bodily processes in a manner that is more insightful, meaningful, and actionable in terms of knowing and working on the body and self (Lupton, 2015, see also Sharon & Zandbergen, 2017). Indeed, self-trackers frequently display a deep dissatisfaction with and distrust of the body and its capacities to sense, feel, and intuit. Biosensors and datafication processes are employed to simultaneously 'look at' as well as 'look beyond' the body because individual perception and consciousness are deemed insufficiently capable of providing stable and reliable insights about the body and self. In other words, the 'body/self is only validated if it appears outside of the body/self, especially in the form of a multiplex data visualisation' (Smith & Vonthethoff, 2017, 11). Moreover, such 'exteriorized' or 'unbodied' data about bodily processes can 'subsume' the experience of embodiment through the outsourcing and perhaps even displacement of bodily intuition, perception, and cognition (Ibidem, 2). This technologically mediated reshaping of conceptualisations of embodiment and health does not, to be sure, operate in a deterministic manner as users remain able to negotiate or even reject such datafied representations of the body and self, or indeed might continue to embrace the insights provided by self-tracking devices and act on them accordingly. However, it does suggest how phenomenological perspectives on the self can be undermined and therefore how the process of datafication can be experienced as disempowering for some users.

Empirical studies of the use of self-tracking among, for example, athletes, find that although self-tracking devices can enhance understanding of one's own body, such devices can also create a distance between an athlete and their bodily sensations as well as 'excessively rationalize' their sports activities (Boldi & Rapp, 2022, see also Pols et al., 2019). Similar to self-tracking for medical uses, the datafication of bodily movements can 'undermine the athlete's confidence' or even jeopardize their 'awareness of sensations' and lead to anxiety and worries, particularly when the information provided does not correspond with an athlete's self-perception (Boldi & Rapp, 2022, 199). By potentially reducing athletes' awareness of bodily sensations, self-tracking can hamper self-knowledge and lead to a sense of loss of control because its abstract and numerical representation of the body cannot 'integrate into a coherent image [...] the body complex nature made up of perceptions, proprioceptive sensations, and self-representations' (Ibidem, 190, see also Roberson's contribution to this volume).

Emergent studies on self-tracking practices in FemTech have similarly made claims that problematize the ability of such devices to straightforwardly produce self-knowledge and enhance bodily control. For example, the claim that menstruation tracking allows users to 'know' and 'demystify' their body strongly suggests that users are currently in a state of 'embodied ignorance' that can only be solved by means of self-tracking technologies (Healy, 2021, 4). Moreover, the outsourcing of knowledge production to datafication processes can 'undermine female self-analysis' and obstruct women's abilities to 'narrate or claim understanding over their own bodies' both individually as well as collectively (Ibidem, 8). That FemTech tracking devices can hamper rather than facilitate self-knowledge is particularly apparent when devices and apps are unable to produce patterns and predictions that make sense to users or that do not align with their expectations and pre-existing self-knowledge. This can give rise to feelings of confusion and even failure, but also cause users to blame their own 'irregularities' or to feel as if they are 'abnormal' or 'not textbook' (Hamper, 2020, 22–23, see also Della Bianca, 2021, 15–16).

Another potential objection to the use of FemTech products concerns the usefulness of tracking devices and the data they produce. For example, many users find that apps are frequently inadequate at accurately predicting menstrual cycles, particularly irregular ones, as well as insufficiently able to accommodate both routine as well as larger life changes, such as switching between methods of birth control or falling pregnant. Although such issues generally arise from flawed assumptions on the part of app developers about the stability and regularity of women's lives, predictions are also inaccurate because 'people often forget to log their period' (Epstein et al., 2017, 6882).

Yet, another observation that casts doubt on the ability of menstrual-tracking technologies to produce actionable and empowering self-knowledge is that they reduce complex embodied and psychosocial experiences to biological processes over which users have little or no control. Kressbach (2021), for example, argues that menstrual-tracking and fertility apps 'reinforce discourses of menstrual concealment' and 'bodily alienation'. By analysing the daily log interfaces and analytics sections of such apps, Kressbach asserts that these not only encourage users to understand their lives and bodies predominantly through their menstrual cycles, but also that they 'frame the body as an unruly and uncontrollable cause of a range of complex emotional and physical experiences' (Ibidem, 243). More specifically, the design and interface of menstrual-tracking apps appear to open up the taboo of menstruation as much as they close this down by visually abstracting from the bodily process and creating a 'mediated distance' between the user and their body. Ovulation and period-tracking apps such as Glow and Flo, for example, are notorious for their stereotypically pink interface design and use of 'feminine' language or euphemistic iconography (Epstein et al., 2017; Healy, 2021).

Like other studies, Kressbach agrees that menstrual tracking can allow users to identify patterns and relationships between their cycles as well as bodily or emotional changes, and therefore to manage and anticipate their daily life by making small adjustments to their habits and behaviours. However, self-tracking apps are only able to draw superficial correlations between cycles and symptoms, such as stress or anxiety, despite their best efforts at suggesting the existence of clear and causal relationships between them. In effect, Kressbach argues, this neglects the effect that a range of social factors might have on such symptoms, and frames them as being produced by individual bodily processes only. In other words, the analytic results provided by menstrual-tracking apps appear to draw causal relationships between menstrual cycles and users' embodied experiences as well as visually represent these insights as 'transparent self-knowledge' using the 'rhetoric of science', but these apps ultimately reduce complex psycho-social dynamics to biological explanations. Although this biomedical understanding of menstruation can be seen as crucial for acknowledging its potential adverse health effects and for channelling medical attention and resources towards issues such as Pre-Menstrual Syndrome, it also risks 'bodily alienation' by situating 'the body as a thing separate from the self' and by framing emotional experiences as being caused by bodily processes that are driven by 'unruly' hormones that cannot be controlled (Ibidem, 254). The self-knowledge produced by menstrual-tracking apps can therefore render the body as an entity that is largely determined by the disruptive effects of uncontrollable biological processes and that can only be understood through these very technologies, thus ignoring the role that social context plays as well as relinquishing individual agency and responsibility. The biomedicalization of knowledge about menstruation through self-tracking technologies can therefore threaten the sense of control that users have over their bodies rather than enhance it.

From this discussion of existing studies on the use of self-tracking devices and apps, and particularly of menstrual- and fertility-tracking technologies developed by FemTech companies, it appears that these technologies can assist in the production of self-knowledge about the body and self, and thus also grant a greater sense of control over one's body and health—and yet there are significant limitations too. These various forms of knowledge and control are only facilitated for some users, namely those who can recognize their own bodily experiences as it is represented by their data, and moreover, these insights are provided with significant trade-offs. Acquiring self-knowledge through self-tracking appears to require an externalization of information about the embodied self, which is subsequently quantified and visualized back to the user. This process can provide some users with insights about their own bodily functions, feelings, and habits in a manner that is considered valuable, actionable, and empowering, but for others whose embodied experiences and self-perception do not align with their datafied selves this can lead to feelings of ambivalence, confusion, anxiety, and disempowerment. The somewhat ambiguous picture that emerges from our discussion of self-tracking and FemTech technologies reflects the multiple positionalities of users and how their various socio-cultural beliefs, personal experiences, and individual capabilities inform the context in which such technologies are valued or rejected. In any case, it is clear that the use of self-tracking technologies does not necessarily or unproblematically result in greater self-knowledge and control over one's body and health.

FemTech Knowledge and the Limitations of Data Sovereignty

What should we make of the issues and trade-offs in the forms of knowledge and control provided by FemTech? What is next beyond critiques and current challenges we have discussed so far? An approach that has emerged in the literature as a way of addressing some of these issues is that of 'data sovereignty'. Data sovereignty is a framework in which individual users should be able to exert sovereignty over their data, thus being aware of the different uses of their personal data by other individuals and organisations as well as capable of stopping unwanted flows and uses of data (Hummel et al., 2021). As such, the idea is that individual users as data sovereigns will have more power to negotiate the use and commercialisation of their personal data with big tech companies, for instance by selling them for profit (Hummel et al., 2020). In critical discussions of FemTech, Anita Gurumurthy and Nandini Chami have argued that data sovereignty can be a way of dealing with some of the criticisms of FemTech, for instance on issues such as privacy and data sharing, exploitation and digital capitalism, discrimination and exclusion (Gurumurthy & Chami, 2021). We agree that more data sovereignty for individual FemTech users would be a positive and welcome improvement for several of the aforementioned issues and risks associated with the increasing implementation of this technology. But what would data sovereignty look like for FemTech and what can it do?

In this section, we discuss the concrete application of data sovereignty to the context of health data, and particularly FemTech products and services, and argue that this creates significant challenges. In order to present these challenges, we turn to the growing body of work that in the last decade has looked at the epistemic, political, and social roles of data and big data in the health and scientific context. This line of work—often referred to as 'data studies' (Iliadis & Russo, 2016; Kitchin & Lauriault, 2018; Leonelli & Tempini, 2020)—involves interdisciplinary approaches from the sociology of science and science and technology studies, philosophy of science and technology, history of science and technology, and more. Philosophical perspectives on the epistemic role of data in the sciences will be particularly relevant for our work in this section: As we have seen, FemTech products are presented as ways to empower users through knowledge, which can take the form of self-knowledge (see previous section) or biomedical and health knowledge, which raises questions on the extent to which these knowledge processes can be governed through data sovereignty. In answering these questions, we argue that the application of data sovereignty to FemTech faces issues regarding the relational features of health data, the need to access the contextual properties of data, and the focus on individualistic and commercial aspects of property. As such, we present data sovereignty as a critical but also problematic issue for FemTech, and sketch out an expanded approach to data access and governance as a forward-thinking conclusion for discussions on what's next for FemTech regulation and use.

The body of work on data-intensive methods in the sciences is particularly significant to studying FemTech and data sovereignty. In this context, empirical studies of the epistemic role of data in the scientific and biomedical context have discussed the relational and contextual nature of data (Leonelli & Tempini, 2020), showing that their value as a source of knowledge is defined by their ability to move and travel between different sites (Latour, 1999) and is expanded by the work needed to make data accessible and reusable for travel (Leonelli, 2009). For example, in the life sciences, substantial work is dedicated to packaging biological data for travel, including labelling, cleaning, and curating data so that they can travel from the initial point of creation and collection; in turn, this work can expand the use of data as knowledge across different areas of research and types of phenomena (Leonelli, 2014). In this sense, the epistemic value of data as evidence, representation, knowledge is not only due to their intrinsic and physical properties, but also a result of the contextual and relational features of the specific situations in which the data are used (Leonelli, 2016). Intrinsic features of data—such as their format, consistency, and resemblance to the phenomena that they represent—clearly matter for the use of data as knowledge, but equally important are the technological, material, and social features of the specific context in which data is re-used. For example, consider menstruation data collected through fertility-trackers, which can be used to develop knowledge on individual menstruation patterns. These data have intrinsic features that make them a particularly useful source of evidence for understanding menstrual cycles, for instance, by underscoring that data may be symmetrical to specific patterns of menstrual cycles. However, the use of these data for knowledge about menstrual cycles is dependent on other factors too: for instance the extent to which comparable data and models about menstrual cycles on 'normal' cycles are available, how computational tools and heuristics fit with the features of the data, and to what extent it is possible to access metadata about individual features of the specific user. These contextual and relational features of data are perhaps particularly pressing in the health context, as differences in the ways in which data are used in a specific context can lead to substantially different types of knowledge—for example, without comparable data about 'normal' menstrual cycles the use of FemTech for (self-)knowledge might not be possible (Fiske et al., 2022).

Taking these results on board, where do they leave us with respect to data sovereignty as a solution to the limitations of FemTech knowledge? A first problem we want to emphasize is that the contextual and relational features of health data make it difficult to govern them through individual sovereignty. According to the data sovereignty framework, one way in which one can 'fix' the critical aspects of FemTech is to focus on the starting point of knowledge processes involving FemTech data. Following FemTech narratives of empowerment, more data on issues that are particularly pressing for female health can lead to more knowledge on these issues and thus empower women in issues related to their health and beyond. In applying the data sovereignty approach to this linear model that connects data, knowledge, and empowerment, the idea seems to be that access to and property of personal data can prevent possible misuse and re-establish possibilities of facilitating knowledge and empowerment (Gurumurthy & Chami, 2021). We agree that individual property of data can prevent several cases of misuse, including some of those we have discussed so far. Considering, for instance, misuses of personal FemTech data for profiling, advertising, and exploitation, these seem to be cases where data sovereignty would probably prevent misuse. In addition, data sovereignty can help more general uses of FemTech for the production of self-knowledge, for instance by helping users make sense of the data and by potentially decreasing the distance between what is represented by FemTech tracking devices and one's bodily sensations.

However, the contextual and relational aspects of data are such that access to and property of data is often not enough. As we have seen, contemporary studies on the use of large datasets as a basis for knowledge processes in the sciences frame data as contextual and relational entities, where features of the context where data are used and the relations connecting data to this context matter as much as the data themselves. Similarly, we argue that individual users and customers of FemTech will need access to these contextual properties in order to understand the ways in which data are analysed, labelled, and interpreted, and thus to be able to use them as the basis for developing (self-)knowledge. Consider, for instance, recent studies of the ways in which individual users such as heart patients use wearable technologies as a basis to develop self- and biomedical knowledge about their health (Lomborg et al., 2020). In these cases, a lack of information on the ways in which the data are collected, analysed, interpreted by wearable technologies constitutes a barrier for users who want to use data for knowledge of their health. Limited information about the contextual features of data is an obstacle for the use of wearable technology as a basis for knowledge production, and, moreover, can become a source of doubt and anxiety as well as lack of trust in the data. As we have seen in the previous section, the distance between measurements and data collected by FemTech products on, for example, sleep patterns and the embodied experience of how long the user has slept, can create doubt that prevents the use of data as a basis for knowledge (Lomborg et al., 2020).

The problem of transparency and lack of contextual information is shared between FemTech and other digital health technologies. Often individual users do not have direct access to the personal and health data that FemTech products and services collect on them, but often there is also a lack of transparency and understanding on the ways in which data are collected, labelled, analysed and used by these services and devices. For example, basic yet crucial assumptions for data analysis that are employed about, for example, what counts as a normal or standard menstrual cycle are often not made clear or explicit to individual users of FemTech menstrual-tracking apps (Hamper, 2020). In turn, in cases where issues of transparency and anxiety related to the data are involved, approaches from the perspective of data sovereignty can help, but only to a certain extent. Property and access to data from sleep or menstrual-tracking devices are significant for allowing individual users to develop their own understanding and knowledge. But on their own, ownership and access are not enough: Without contextual information on the ways in which their personal data is related to assumptions, analyses, interpretations, and so on, it can be very difficult to check the accuracy, quality, and validity of the data as a basis for self-knowledge and beyond (Canali et al., 2022). In thinking about what data sovereignty might mean and could do in the FemTech context, ensuring that users can have access to and be individual owners of their personal data is an important starting point—yet consideration of the contexts in which data are created, collected, and used is necessary. Access to these contextual properties of data are crucial to govern their journeys and possible misuses and prevent new ethical issues, thus also following one of the principles of data feminism as presented by Catherine D'Ignazio and Lauren Klein: 'Data feminism asserts that data are not neutral or objective. They are the products of unequal social relations, and this context is essential for conducting accurate, ethical analysis' (D'Ignazio & Klein, 2020, 18).

A final point to highlight in relation to data sovereignty and FemTech concerns a more practical consequence of the data sovereignty framework. While data sovereignty seems to align well with feminist proposals towards individual and bodily sovereignty, we argue that an expanded notion of sovereignty and access is needed to include the ability to be represented in decisions of public value and benefits and to help develop contextually relevant and democratically accountable data systems (Gurumurthy & Chami, 2021). The limitation we see in this direction is that the data sovereignty framework could be seen as a way to focus on mostly individualistic and commercial aspects of property. Individual property can be a helpful tool to use when trying to counter the misuse of personal FemTech data, but could also lead users to sell their personal data for specific services and benefits. In this sense, for instance, data collected by menstrual FemTech apps and devices would be individually owned by users, who could then freely choose to sell them in order to, for example, receive personalized analyses of their menstrual cycles, but potentially also for marketing purposes or profit. These proposals seem to go into a direction that is highly individualistic, framing individual users mostly in terms of consumers and customers and as uniquely responsible for data journeys, thus potentially exacerbating existing or creating additional inequalities between those who need to sell their data and those who do not (Prainsack & Forgó, 2022; Schüll, 2016). In reaction to these issues, some have recently argued for an approach to data governance in which health data is a collective form of property, which can strengthen collective control and ownership of data, ensure that benefits and costs of digital practices are distributed collectively, and promote solidarity in the collective sharing of data for research and beyond (Prainsack et al., 2022; Staunton et al., 2021). On the basis of the considerations discussed in this section, we similarly argue that an expanded conceptualization of access should lie at the basis of critical approaches to FemTech (which can also inform new regulatory approaches), namely a notion of access that is focused as much on access to the data themselves as the contextual properties and relational elements of data use, and one that poses crucial questions about who has access and responsibility both as individuals or communities.

Conclusion

This chapter has critically interrogated the assertion that FemTech products and services can benefit the production of (self-)knowledge and therefore foster individual as well as collective control and empowerment over women's health. From our discussion of the ethnographic literature on self-tracking practices and FemTech products, it has become clear that menstrual- and fertility-tracking technologies can assist some users in the production of self-knowledge about the body and self, and thus grant them a greater sense of control over their body and health. However, the production of knowledge through self-tracking devices requires an externalization of information about the embodied self and can potentially distance users from their own embodied perceptions and experiences. Although some users consider the mediated process of knowledge production as providing valuable and actionable insights, and thus also creating a greater sense of control over one's health, for others the opposite is true. For those whose embodied experiences and self-perception do not align with their datafied selves, the usage of FemTech self-tracking devices can lead to feelings of ambivalence, confusion, and disempowerment. Engaging with FemTech self-tracking practices, in other words, does not necessarily or straightforwardly lead to the production of self-knowledge or foster control and empowerment over one's body and health.

On the basis of these results, we have looked at data sovereignty as a possible solution to the limitations of using FemTech data as a basis of self-knowledge. Relying on studies of contemporary uses of large data-sets as a basis for knowledge processes in the biomedical sciences, we have argued that the contextual and relational features of biomedical data raise concern on the extent to which sovereignty can be exerted over FemTech data. At the same time, access to and ownership of FemTech data, as conceptualized within the framework of data sovereignty, are probably not enough to enable users to develop knowledge as a result of their use of FemTech products and services. Finally, we have warned against the individualistic and commercial aspects of data sovereignty, which might lead to unwanted effects such as more discrimination and exploitation of individual users. What we need is an expanded notion of data access that includes access to the contextual and relational features of FemTech data.

In conclusion, it is important to acknowledge how FemTech products are altering our senses as well as our relationship to our bodies and ourselves in a specific even if not yet fully understood manner. Importantly, self-tracking devices do not, and perhaps cannot, monitor the various tacit forms of understanding that arise from experience with one's body and self, and—because they are often perceived as providing more 'objective' knowledge about the body—have the possibility of displacing or replacing this crucial form of self-perception and knowledge. Not everything can be tracked by sensors and therefore measured and quantifiably 'known', and technologies do carry an ability not just to enhance but also obstruct one's sensory capacities. Taking a co-constructive approach can highlight the mutual shaping of technology and our senses, and especially how this process can shift what we consider as normal or natural. Although some users will undoubtedly continue to consider the insights that are provided by self-tracking or FemTech applications as valuable and empowering, and others users will not, it is important to move beyond a dichotomous distinction that frames technologies as either good or bad and users as either empowered or disempowered. As ostensibly true and important as this distinction might initially seem, it is perhaps more helpful to approach the relationship between self-tracking technology and embodiment from a more co-constructive perspective. Such an approach provides a better grasp of who or what is being mutually shaped as well as how this process might be unfolding and on what level, which will ultimately allow us to evaluate such developments more critically.

Finally, if FemTech products are truly supposed to be a tool for empowerment through (self-) knowledge, then this understanding of empowerment needs to extend beyond that of the individual self, and ideally towards a collective concern with women's healthcare that is not informed by biopolitical regimes and dominated by commercial incentives (cf. Gurumurthy & Chami, 2021). If the self knowledge that is presumably generated through FemTech devices and apps is to be conceptualized in terms of both control and empowerment, it might appear that these both lie more firmly in the database of the producer than it is in the hands of the consumer. We need to open up possibilities for users to be empowered as active users of FemTech, not just passive owners of FemTech data and products.

References

Ajana, B. (2017). Digital health and the biopolitics of the Quantified Self. *DIGITAL HEALTH, 3*, 1–18.

Almeida, T., Shipp, L., Mehrnezhad, M., & Toreini, E. (2022). Bodies like yours: Enquiring data privacy in FemTech. *Adjunct Proceedings of the 2022 Nordic Human-Computer Interaction Conference*, 1–5. https://doi.org/10.1145/3547522.3547674

Boldi, A., & Rapp, A. (2022). Quantifying the body: Body image, body awareness and self-tracking technologies. In K. Wac & S. Wulfovich (Eds.), *Quantifying quality of life* (pp. 189–207). Springer International Publishing. https://doi.org/10.1007/978-3-030-94212-0_9

Brown, E. A. (2021). The Femtech Paradox: How workplace monitoring threatens women's equity. *Jurimetrics, 61*(3), 289–329.

Canali, S., Schiaffonati, V., & Aliverti, A. (2022). Challenges and recommendations for wearable devices in digital health: Data quality, interoperability, health equity, fairness. *PLOS Digital Health, 1*(10), e0000104. https://doi.org/10.1371/journal.pdig.0000104

Della Bianca, L. (2021). The Cyclic Self: Menstrual Cycle Tracking as Body Politics. *Catalyst: Feminism, Theory, Technoscience, 7*(1), 1–21.

D'Ignazio, C., & Klein, L. F. (2020). *Data feminism*. MIT Press.

Epstein, D. A., Lee, N. B., Kang, J. H., Agapie, E., Schroeder, J., Pina, L. R., Fogarty, J., Kientz, J. A., & Munson, S. A. (2017). Examining menstrual tracking to inform the design of personal informatics tools. *Proceedings of the SIGCHI Conference on Human Factors in Computing Systems. CHI Conference, 2017*, 6876–6888.

Faubion, S. S. (2021). Femtech and midlife women's health: Good, bad, or ugly? *Menopause, 28*(4), 347–348. https://doi.org/10.1097/GME.0000000000001742

FemTech Analytics. (2021). FemTech Industry 2021 / Q2 Landscape Overview. www.femtech.health

Fiske, A., Degelsegger-Márquez, A., Marsteurer, B., & Prainsack, B. (2022). Value-creation in the health data domain: A typology of what health data help us do. *BioSocieties*. https://doi.org/10.1057/s41292-022-00276-6

Ford, A., De Togni, G., & Miller, L. (2021). Hormonal health: Period tracking apps, wellness, and self-management in the era of surveillance capitalism. *Engaging Science, Technology, and Society, 7*(1), 48–66.

Fox, S., & Spektor, F. (2021). Hormonal advantage: Retracing exploitative histories of workplace menstrual tracking. *Catalyst: Feminism, Theory, Technoscience, 7*(1).

Gambier-Ross, K., McLernon, D. J., & Morgan, H. M. (2018). A mixed methods exploratory study of women's relationships with and uses of tracking apps. *DIGITAL HEALTH, 4*, 1–15.

Gurumurthy, A., & Chami, N. (2021). *Beyond data bodies: New directions for a feminist theory of data sovereignty*. Data Governance Network, 24th Working paper—IT for Change. https://itforchange.net/beyond-data-bodies-new-directions-for-a-feminist-theory-of-data-sovereignty

Hamper, J. (2020). 'Catching ovulation': Exploring women's use of fertility tracking apps as a reproductive technology. *Body & Society, 26*(3), 3–30.

Healy, R. L. (2021). Zuckerberg, get out of my uterus! An examination of fertility apps, data-sharing and remaking the female body as a digitalized reproductive subject. *Journal of Gender Studies, 30*(4), 406–416.

Hummel, P., Braun, M., & Dabrock, P. (2020). Own data? Ethical reflections on data ownership. *Philosophy and Technology*. https://doi.org/10.1007/s13347-020-00404-9

Hummel, P., Braun, M., Tretter, M., & Dabrock, P. (2021). Data sovereignty: A review. *Big Data & Society, 8*(1), 1–17.

Iliadis, A., & Russo, F. (2016). Critical data studies: An introduction. *Big Data & Society, 3*(2). https://doi.org/10.1177/2053951716674238

Kitchin, R., & Lauriault, T. P. (2018). Toward critical data studies: Charting and unpacking data assemblages and their work. In J. Thatcher, J. Eckert, & A. Shears (Eds.), *Thinking Big Data in geography: New regimes, new research* (pp. 3–20). University of Nebraska Press.

Kressbach, M. (2021). Period hacks: Menstruating in the Big Data paradigm. *Television and New Media, 22*(3), 241–261.

Krishnamurti, T., Birru Talabi, M., Callegari, L. S., Kazmerski, T. M., & Borrero, S. (2022). A framework for Femtech: Guiding principles for developing digital reproductive health tools in the United States. *Journal of Medical Internet Research, 24*(4), e36338.

Kristensen, D. B., & Ruckenstein, M. (2018). Co-evolving with self-tracking technologies. *New Media & Society, 20*(10), 3624–3640.

Latour, B. (1999). Circulating reference: Sampling the soil in the Amazon forest. In *Pandora's hope: Essays on the reality of science studies by Bruno Latour* (pp. 24–79). Harvard University Press.

Leonelli, S. (2009). On the locality of data and claims about phenomena. *Philosophy of Science, 76*(5), 737–749. https://doi.org/10.1086/605804

Leonelli, S. (2014). What difference does quantity make? On the epistemology of Big Data in biology. *Big Data & Society, 1*(1), 205395171453439.

Leonelli, S. (2016). *Data-centric biology: A philosophical study*. The University of Chicago Press.

Leonelli, S., & Tempini, N. (Eds.). (2020). *Data journeys in the sciences*. Springer International Publishing. https://doi.org/10.1007/978-3-030-37177-7

Lomborg, S., Langstrup, H., & Andersen, T. O. (2020). Interpretation as luxury: Heart patients living with data doubt, hope, and anxiety. *Big Data & Society, 7*(1).

Lomborg, S., Thylstrup, N. B., & Schwartz, J. (2018). The temporal flows of self-tracking: Checking in, moving on, staying hooked. *New Media & Society, 20*(12), 4590–4607.

Lupton, D. (2015). Quantified sex: A critical analysis of sexual and reproductive self-tracking using apps. *Culture, Health & Sexuality, 17*(4), 440–453.

Lupton, D. (2016). *The quantified self: A sociology of self-tracking cultures*. Polity Press.

Lupton, D. (2019). 'It's made me a lot more aware': A new materialist analysis of health self-tracking. *Media International Australia, 171*(1), 66–79.

Martin, E. (1987). *The woman in the body*. Open University Press.

McEwen, K. D. (2018). Self-tracking practices and digital (re)productive labour. *Philosophy and Technology, 31*(2), 235–251.

McKinsey. (2022). The dawn of the FemTech revolution. Retrieved November 23, 2022, from https://www.mckinsey.com/industries/healthcare-systems-and-services/our-insights/the-dawn-of-the-femtech-revolution

Mehrnezhad, M., Shipp, L., Almeida, T., & Toreini, E. (2022). Vision: Too little too late? Do the risks of FemTech already outweigh the benefits? *Proceedings of the 2022 European Symposium on Usable Security (EuroUSEC '22)*, 145–150.

Mishra, P., & Suresh, Y. (2021). Datafied body projects in India: Femtech and the rise of reproductive surveillance in the digital era. *Asian Journal of Women's Studies, 27*(4), 597–606.

Mopas, M. S., & Huybregts, E. (2020). Training by feel: Wearable fitness-trackers, endurance athletes, and the sensing of data. *The Senses and Society, 15*(1), 25–40.

Neff, G., & Nafus, D. (2016). *Self-tracking.* MIT Press.

Pantzar, M., & Ruckenstein, M. (2017). Living the metrics: Self-tracking and situated objectivity. *DIGITAL HEALTH, 3*, 1–10.

Pink, S., Lanzeni, D., & Horst, H. (2018). Data anxieties: Finding trust in everyday digital mess. *Big Data & Society, 5*(1), 1–14.

Plant, S. (1998). *Zeros and ones: Digital women and the new techno-culture.* Fourth Estate.

Pols, J., Willems, D., & Aanestad, M. (2019). Making sense with numbers. Unravelling ethico-psychological subjects in practices of self-quantification. *Sociology of Health & Illness, 41*(S1), 98–115.

Prainsack, B., El-Sayed, S., Forgó, N., Szoszkiewicz, Ł., & Baumer, P. (2022). Data solidarity: A blueprint for governing health futures. *The Lancet Digital Health, 4*(11), e773–e774.

Prainsack, B., & Forgó, N. (2022). Why paying individual people for their health data is a bad idea. *Nature Medicine.*

Predel, C., & Steger, F. (2021). Ethical challenges with smartwatch-based screening for atrial fibrillation: Putting users at risk for marketing purposes? *Frontiers in Cardiovascular Medicine, 7*, 615927. https://doi.org/10.3389/fcvm.2020.615927

Roetman, S. (2020, October). *Self-tracking 'femtech': Commodifying & disciplining the fertile female body.* Paper presented at AoIR 2020: The 21th Annual Conference of the Association of Internet Researchers. Virtual Event: AoIR. http://spir.aoir.org

Ruckenstein, M. (2014). Visualized and interacted life: Personal analytics and engagements with data doubles. *Societies, 4*(1), 68–84.

Ruckenstein, M. (2022). Charting the unknown: Tracking the self, experimenting with the digital. In M. H. Bruun et al. (Eds.), *The Palgrave handbook of the anthropology of technology* (pp. 253–271). Palgrave Macmillan.

Ruckenstein, M., & Schüll, N. D. (2017). The datafication of health. *Annual Review of Anthropology, 46*, 261–278.

Sanders, R. (2017). Self-tracking in the digital era: Biopower, patriarchy, and the new biometric body projects. *Body & Society, 23*(1), 36–63.

Schüll, N. D. (2016). Data for life: Wearable technology and the design of self-care. *BioSocieties, 1*(1), 317–333.

Schüll, N. D. (2018). Self in the loop: Bits, patterns, and pathways in the quantified self. In Z. Papacharisi (Ed.), *A networked self* (Vol. 5, pp. 25–38). Routledge.

Schüll, N. D. (2019). The data-based self: Self-quantification and the data-driven (good) life. *Social Research International Quarterly, 86*(4), 909–930.

Sharon, T., & Zandbergen, D. (2017). From data fetishism to quantifying selves: Self-tracking practices and the other values of data. *New Media & Society, 19*(11), 1695–1709.

Shipp, L., & Blasco, J. (2020). How private is your period?: A systematic analysis of menstrual app privacy policies. *Proceedings on Privacy Enhancing Technologies, 2020*(4), 491–510. https://doi.org/10.2478/popets-2020-0083

Smith, G. J., & Vonthethoff, B. (2017). Health by numbers? Exploring the practice and experience of datafied health. *Health Sociology Review, 26*(1), 6–21.

Staunton, C., Barragán, C. A., Canali, S., Ho, C., Leonelli, S., Mayernik, M., Prainsack, B., & Wonkham, A. (2021). Open science, data sharing and solidarity: Who benefits? *History and Philosophy of the Life Sciences, 43*(4), 115.

Vallor, S. (2016). Chapter 8: Surveillance and the examined life: Cultivating the technomoral self in a panoptic world. In *Technology and the virtues*. Oxford University Press.

Van Dijck, J. (2014). Datafication, dataism and dataveillance: Big Data between scientific paradigm and ideology. *Surveillance and Society, 12*(2), 197–208.

Wajcman, J. (1991). *Feminism confronts technology*. Penn State Press.

Wajcman, J. (2004). *TechnoFeminism*. Polity.

Wilkinson, J., Roberts, C., & Mort, M. (2015). Ovulation monitoring and reproductive heterosex: Living the conceptive imperative? *Culture, Health & Sexuality, 17*(4), 454–469.

14

Conclusion: Can the "Fempire" Strike Back?

Lindsay Balfour

This volume has brought together research from all over the globe to ask the question—who is FemTech for? Significantly, the chapters here have shown that future research and innovation into the sector requires deeper thinking on issues of access, intersectionality, and equity. However, they have also demonstrated the various ways in which FemTech is *flourishing* at the so-called "margins." Unlike Western and Northern markets, which are no doubt growing exponentially but where the baseline user remains the same—white, heterosexual, and middle to upper class—it is the Global South that is challenging the status quos of digital health and widening our scope of what feminine technologies mean, and include, and disrupting the market with regard to gender and sexuality, race, class, and ability. Much like Seddig argues in her chapter on the "silicon Savannah," there is much potential in these "high need, low resource" communities. But this is not to discount, of course, the realities of those marginalized in and within white, western communities, as Roberts and Roberson note, respectively, in their chapters on AI interventions for

L. Balfour (✉)
Centre for Postdigital Cultures, Coventry University, Coventry, UK
e-mail: Lindsay.Balfour@coventry.ac.uk

L. Balfour (ed.), *FemTech*, https://doi.org/10.1007/978-981-99-5605-0_14

autoimmune disease, and the surveillance of black, female bodies in sport. Indeed, even in America, where FemTech investments are highest (FemTech Analytics, 2021), there is much need to consider how the industry could benefit those traditionally excluded from technological health innovation. Within heavily industrialized nations, race, class, and gender converge in ways that make access to potentially transformative tools infinitely more complex.

Yet, while there is temptation to separate FemTech into its Northern and Global counterparts, or the essentialized "have" and "have nots," we also need to recognize and consider the paradoxes within the global eco-system. How does discussion on intersectional access and inclusion work in regions like East Asia, for example, where investments into FemTech are growing exponentially but stigmatization, reproductive surveillance, and rigid conceptions of gender and femininity still reign? To what extent is FemTech truly disrupting such inequalities? Moreover, how do we account for diversity *within* regional markets, where, as Mishra et al. and Khan and Farrah detail in chapters 5 and 9, the gaps are not so much cultural or regional as they are a reflection of the rural/urban divide and broader concerns around class and caste, and digital access and literacy. If anything, the work presented here reveals FemTech to be an expansive, sometimes contradictory, and diverse landscape. This volume has been neither entirely celebratory, nor entirely critical of the FemTech ecosystem, but it has asked, at many points throughout, just how innovative feminine technologies are if they risk perpetuating the same inequalities and assumptions?

Science and Technology Studies as Critical FemTech Intervention

Given such complexity, Science and Technology Studies, and Feminist technoscience in particular, remains a useful lens through which to interrogate intersectional justice within a health ecosystem that has an inevitable digital future. As the Introduction to this volume argued, Feminist STS is critical to the movement to achieve gender justice and if STS is an exploration of the social, historical, and cultural consequences of science and technology, then the emergence of the digital health milieu certainly fits within that scope. The interrogation of intersectionality is certainly not new and has always drawn on Feminist theory to displace not only gendered inequalities, but the assumptions and naturalizations around "woman" as a fixed or stable category and the powerful hierarchies or race and class that circulate even within the marginality of gender relations. Feminist STS advocates for a flexible relationship between gender and technology, one that "co-evolves" rather than remains entrenched in old patterns and theories (Burt-D'Agnillo, 2022: 16). As Burt-D'Agnillo argues, "a feminist technoscience lens studies and emphasizes the functional and fluid relationship between gender and technology" (2022: 16). Beyond this, an intersectional approach contributes to a deeper reflection of how STS maps onto FemTech, by considering how gender operates in relation to other forms of oppression. When applied to FemTech then, we are reminded that digital health products created with "women" in mind may reflect cultural change but do not necessarily create it. In other words, FemTech must remain attend to socio-cultural intersectionality; equitable transformation must happen through feminist politics where technology is not the agent but, rather, the tool (Wajcman, 2007: 288). While the chapters here may critique forms of gendered and racialized surveillance, the essentialism of women's bodies, or the reproduction of myths around beauty and femininity, these are reflections of the wider cultural relationship between patriarchy, capitalism, and race. As such, FSTS not only places technology within its wider socio-cultural context, but also challenges the zero-sum game of digital health in which innovation is privileged over justice and ethical social change. Included within this STS lens is a recognition of what science and medicine have left out—whose needs have gone unnoticed, what users have been excluded, and how identities have been forged and disavowed in the pursuit of health innovation. This volume has explicitly raised those absences here in an effort to expose hidden injustice and make visible the ways in which it is being overcome.

At the same time, FSTS has important implication for research and how we conduct analyses of cultural phenomena with often intimate implications. In her article for *Science and Culture* (2010), Chikako Takeshita reflects on what it might mean to *embody* Feminist Technoscience in situations where the researcher if often research subject at the same time. Detailing the intimate experience of subscribing to feminine technologies while intellectually critiquing them, Takeshita writes:

> Reflecting on my own embodiment of the IUD while conducting academic research on the same technology helped me understand how social and historical conditions constructed my reproductive choice as an American consumer of the device and how such 'choice' is constrained by the scientific community's willingness to develop birth control methods, medical practices, and corporate profitability. Personally enjoying the IUD and benefiting from studying it academically, I faced a moral dilemma between my own empowerment and the disempowerment that many other women experienced in relationship to this technology. (2010: 38)

As Takeshita infers, within the reflexive methodologies of STS research, the role of the researcher is never fully divorced from the "texts" or phenomena that are studied. In this case, the reflection on the contradictions between finding utility in a FemTech device and the reality that such options are not available to all women is an unsettling point of conflict. Takeshita credits STS "training" as offering the ability to "analyze technologies as products of social relationships that are not politically innocent (55). Many chapters in the follow have followed that example, with reflexive, anecdotal, and engaged research that addresses the challenges of interweaving the personal and the political.

The body–machine assemblage has never been more ubiquitous, and Feminist Science and Technology Studies is needed to critically reflect on the intersections of gender, health, and technology, not to mention the complex challenges of inclusion and oppression woven therein. As the introduction to this chapter explores, feminist theory has long been associated with the critique of the traditional relationship between gender and science, exposing the "natural" or taken-for-granted ways in which science has negated women's importance—whether as researchers or research subjects. Yet, even within an industry such as FemTech, which aims to fill in this absence, STS is needed to recognize not only the medical consequences of the gender gap, but the social and cultural consequences of excluding other forms of oppression that the industry has yet to take into account.

Future Challenges and Directions for Research

While the chapters included here raise some significant questions for the current FemTech landscape, and the challenges to come, there remain several areas which demand further research and reflection. Despite intersectional and inclusive transformation occurring in the Global South, for instance, investment remains focused on primarily Western markets (FemTech Analytics, 2021), and despite the potential for health technologies to radically alter gender inequalities and increase reproductive health outcomes, underserved regions will not benefit from the "trickle down" approach employed in other technology sectors. Reused and second-hand devices, "knock-off" mimics of market-leading products, and the tendency to view investment as charity have long been the delivery mechanisms of bringing digitalization to the Global South. FemTech, however, has the opportunity to develop in the opposite direction—with investment and design taking Africa, South Asia, South America, and the Middle East as examples rather than afterthoughts. The UN Women's Innovation Strategy could be used as a helpful model here, as it advocates for an "innovation market that advances gender equality and empowerment of women and girls" (UN Women, 2017). Intersectional equity within the FemTech market will only be achieved if women themselves have ownership over the building blocks of the industry, from investment, to design, to infrastructure and ICT development.

Secondly, despite the growing technological affordances of previously unconnected or underserviced regions, substantial taboos remain around women's health and processes such as menstruation, sex, pregnancy, and nonconfirming gender identity and sexual wellness (see Schweizer et al., 2023; Bobel & Fahs, 2020; Mishra et al., this volume). As such, more investigation is needed into how FemTech and intimate health operate in diverse regional contexts and with varying cultural politics. At the same time, intimate health technologies offer a significant pathway to gender equality and reproductive justice globally. As Tuli et al. (2022) optimistically project, period tracking can be avenue toward the emancipation of those who menstruate and "make possible a period-positive future for those in the Global South." In 2019, the World Economic health Forum identified three roadblocks to menstrual hygiene around the world: lack of awareness, lack of acceptance, and lack of access (Gopalan, 2019). FemTech has a potentially world-changing role to play in all three challenges, using digital tools to bring discreet, medically accurate, and accessible information to women and girls who might not receive the education and care they need via traditional methods such as family knowledge sharing and school-based learning. At the same time, taboos and stigmas are not limited to menstruation and reproductive health; in many parts of the world, where nonconfirming gender and sexuality remain not only silenced but often persecuted, FemTech has opportunity to meet the needs of those suffering under cultural, regional, and religious healthcare regimes, including those that occur within affluent Western contexts as well. This is not only a health issue, but a human rights one, and while the potential extent of FemTech's reach into such challenges remains to be seen, it is clear that more research is needed to determine how digital health can expand to address a broader remit of health and gender inequalities around the globe.

Finally, as many chapters in this volume identify (Jules, Roberson, Monteleone and Day, Canali and Hesselbein), surveillance remains a critical challenge that will be difficult to overcome within a market ecosystem that is sustained, and often financed, by third-party information sharing. Indeed, as Canali and Hesselbein point out, it is "[the] body itself, [that] provide[s] the data that are being collected, counted, and analysed, and these outputs are subsequently used as the basis upon which FemTech products can be manufactured and marketed." Through intimate platforms such as menstruation or ovulation apps, both state and corporate biopower operate at their peak, whereby gender and surveillance converge to produce and regulate the reproductive body. Such intimate forms of surveillance and data tracking will continue to be a significant challenge for the FemTech industry. This is nothing new of course; while not writing on feminine technologies specifically, Deborah Lupton—pioneer of studies of the "quantified self"—identified over a decade ago, how "various kinds of social relations and interactions, including power relations, are created in and through surveillance technologies…[that are] part of the production of the citizen in neoliberal societies" (Lupton, 2012: 235). Yet, for FemTech to operate as a truly inclusive ecosystem, it will need to think more critically not just about the kinds of data it collects—some of which is, to be fair, necessary for the health function of the app—but also about whose data is being privileged (and excluded) and how the intimate nature of surveillance disproportionately affects those already marginalized by factors such as race and class. Added to this challenge is the lack of consistency around privacy law (Taylor, 2020–2021; Alfawzan et al., 2022), where FemTech—a global enterprise—is subject to often local regulations. Things like privacy law and quality assurance therefore become muddled when a product is created in one legal context, but then taken up in another. There are, to be sure, laws that govern the use of personal data, such as General Data Protection Regulation (GDPR) in the EU, Data Protection Act (DPA) in the United Kingdom, the (Health Insurance Portability and Accountability Act) HIPPA in the United States, and the Personal Data Protection Bill (PDPB) in India, among many others. A transnational industry that is bound by local regulations poses serious challenges for digital health, particularly for users who are subject to confusing and jargon-laden terms and conditions that they do not understand. This becomes even more acute in the case of urgent health crisis, where users (particularly those accessing digital health in abusive, coercive, outlawed, or stigmatized scenarios) do not have the time or emotional bandwidth to closely read lengthy privacy policies. Following the arguments made in this volume then, the question of how such laws are made, and who they truly protect, demands further interrogation.

One final challenge, perhaps the most difficult of all, is the potential misuse of FemTech applications. As much as this volume documents both the ethical and material problems of (self) surveillance and the dangers of data from such platforms being sold to third parties, such data can also be leveraged in even more dangerous ways. One such way, as briefly hinted at in the introduction, is the threat of intimate health data being used, in the aftermath of *Roe v. Wade*'s overturn, to prosecute now-outlawed forms of reproductive care. Concerns that personal information such as search and location histories and appointment bookings saved into digital calendars could be subpoenaed are very real, and perhaps more alarming than the selling of data to social media for the purpose of algorithmically developed targeted advertising. Moreover, intimate data can potentially be used as a tool for violence and intimate partner abuse. Here, surveillance occurs in the domestic sphere and, rather than being leveraged by capitalism or government, it is used to facilitate control and tracking within violent relationships. One example of this is the use of menstruation or ovulation data as forms of reproductive coercion or punishment. If, for instance, one partner is secretly using a tracking app to avoid pregnancy, while their partner wants pregnancy to occur, what was once a useful health tool potentially turns into a weapon. Once again, the capacity for harm in such scenarios is often exacerbated by intersectional marginalization and domestic vulnerabilities, as well as in the cases of stigma and taboo discussed above. As the UN Innovation for Gender Equality report (2019) outlines "Not only are women under-represented across core innovation sectors, including science, technology, engineering and mathematics, but new technology brings risks of bias and possibilities for misuse, creating new human rights challenges for the 21st century." In other words, FemTech products for women have the potential to cause harm even while they purport to increase positive health outcomes, and such concerns need to be reflected in new research that considers the intersections between gender, health, technology, and violence.

Why Intersectionality? Why Now?

At its core, this volume interrogates the disproportional effects that the FemTech ecosystem has for marginalized and underserved populations who suffer within healthcare systems that do not meet their needs, and for reasons that often have much to do with race, class, sexuality, ability, and more. The question "who is FemTech for?" is not to discount the transformative and innovative ways in which women's health in particular has been democratized, globalized, and made available in situations where conventional healthcare has failed. It is, however, to suggest that further consideration of intersectional oppression, privacy sand safety, and regional and cultural difference is imperative to establishing an industry that is truly revolutionary for all who need it. Science and Technology Studies thus provides a critical lens through which to tackle these challenges, drawling on traditional concepts of feminist technoscience to identify gaps in both the research and in the market, while continuing to ensure that the social and cultural contexts of health and technology remain at the forefront of innovation.

The three sections offered here are by no means an exhaustive review of the FemTech landscape, yet they represent three critical areas of intervention. The first is the need to draw on feminist theory in interrogations of digital health and to question latent discourses of beauty, biological essentialism and normative gender and sexuality. Part Two reminds us of the imperative to consider FemTech innovations at the margins, not only as regions of "high need" but as loci of transformative digital health practice. Indeed, the women's march inspired phrase "the Fempire strikes back"[1] has significant resonance here, not only to designate the intent of women to reclaim power in culture and politics, but also to do so from the margins or areas previously under the control of powerful empires. Health care can be considered one such empire, and the phrase, while borrowed in this case from the fictional *Star Wars* franchise, also recalls the seminal 1989 volume by Bill Ashcroft, Gareth Griffiths, and Helen Tiffin, *The Empire Writes Back*, the title here also an homage to Salman Rushdie's 1982 essay "The Empire Writes Back with a Vengeance." Both texts describe the emergence and recognition of postcolonial writing as a resistance to colonial rule as well as the displacement of the histories and cultures of empire. In "the Fempire strikes back," then both feminism and anticolonialism work together to produce a new narrative of intersectional politics that resist the notion of white western nations being the center of social, political, and cultural power. Likewise, the chapters that make up the largest section here "write back" to the dominant centers of digital health, advocating for a FemTech of, by, and for the so-called margins, and recognizing the significant contributions, both technological and theoretical, that the digital health ecosystems of the Global South afford. Finally, the third section on this collection has endeavored to ask the question "what next?" What is the future of FemTech, and what challenges still remain? And, as Stuifzand and Smit explore in their chapter,

---

[1] In 2017, fuelled by actress Carrie Fisher's role as Princess Leia and real-life death while making Star Wars: The Rise of Skywalker, feminist marches worldwide included signs of homage to the star, and included slogans such as "A Woman's Place is in the Resistance," "The Female Force Awakens," and "The Fempire Strikes Back" (Knopf, 2019).

what methods might be used to address these challenges, particularly as the breadth of FemTech across media, platforms, software, and hardware necessitates a varied approach to the data.

The volume thus remains necessarily open-ended. What is clear, however, is that FemTech is on a precipice—primed for exponential growth that could come as a huge benefit to women worldwide, or could come at a cost. The insights offered here thus issue not a blueprint for success, but a critical reflection and urgent prompting to think far more deeply about how we might catalyze the burgeoning industry of FemTech for growth that is safe, feminist, equitable, and inclusive. We argue that intersectional justice must be the foundation of the industry rather than an afterthought considered only once innovation is achieved. FemTech in the Global South is an opportunity to "get it right"—and given the histories and contemporaries of oppression, marginalization, and resource extraction, not to mention the forms of intersectional injustice that exist *within* dominant and affluent markets—it is imperative that we do.

References

Alfawzan, N., Christen, M., Spitale, G., & Biller-Andorno, N. (2022). Privacy, data sharing, and data security policies of women's mHealth apps: Scoping review and content analysis. *JMIR mHealth and uHealth, 10*(5).

Bobel, C., & Fahs, B. (2020). From bloodless respectability to radical menstrual embodiment: Shifting menstrual politics from private to public. *Signs, 45*(4).

Burt-D'Agnillo, M. (2022). FemTech: A Feminist Technoscience Analysis. *The iJournal, 8*(1).

FemTech Analytics. (2021). FemTech Industry Landscape Overview. https://www.femtech.health/femtechoverview-q4-2021

Gopalan, M. (2019). There are 3 barriers blocking good menstrual hygiene for all women. Here's how we overcome them. *World Economic Forum.* https://www.weforum.org/agenda/2019/11/menstruation-in-different-cultures-period-taboos/

Knopf, C. M. (2019). Carrie Fisher sent me: Princess Leia as an avatar of resistance in the Women's March. *Unbound: A Journal of Digital Scholarship Realizing Resistance: An Interdisciplinary Conference on Star Wars, Episodes VII, VIII & IX.*

Lupton, D. (2012). M-health and Health Promotion: The digital cyborg and surveillance society. *Social Theory & Health, 10*, 229–244.

Schweizer, C., Böhm, M., & Paudel, R. (2023). How menstrual discrimination is approached by menstrual movements in the Global North and the Global South. *Dignified Menstruation.org.* https://dignifiedmenstruation.org/wp-content/uploads/2022/11/Menstrual-Movement-Global-Mapping.pdf

Takeshita, C. (2010). The IUD in me: On embodying feminist technoscience studies. *Science as Culture, 19*(1).

Taylor, A. (2020–2021). Fertile ground: Rethinking regulatory standards for Femtech. *UC Davis Law Review, 54.*

Tuli, A., et al. (2022). Rethinking menstrual trackers towards period-positive ecologies. *Proceedings of the 2022 CHI Conference on Human Factors in Computing Systems, 238.* https://doi.org/10.1145/3491102.3517662

UN Women. (2017). Making innovation and technology work for women. https://www.unwomen.org/en/digital-library/publications/2017/7/making-innovation-and-technology-work-for-women

UN Women. (2019). Innovation for gender equality. https://www.unwomen.org/sites/default/files/Headquarters/Attachments/Sections/Library/Publications/2019/Innovation-for-gender-equality-en.pdf

Wajcman, J. (2007). From women and technology to gendered technoscience. *Information, Communication & Society, 10.* https://doi.org/10.1080/13691180701409770

Index[1]

---

[1] Note: Page numbers followed by 'n' refer to notes.